Frontiers in Clinical Neurosurgery

Edited by Xianli Lv, Guihuai Wang, James Wang and Zhongxue Wu

Published in London, United Kingdom

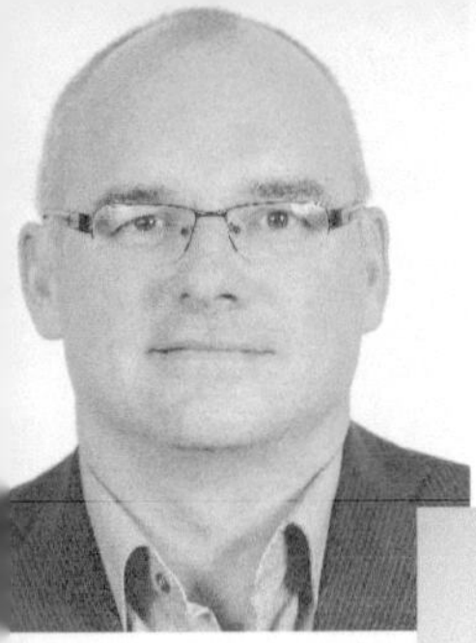
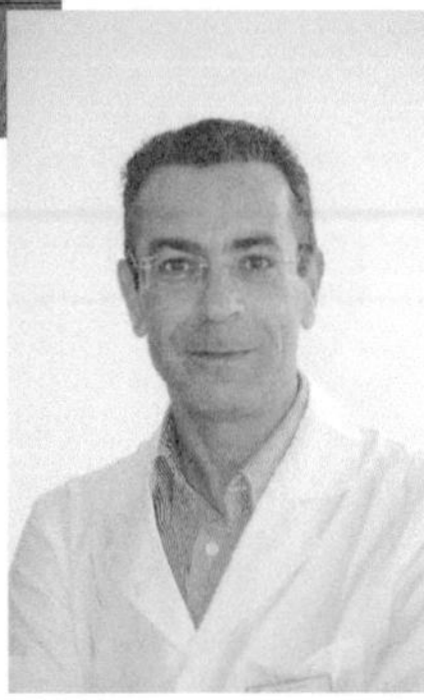
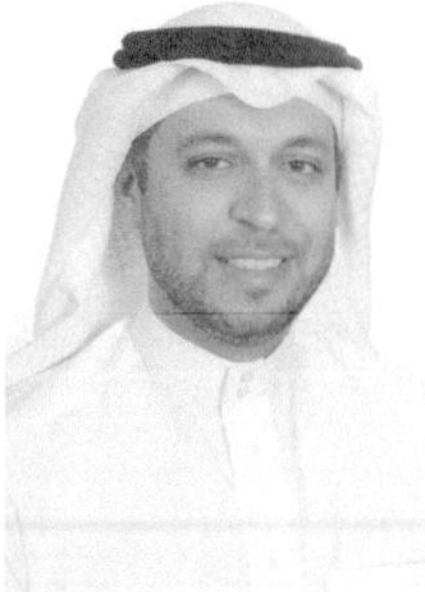
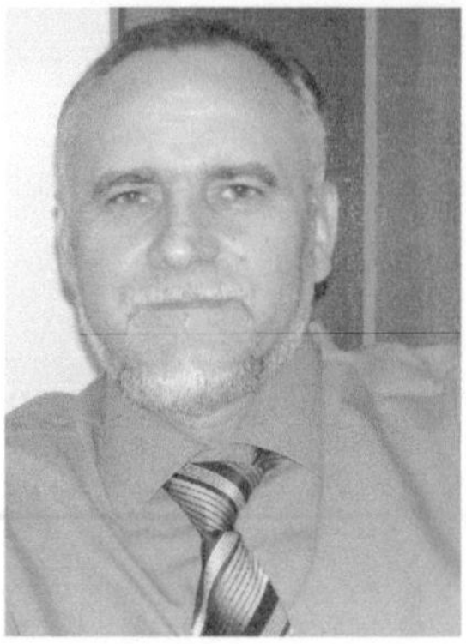
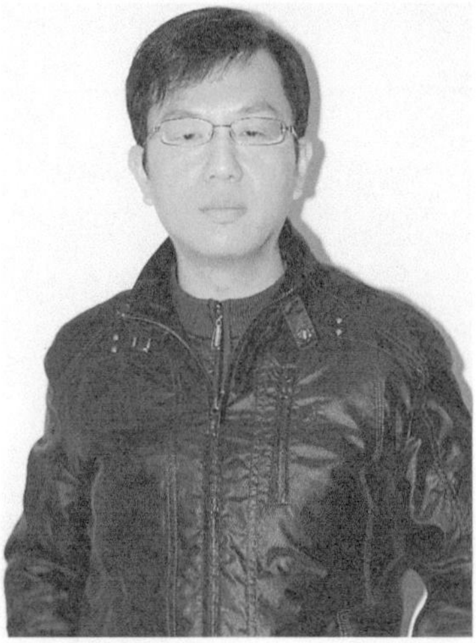
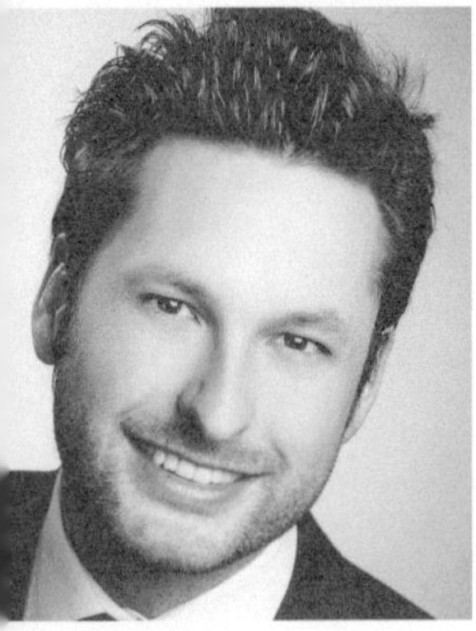
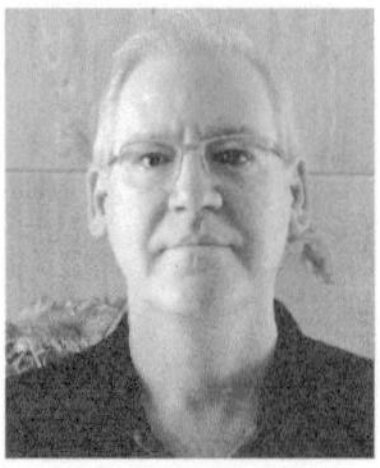

IntechOpen

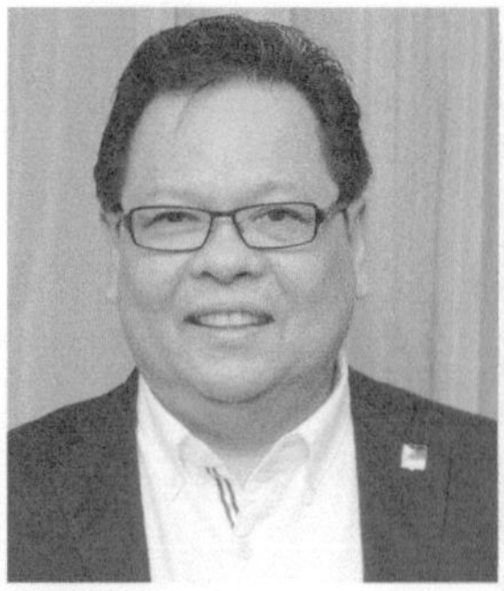
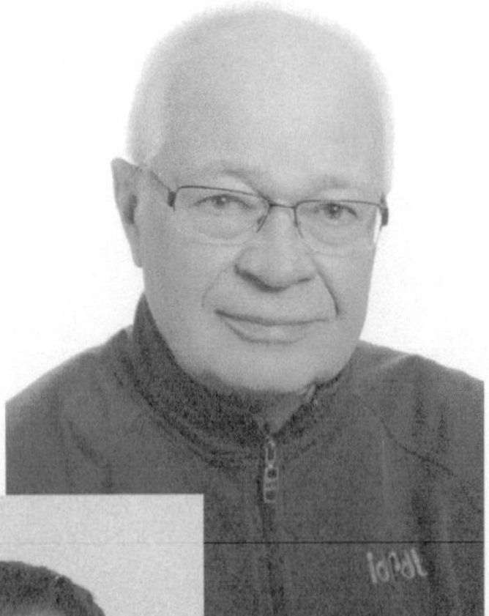
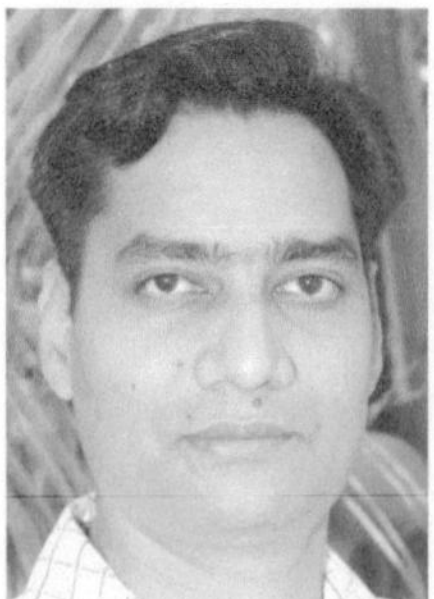
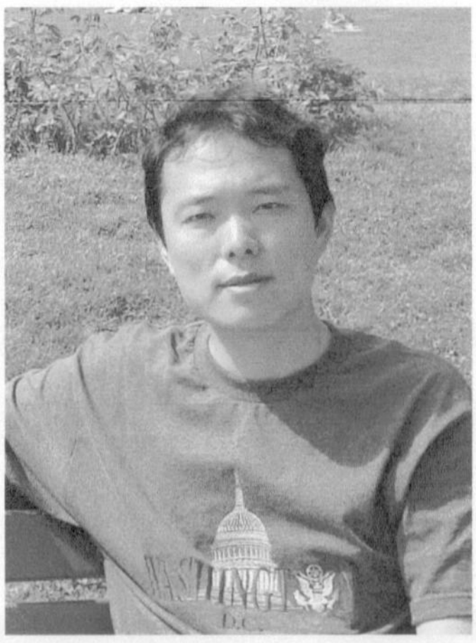
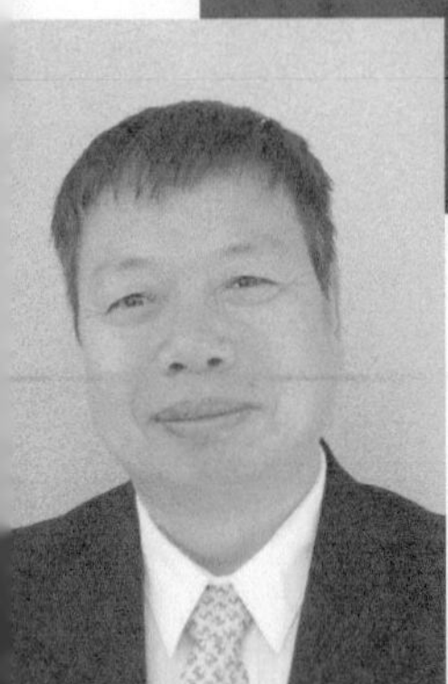
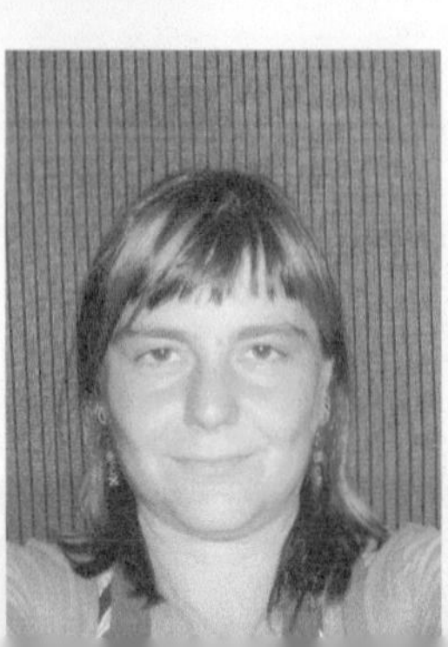

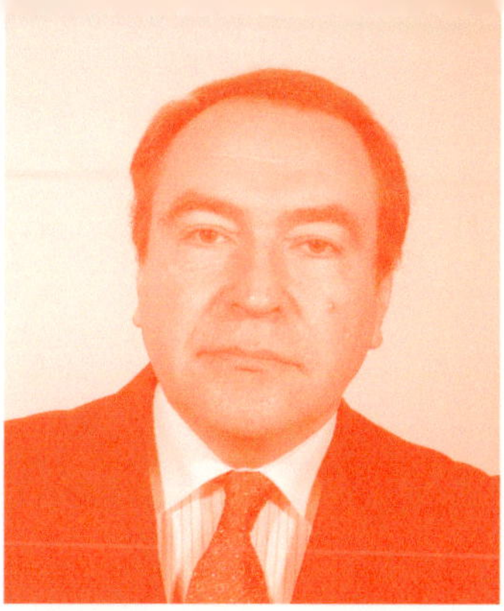
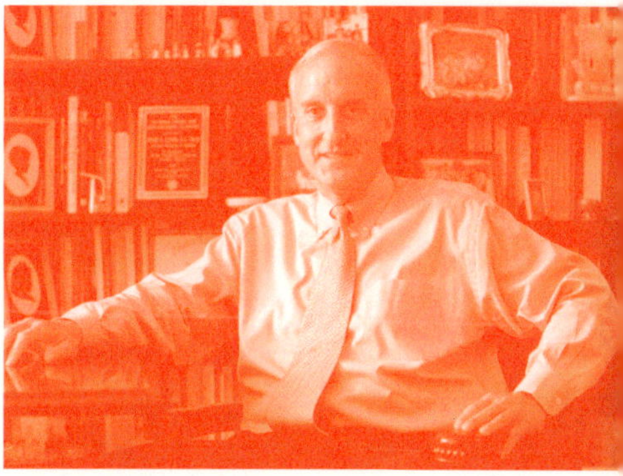
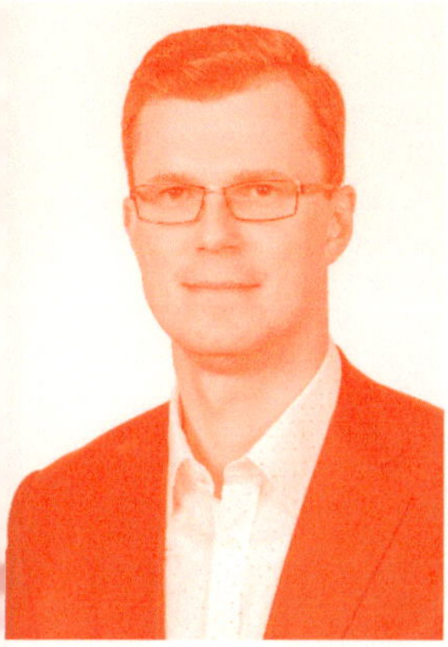
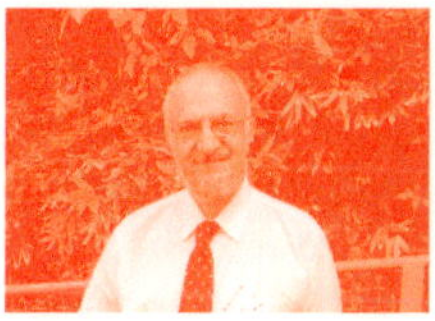
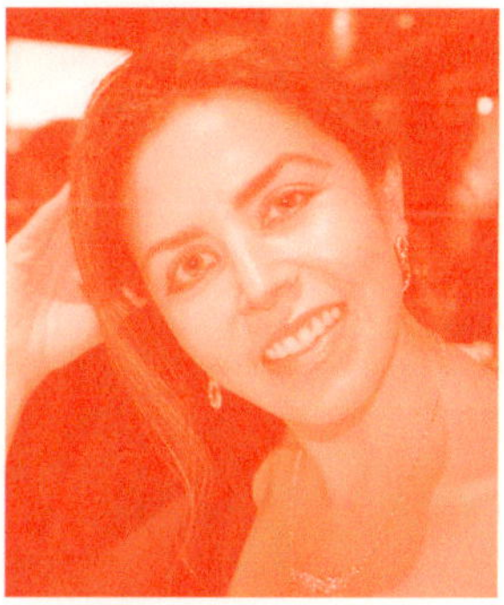

Supporting open minds since 2005

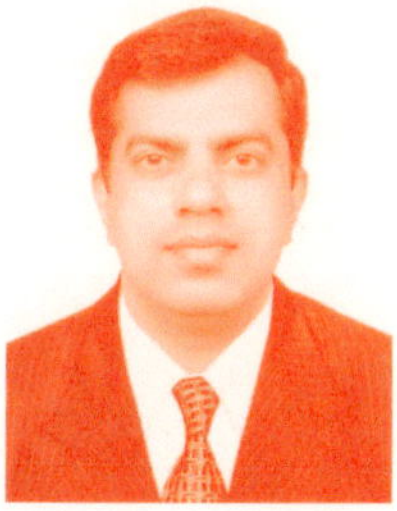
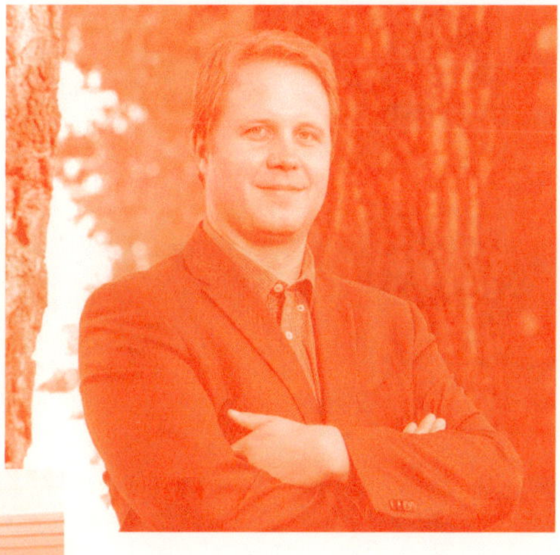
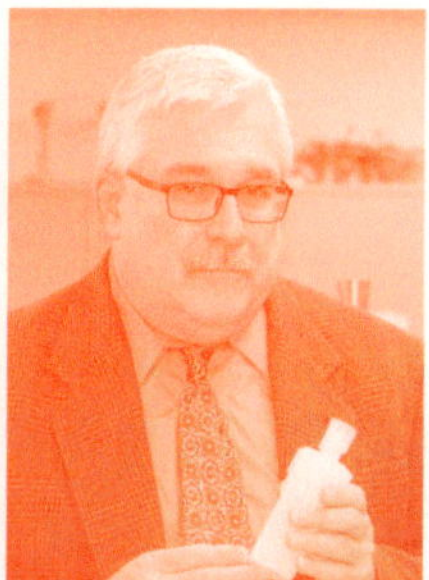
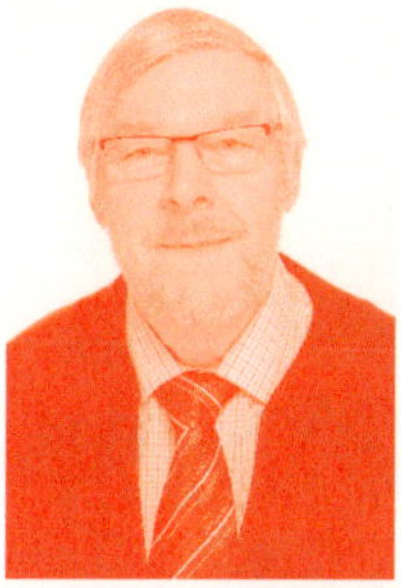
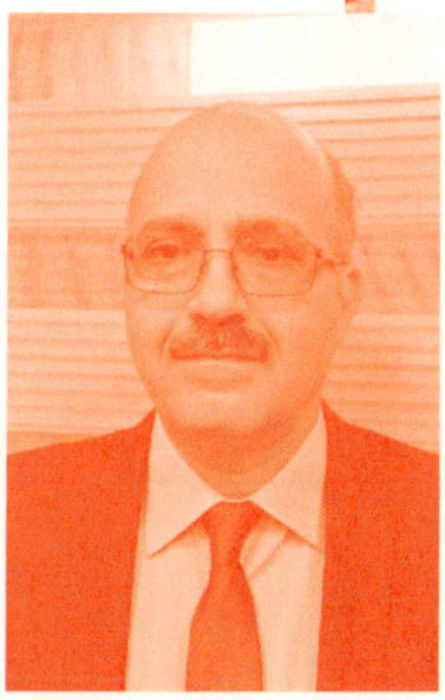
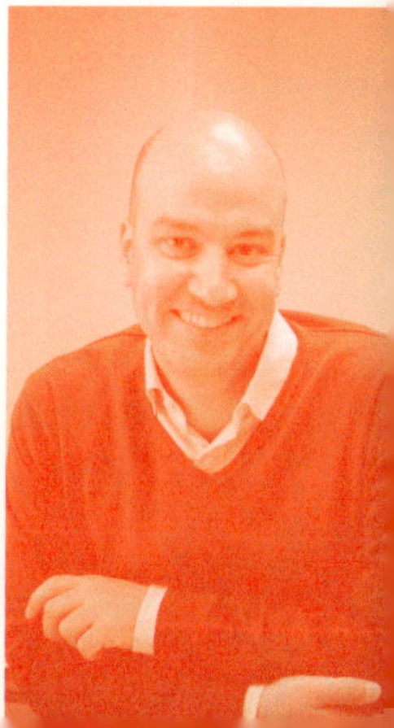
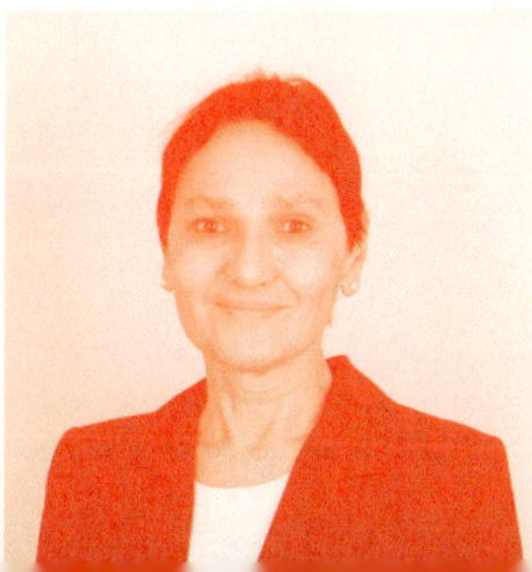

Frontiers in Clinical Neurosurgery
http://dx.doi.org/10.5772/intechopen.92911
Edited by Xianli Lv, Guihuai Wang, James Wang and Zhongxue Wu

Contributors
Tryggve Lundar, Bernt Johan Due-Tønnessen, Francesco Maiuri, Sergio Corvino, Elia Guadagno, Marialaura Del Basso De Caro, Lydia Kaoutzani, Scott Rahimi, José Damián Carrillo-Ruiz, Jose Luis Navarro-Olvera, Francisco Velasco, Francisco Villegas, José Rodrigo Carrillo-Márquez, Luis García-Muñoz, Jesús Quetzalcoatl Beltrán, Ekkehard Matthias Kasper, Fred Lam, Hanan Algethami, Rafael Rojas, Gustavo Parra-Romero, Stephanie Heres-Becerril, Gustavo Aguado-Carrillo, David Trejo, Xianli Lv, Krishna Kumar, Anandh Balasubramaniam, Pradeep K, Nitin Manohar, Khandkar Ali Kawsar, Ethan Sissman, Themistocles Protopsaltis, Rajab Al-Ghanem, Michael L. Levy, Usman A. Khan, Robert C. Rennert, Jillian H. Plonsker, Gary Senecal, Patrick Whitehead, Kleber Gonzalez Echeverría

First published in London, United Kingdom, 2021 by IntechOpen
IntechOpen is the global imprint of INTECHOPEN LIMITED, registered in England and Wales, registration number: 11086078, 5 Princes Gate Court, London, SW7 2QJ, United Kingdom
Printed in Croatia

British Library Cataloguing-in-Publication Data
A catalogue record for this book is available from the British Library

Additional hard and PDF copies can be obtained from orders@intechopen.com

Frontiers in Clinical Neurosurgery
Edited by Xianli Lv, Guihuai Wang, James Wang and Zhongxue Wu
p. cm.
Print ISBN 978-1-83968-686-3
Online ISBN 978-1-83968-687-0
eBook (PDF) ISBN 978-1-83968-688-7

For EU product safety concerns:
IN TECH d.o.o., Prolaz Marije Krucifikse Kozulić 3, 51000 Rijeka, Croatia, info@intechopen.com or visit our website at intechopen.com.

Meet the editors

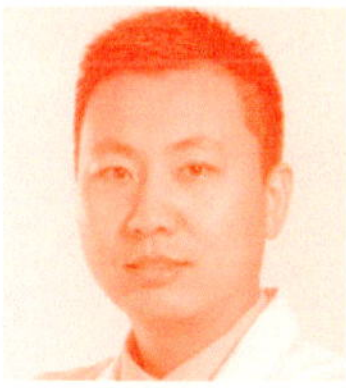

Dr. Xianli Lv, MD, is an Associate Professor of Endovascular Neurosurgery, Department of Neurosurgery, Beijing Tsinghua Changgung Hospital, School of Clinical Medicine, Tsinghua University, China. His research focuses on interventional therapy of intracranial aneurysm, cerebral arteriovenous malformation, intracranial dural arteriovenous fistula, spinal vascular malformation, and pediatric cerebrospinal vascular malformations. He is an editorial member of the *Journal of Interventional Neuroradiology*, *Journal of Stroke and Vascular Neurology*, *Journal of Neuroradiology*, and *The Neuroradiology Journal*. He is also a deputy editor of *Frontiers in Neurology* and *Neuroscience* Informatics. Dr. Lv is a senior member of the World Federation of Interventional Therapeutic Neuroradiology (WFITN) and a consultant for BALT, Montmorency, France.

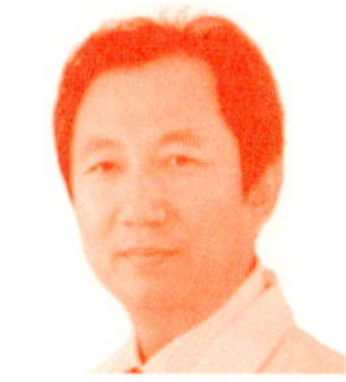

Dr. Guihuai Wang is a professor and director in the Department of Neurosurgery, Beijing Tsinghua Changgung Hospital, School of Clinical Medicine, Tsinghua University, China. He serves as the chairman of the Spinal Cord and Spine Expert Committee of the Neurosurgeon Branch of the Chinese Medical Doctor Association, the deputy chairman of the Neuro-Oncology Committee of the Chinese Anti-Cancer Association, and the deputy chairman of the Spinal Cord and Peripheral Nerve Repair Materials and Application Professional Committee of the Bone Repair Materials and Devices Branch of the Chinese Society of Biomaterials. He is also deputy secretary-general and a member of the Standing Committee of the First Committee of the Neuro-Tumor Branch of the Chinese Society of Neuroscience, a member of the World Federation of Neurosurgery, and an editorial board member of *Translational Neuroscience and Clinics*.

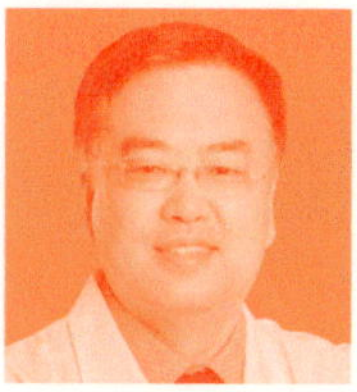

Dr. James Wang is a Professor of Neurosurgery, Beijing Tsinghua Changgung Hospital, School of Clinical Medicine, Tsinghua University, China. He is also a professor in the Neurosurgery Department, University of Washington, Seattle, USA. He graduated from Beijing Capital Medical College in 1986 with a master's degree in Medicine. In the same year, he studied in the United States, received credentials from the US Education Commission for Foreign Medical Graduates (ECFMG) in 1990, and became an American neurosurgeon in 1993. He was a resident of neurosurgery at Ohio State University School of Medicine from 1993 to 1999 and completed a seven-year residency degree in 1999. From 2002 to 2009, he served as the chief physician of neurosurgery at Washington School of Medicine. From 2010 to 2014, he served as Associate Professor of Neurosurgery at the University of Washington School of Medicine, and chief physician of neurosurgery at the Institute of Neurology, Swedish Hospital. Since 2015, he has been the chief physician of neurosurgery at the University of Washington Affiliated Hospital and associate dean of the Institute of Clinical Neurosciences, Tsinghua University.

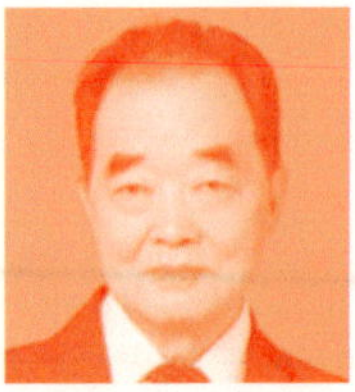

Dr. Zhongxue Wu is a vice director, Beijing Neurosurgical Institute (BNI), and a founding member of the Chinese Societies of Neurosurgery. He is also the recipient of "Medal of May Day." He is an expert with outstanding contributions from the Ministry of Health. He has won several awards including an award for National Outstanding Medical Worker and Young and Middle-aged Experts with Outstanding Contributions by the Ministry of Health. He has presided over major medical science and technology research support projects by the National Natural Science Foundation of China and the Ministry of Health. He has published nearly 200 academic papers in national and international journals. He engaged in neurointervention work for more than twenty years and has trained three master's students and eighteen doctoral students.

Contents

Preface

This book covers humanism in neurosurgery; social support for patients with brain injury; preoperative, intraoperative, and postoperative evaluation and treatment decision-making for brain tumors; the application of neuroendoscopy; the treatment of pediatric skull base tumors and hydrocephalus; and endovascular neurosurgery and neurosurgical treatment of ischemic stroke.

The book is divided into five sections. We believe that medical ethics and humanism should be mastered by all neurosurgeons and neurologists to serve our patients well, therefore we address these philosophical topics in Section I, which consists of two chapters: "Medical Humanism in Neurosurgery" and "Social Support, Identity, and Meaning: A Phenomenological Analysis of Post-Concussion Syndrome." This section provides readers with training, lectures, role modeling, and interpersonal communication training in competency, literature, and humanities studies, teaching neurosurgeons the core values of medical humanism. The level of social support can play an important role in improving and/or exacerbating the physical and psychological difficulties of patients with traumatic brain injury and post-concussion syndrome.

Section II focuses on brain tumors, including the development of imaging evaluation and surgical techniques in modern brain tumor surgery. In the past thirty years, functional neuroimaging such as fMRI, DTI, MRP, MRS, AS-PET-CT, SPECT, and TMS have been developed as non-invasive tools to visualize the inner brain and spinal functional morphology. Chapters 3 and 4 demonstrate that the preoperative and intraoperative application of fMRI- and DTI-based navigation can assist the safest possible removal of brain tumors. Chapter 5 outlines the interdisciplinary work of neurosurgeons, neuroanesthesiologists, and neuropsychologists in the management of brain tumors in awake patients. Chapter 6 discusses the pathological and surgical features of diffuse-multicentric versus local-peripheral recurrence of meningiomas. Chapter 7 introduces the evolution of neuroendoscopy to readers.

Section III introduces the developmental status of endovascular neurosurgery and neurosurgical treatment of ischemic stroke. Section IV covers neurosurgical treatment of spasticity due to brain and spinal cord injuries and puts forward a proposal that points to the possible path to treat spasticity in the future. This section also introduces the treatment of cervical deformity and the necessary steps that should be taken to minimize the risk of distal junctional kyphosis (DJK) post-operatively. Section V is on pediatric neurosurgery. The authors generously share their experience in managing surgical lesions of the pediatric skull base and long-term shunt-dependency in children treated for idiopathic intracranial hypertension with CSF diversion.

We would like to thank all the authors for their contributions. We would also like to acknowledge the encouragement, motivation, and assistance from the Beijing Municipal Administration of Hospitals Incubating Program (PX2020039), Beijing, China, and Tsinghua Precision Medicine Foundation (20219990008), Tsinghua University, Beijing, China. We are grateful to Author Service Manager Romina Rovan at IntechOpen for her dedication and hard work to ensure the smooth publication of this book. Finally, we owe a debt of gratitude to Professor Zhongcheng

Wang, academician of the Chinese Academy of Engineering and the founder and pioneer of Chinese neurosurgery, for without his tireless efforts over the decades Chinese neurosurgery would not be what it is today.

Xianli Lv, Guihuai Wang, James Wang and Zhongxue Wu
Neurosurgery Department,
Beijing Tsinghua Changgung Hospital,
School of Clinical Medicine,
Tsinghua University,
Beijing, China

In Memoriam

In Memoriam Academician Zhongcheng Wang (20th, Dec, 1925-30th, Sep, 2012)

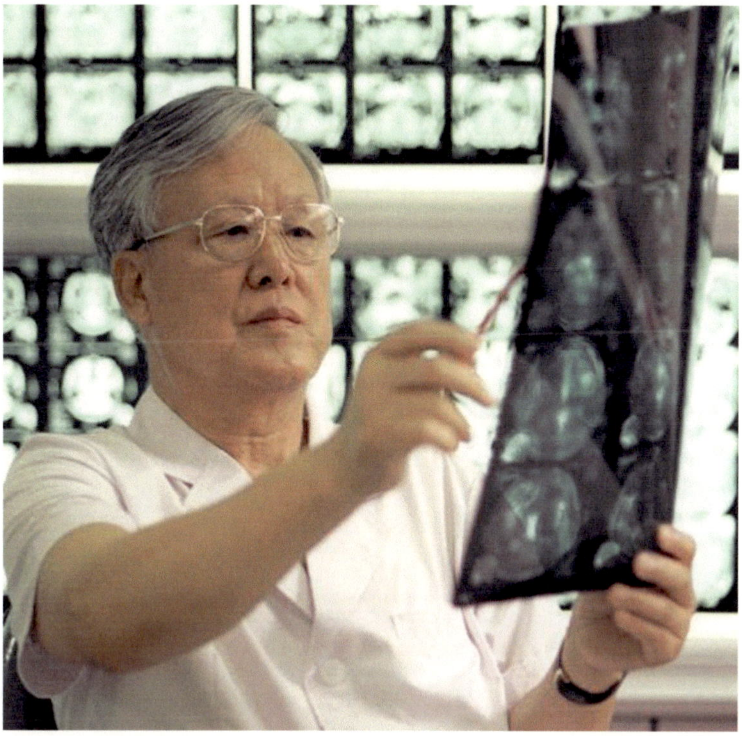

Professor Zhongcheng Wang, academician of the Chinese Academy of Engineering, the founder and pioneer of Chinese neurosurgery, without his decades' long tireless effort, Chinese Neurosurgery won't be what it is today.

Section 1

Philosophical Issues

Chapter 1

Medical Humanism in Neurosurgery

Rajab Al-Ghanem

Abstract

Patient-centered care means organizing health care that is respectful and responsive to the patient needs, preferences, and values, and ensuring that the patient values guide all clinical decisions. Teaching of medical humanism becomes a necessity to help neurosurgery residents in their future practice to do what they are already doing but in a more humanistic and empathic attitudes. A training programme to teach medical humanism core values through lectures, role modeling, and training in interpersonal skills, literature and humanities study can improve attitudes and behaviors. A set of 10 medical humanism values relevant to contemporary challenges, research, and practice of neurosurgery practice that can help residents and practicing physicians to maintain humanism behaviors in their practice are presented. A humanistic neurosurgeon provide a skilled, compassionate, and empathic care to her/his patients, and demonstrates respect for their values, autonomy, beliefs and cultural backgrounds. Neurosurgery is an apprenticeship profession, where humanism values can be taught and behaviors associated with humanism can be learned.

Keywords: humanism, medical education, neurosurgery, patient-centered care, professionalism, values

1. Introduction

Patient-centered care means organizing health care to serve the patients. In this context, and in order to respond to the new demands of society for the reliability of doctors in the 21st century and seeking greater adaptation and development of professionals, Competence Based Training (CBT) was developed [1]. Humanism in medicine, a central aspect of professionalism, combines scientific knowledge and skills with respectful, compassionate care that is sensitive to the values, autonomy, beliefs and cultural backgrounds of patients and their families.

According to Jean-Paul Sartre, "humanism is a theory which upholds man as the end-in-itself and as the supreme value". Man is the point-of-care, the thing-of-focus, and the centerpiece of our attention. Medical humanism, or humanistic medicine, is an interdisciplinary field which aims to address problems in health care. According to The Arnold P. Gold Foundation, it is "characterized by a respectful and compassionate relationship between physicians and their patients" centered on several ideals, including integrity, excellence, compassion, altruism, respect, empathy, and service [2].

Humanism represents the basis of medicine throughout history, beginning from the time of Hippocrates and the development of the Hippocratic Oath.

Medicine has been regarded as a moral profession and carried out in accordance with a set of morals and ethics [3]. The first conference concerned with humanism, was held at Chicago University in 1933, recommended considering humanistic science as the basis of morality and decision-making in medical practice.

The past four decades showed great advances in medical knowledge and new technological devices have been extensively incorporated into medical practice. Physicians emphasized on the disease, use of technology, laboratory investigations, treatment and physical recovery. They ignore patient psychological status, ethical and social cultures. These events abolished medical humanistic spirit. Such dehumanized medicine appears to have no past, no cultural language and no philosophy.

Sir William Osler (1837–1901), considered as the father of modern medicine, advised ¨Listen to the patient. He is telling you the diagnosis¨. Sir Osler also stated that (it is much more important to know what sort of person has a disease, than to know what sort of disease a person has) [3]. Marañón's words provide us with the following reflection "... a mere diagnostic system, deduced exclusively from analytical data, dehumanized, independent of direct and endearing observation of the patient, carries the fundamental error of forgetting the personality, which is so important in etiologies and to stipulate the prognosis of the patient and teach us, doctors, what we can do to alleviate his sufferings" [4].

Humanism is an essential component of the art of Neurosurgery that allows the science of Neurosurgery to prosper. Without humanism, medicine is no longer; without medical science, medical humanism has no vehicle. The practice of Neurosurgery is both a science and an art. Contemporary Neurosurgery is based on scientific rigor but good medical practice should be 'an art that uses science as one of its tools'. It is the art of Neurosurgery that facilitates teamworking, communication, partnership with patients and maintenance of trust—key elements of professional guidance on good medical practice—whereas science upholds evidence-supported practice.

2. Humanism core values in neurosurgery

The young resident begins the residency full of dreams and desires to take care of patients, full of idealism; and by a process that has not been explained sufficiently ends up becoming indifferent to human suffering, gets used to the disease, unleashes the sufferer and becomes "dehumanized". The question is: what skills and qualities do neurosurgeons need to practice a humanistic patient-centered care?

Knowing how to care for the sick in all their human dimensions is the main challenge facing medical education today. This is the construction of a new medical humanism capable of harmonizing the care that the patient needs. A training programme was conducted to teach medical humanism core values through lectures, role modeling, and training in interpersonal skills, literature and humanities study. Improvements in medical humanism attitudes and behaviors were attained after successfully completing the course through lectures, role modeling, and training in interpersonal skills, literature and humanities study. A humanistic neurosurgeon provides a skilled, compassionate, and empathic care to her/his patients, and demonstrates respect for their values, autonomy, and cultural backgrounds. Neurosurgery is an apprenticeship profession, where medical humanism can be taught and behaviors associated with humanism can be learned.

A set of 10 humanistic values that can help residents and practicing physicians to maintain humanism behaviors in their practice are presented here [5]. A proposal of a new model of medical humanism in neurosurgery, resulting from harmony that perfectly combines the science of modern neurosurgery with the art of care, which involves understanding the sick as a person, focusing on the patient.

1. The utmost important rule in Medicine: *Aeger Primo*, "The Patient First" [5]. The patient-centered perspective suggests physician-patient relationship, communication and relational skills and techniques are a core professional competence to be used by clinicians. Placing patients first adds important dimensions to how we judge the success and failure as neurosurgeons.

2. Every patient is a unique human being: In patient-centered medicine, the patient has to be understood as a unique human being. "Treat the patient, not the disease". The biopsychosocial model challenges the neurosurgeon to address both the biological as well as psychosocial dimensions of illness; care the needs of the patient [6]. The practice of neurosurgery that reflects humanism values involves physician– patient interactions during which the patient is seen as a unique individual who should be treated with dignity and respect.

3. The practice of Neurosurgery is both a science and an art. Carefully planning the surgical procedure is accomplished by a thorough preoperative assessment and a comprehensive treatment plan, review the anatomy and follow a careful and aseptic technique, the most basic principle of surgery. The supreme rule of the Greek medical ethics (Hippocrates): opheléein ê mê bláptein, "first to be useful, then do no harm".

4. Some neurosurgical conditions have no satisfactory solutions: To be honest but not brutal, to offer hope always and if we cannot cure, we can help, are some useful principles in guiding patients through their process when faced with catastrophic disease that has no satisfactory solution [7]. Some diseases are incurable; it's attributed to Hippocrates that in Medicine we are called "to cure sometimes, to relieve often, and to comfort always". The neurosurgeon must remember that any outcome estimates are statistical probabilities based on large groups of patients and do not predict how any given individual patient will respond.

5. Neurosurgery, as much as Medicine, is a service profession and the commitment to serve our patients is a hallmark of humanistic physicians. The Gold Foundation defines service as "the sharing of one's talent, time, and resources with those in need; giving beyond what is required" [8].

6. The humanistic neurosurgeon demonstrates the following attributes: Integrity, clinical excellence, compassion and collaboration, altruism, respect and resilience, empathy and service to her/his patients.

7. To participate in biomedical research and the advancement of neurosurgery and medicine. We, as a community of learners and knowledge builders, can and must develop meaningful methods of learning and improvement in practice [9]. We must find ways to make continuous learning and improvement an integral part of our workday, just as much as our neurosurgical procedures themselves.

8. To maintain an open, flexible and life-long learning-oriented mentality. Carl Rogers, a humanist psychologist, stated the goal of modern education:

The only man who is educated is the man who has learned how to adapt and change—the man who has realized that no knowledge is secure and that only the process of seeking knowledge gives a basis for security. The goal of education, if we are to survive, is the facilitation of change and (life-long) learning.

9. To be skeptical: scientific knowledge, the methods and results must be continuously scrutinized for possible errors. It is difficult for the medical literature to exceed 50% (17–85%) of correction, on average. Understanding of the methodology and application of evidence-based medicine (**Figure 1**) is needed to correctly interpret the literature on causation, prognosis, diagnostic tests and treatment strategies.

10. Neurosurgery is a teamwork: preparation, effective communication and respect are essential elements that affect both patient outcomes and the work environment. Good leadership knowledge and skills are crucial to team success and, more important, patient outcomes.

The humanities incorporated in the academic training process are an important resource that allows developing the human dimension of the physician. In coexistence with these realities, the humanities help and, above all, they educate. Educating is much more than training skills: involves creating a thoughtful attitude and a continuing desire to learn.

Teaching medical humanism today implies facing the challenge of promoting a true philosophical reconstruction of the physician, which is the anthropological position. And thus building "bifocal" neurosurgeons, who are capable of caring to their patients with a professional, technical and humanistic competence, in harmony, taking advantage of the best that progress offers them, to serve them in their physiological and human needs (**Table 1**).

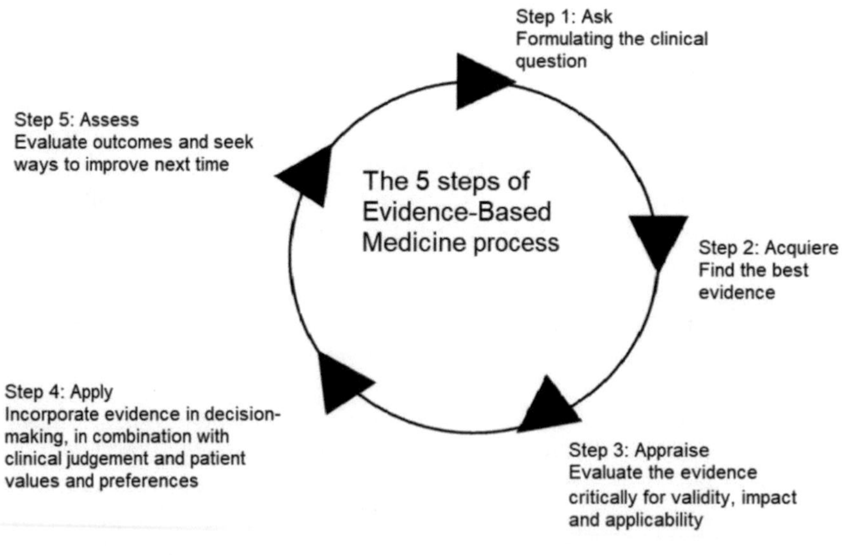

Figure 1.
The 5 steps of evidence-based medicine process (5 A's) based upon the Sackett et al. model [10]. Integrating the best available evidence with clinical expertise (proficiency and judgment) and patient values, beliefs and preferences.

• Attitudes:	Humility Curiosity Standard of behavior Humanism as medically important for the patient. Humanism as important for the physician. Role of physician as treating more than just the disease.
• Habits regularly practiced by physicians	Self-reflection Seeking connection with patients Teaching/role modeling humanism Striving to achieve balance Mindfulness and spiritual practices
• Deliberate, intentional work at habits to sustain humanism. • Develop communication and learning skills to work with families: Caring for the patient and his family. • Comprehensive training as a person: Humanistic training of the physician. • Leadership and management learning: Acquiring leadership knowledge and skills. • External/environmental support: Physician colleagues, nurses and learners are important. • Humanism as antidote to burnout: Treating patients humanistically can be "the antidote" to burnout.	

Table 1.
Factors that help sustain humanism in medical education and patient care (modified from Chou CM et al. [11]).

3. Connecting professionalism to humanism

Humanism and professionalism, to some authors, identify two different ethos of physician practice and emerge from divergent visions for the physician–patient relationship (**Table 2**) [12].

Humanism conveys a deep respect to humans individually, and to humanity collectively, and concern for their general welfare and flourishing. The hallmarks of humanism are its universality, its egalitarianism, and its scope. Its concerns, on the one hand, and obligations, on the other, apply to all humans equally; its training ground, for the most part, is experience—as a human and with humanity; and its ultimate vision is for human welfare, as broadly conceived as possible.

Professionalism, in contrast, is a socially constructed, local phenomenon. Professionalism raises expectations for professional behavior to the level of ideology, encouraging all members to embrace the traditions of the profession and to be as "professional" as they can. However, promoting professionalism -competence and excellence- does not mean to train technicians. No profession will be exercised competently if technical skills are not subordinate to a broader cultural training that encourages cultivating the spirit, the humanistic dimension. So, it is necessary to incorporate the humanistic dimension in the teaching of professionalism.

Nurturing the humanistic predispositions of residents seems to be the key to ensuring that future neurosurgeons manifest the attributes of professionalism,

Characteristic	Humanism	Professionalism
Types of values	Universal (Apply to all humans equally)	Local (A socially constructed, local phenomenon)
Sources of learning	Human experience	Socialization into profession
Motivation	Human welfare	Strengthening of professional identity
Primary duty	To other humans; to society	To the professional group
Cognitive basis	"Postconventional thinking": Judging behavior through deliberation about universal values.	"Conventional thinking": Judging behavior by comparison with the accepted social norms of a specific group.

Connecting professionalism to humanism: nurture the humanistic dimension to promote professionalism.

Table 2.
Humanism and professionalism characteristics (modified from Goldberg JL [12]).

as professionalism and humanism share common values and that each can enrich the other [13, 14]. The teaching of humanism values is recognized as an essential component of medical education and continuing professional development of physicians [15]. The application of humanism values in medical care can benefit residents, clinicians and patients [16]. The study of humanism values has a solid research base. Research has demonstrated that behaviors that are associated with humanism values improve practice and patient outcomes. The teaching of humanism values can be integrated into formal learning experiences and clinical settings, incorporating empathy, nurturing dignity, respect and confidentiality and fostering role modeling [5, 17].

The fast scientific advances require, to maintain the equilibrium, an expansion of the scope of the medical humanism, that is, a medical humanism at the height of scientific advancement. And it would be this extension of humanism, adapted to the present day, in a modern version, which would lack the process of medical education. If this humanistic update is not made, it would fall into a disproportion that would be reflected in neurosurgeons technically trained, but with serious humanistic deficiencies. We will have deformed physicians, with hypertrophy of technical knowledge, without balance, which naturally does not conquer the confidence of the patient who expects a balanced doctor. Therefore, the function of the University and the training institutions would be to expand the humanist concept in modern views, opening horizons and new prospects. And, to achieve this, the methodology and the systematic learning how to do things, when these things are many and they are wrapped in high technology and commanded by a fast scientific progress. Thus building "bifocal" neurosurgeons, who are able to care for their patients with professional, technical and humanistic competence, in harmony, taking advantage of the best that progress offers, to serve them in their physiological and human needs and beliefs.

Humanism is, therefore, a source of knowledge that the neurosurgeon uses for his/her profession. A knowledge as important - neither more nor less - such as those acquired by other ways that help him in his desire to take care of the human being who is sick. They are different routes that find in the person –the realm of medical care- their common goal and allow, with mutual coexistence presided over by respect, the union of forces, synergy in the active will to heal. Humanism in Neurosurgery it is not a temperamental issue, an individual taste, not even an interesting complement. All that would be to place "humanistic attitudes" in the balance, to compensate for the excesses of science. Humanism is, for the neurosurgeon, a true work tool, not a cultural appendix; it is a scientific attitude, weighting, the result of a conscious effort of learning and a method. It is necessary for the neurosurgeon to have a correct balance, a bifocal perspective, that manages to combine in an artistic symbiosis the attention to the disease – with all the technical evolution – and to the patient who feels sick - with the vital understanding that requires. This is, in practice, the person-centered medical care, the most accurate synthesis of the physician practicing science and art simultaneously.

4. Conclusion

Therefore, it is not enough to recommend training in medical humanism, but rather it is necessary to find a formal curricular space, that is, it is necessary to dedicate time and resources. Acknowledge and address the hidden curriculum, while sustaining a vision that incorporates humanism values. Nurturing the development of humanistic values in neurosurgery residents requires individual and institutional appreciation, recognition and commitment. A successful training programme turns residents into professionals prepared for the exercise of the art and science of Neurosurgery, by means of an active learning, where the patient is the focus of health care. A humanistic neurosurgeon provides a skilled, compassionate, and empathic care to her/his patients, and demonstrates respect for their values, autonomy, beliefs and cultural backgrounds. Neurosurgery is an apprenticeship profession, where humanism values can be taught and behaviors associated with humanism can be learned. We present a set of 10 medical humanism core values that can help residents and practicing physicians to maintain humanism behaviors in their practice. A proposal of a new model of medical humanism in neurosurgery, resulting from harmony that perfectly combines the science of modern neurosurgery with the art of care, which involves understanding the sick as a person, focusing on the patient.

In conclusion, to train a neurosurgeon who treats patients rather than diseases, and who lives the values of humanism.

Conflict of interest

The author declares no conflict of interest.

Author details

Rajab Al-Ghanem
Department of Neurosurgery, University Hospital of Jaén, Spain

*Address all correspondence to: ral_ghan@yahoo.es

References

[1] Lobato RD, Jiménez Roldan L, Alen JF, Castaño AM, Munarriz PM, Cepeda S, et al. Competency-based Neurosurgery Residency Programme. Neurocirugia. 2016; 27:75-86.

[2] Gold A, Gold S. Humanism in medicine from the perspective of the Arnold Gold Foundation: Challenges to maintaining the care in health care. J Child Neurol. 2006;21: 546-549.

[3] Hulail M. Humanism in medical practice: what, why and how?. Hos Pal Med Int Jnl. 2018;2(6):336-339. 10.15406/hpmij.2018.02.00119.

[4] Marañon G. La Medicina y nuestro tiempo. Madrid: Espasa Calpe;1954.

[5] Al-Ghanem R, Abdullah El-Rubaidi O. Medical humanism values for neurosurgery resident. Neurocirugia (Astur). 2020 Mar-Apr;31(2):103-104. Spanish. doi: 10.1016/j.neucir.2019.08.002. Epub 2019 Oct 13. PMID: 31615692.

[6] Engel GL. The Biopsychosocial Model and Medical Education. Who Are to Be the Teachers? N Engl J Med. 1982;306:802-805.

[7] Shetter AG. The fundamentals of patient assessment: The importance of the examination and the patient relationship.Clin Neurosurg. 2004;51:26-29.

[8] Kesselheim JC, Cassel CK. Service: An essential component of graduate medical education. N Engl J Med. 2013;368:500-501.

[9] Asher AL. Enlightened learning in a knowledge society. 2008 Congress Of Neurological Surgeons Presidential Address. Clin Neurosurg. 2009;56:2-8.

[10] Sackett DL, Strauss SE, Richardson WS, Rosenberg W, Hayes RB. Evidence-based medicine: how to practice and teach EBM. 2nd ed. New York: Churchill Livingstone; 2000.

[11] Chou CM, Kellom K, Shea JA. Attitudes and habits of highly humanistic physicians. Acad Med. 2014 Sep;89(9):1252-1258.

[12] Goldberg JL. Humanism or professionalism? The White Coat Ceremony and medical education. Acad Med. 2008 Aug;83(8):715-722. doi:10.1097/ACM.0b013e31817eba30. PMID: 18667880.

[13] Cohen JJ. Viewpoint: linking professionalism to humanism: what it means, why it matters. Acad Med. 2007 Nov;82(11):1029-1032.

[14] Swick HM. Viewpoint: professionalism and humanism beyond the academic health center. Acad Med. 2007 Nov;82(11):1022-1028.

[15] Liaison Committee on Medical Education. 2004. Functions and structure of a medical school standards for accreditation of medical education programs leading to the M.D. degree. Washington, D.C.: Liaison Committee on Medical Education.

[16] Robbins J, Bertakis K, Helms L, Azari R, Callahan E, Creten D. 1993. The influence of physician practice behaviors on patient satisfaction. Fam Med 25:17-20.

[17] Cohen LG, Sherif YA. Twelve tips on teaching and learning humanism in medical education. Med Teach. 2014 Aug;36(8):680-684.

Chapter 2

Social Support, Identity, and Meaning: A Phenomenological Analysis of Post-Concussion Syndrome

Gary Senecal and Patrick Whitehead

Abstract

After a traumatic blow to the head, it is common to experience difficulty focusing, disorientation, dizziness, nausea, sensitivity to light and sound, and often loss of consciousness. These symptoms often persist for several weeks following the concussion before diminishing completely. Post-concussion syndrome (PCS) refers to the persistence of concussion symptoms beyond the normal two-week window. For some, symptoms can continue for several months to several years, even further manifesting into depression, anxiety, and substance abuse in time. Though the American Psychiatric Association's (APA) Diagnostic and Statistical Manual of Mental Disorders (DSM) has continued to grow with each new version, PCS has not been included in its most recent iteration. An acquired brain injury rehabilitation specialist can be recommended for TBI, and a clinical psychologist or psychiatrist can be recommended for Acute Stress Disorder. The authors commend this reclassification because it recognizes that brain injuries are to be studied by neurologists and other medical specialists while transformations to one's existence are to be studied by psychologists. Nevertheless, while the present analysis aims at PCS in the latter (psychological) sense, it is worth mentioning that acquired brain injury (ABI) specialists have found it appropriate and even necessary to adopt an existential-phenomenological perspectives to more fully conceptualize this phenomenon. This study utilized the Interpretive Phenomenological Analysis (IPA) and arranged case studies with three athletes who had been forced to retire from sport due to major TBI's and prolonged PCS. Authors identified common themes across each interview and used free imaginative variation to describe the dimensions of the PCS experience. Specifically, the way participants were able to cope with the loss of identity and meaning after sport, as well as their perceived level of social support in the aftermath of TBI and PCS, played major roles in ameliorating and/or exacerbating both somatic and psychological difficulties associated with TBI and PCS.

Keywords: traumatic brain injury, post-concussion syndrome, phenomenology, identity, athletic retirement

1. Introduction

After a traumatic blow to the head, it is common to experience difficulty focusing, disorientation, dizziness, nausea, sensitivity to light and sound, and often loss of consciousness. These symptoms often persist for several weeks following the concussion before diminishing completely. Post-concussion syndrome (PCS) refers to the persistence of concussion symptoms beyond the normal two-week window. For some, symptoms can continue for several months to several years.

Though the American Psychiatric Association's (APA) *Diagnostic and Statistical Manual of Mental Disorders* (DSM) has continued to grow with each new version, PCS has not been included in its most recent iteration. The *DSM-5* task force explains, "[s]ymptoms previously termed *postconcussive* (e.g., headaches, dizziness, sensitivity to light or sound, irritability, concentration deficits) can occur in brain-injured and non-brain injured populations, including individuals with acute stress disorder" ([1], p. 286). The argument is that the causal linkage between traumatic brain injury (TBI) and PCS breaks down because the symptoms of PCS are either a variation of Acute Stress Disorder or TBI. An acquired brain injury rehabilitation specialist can be recommended for TBI, and a clinical psychologist or psychiatrist can be recommended for Acute Stress Disorder. The authors commend this reclassification because it recognizes that brain injuries are to be studied by neurologists and other medical specialists while transformations to one's existence are to be studied by psychologists.

While the present analysis aims at PCS in the latter (psychological) sense, it is worth mentioning that acquired brain injury (ABI) specialists have found it appropriate and even necessary to adopt an existential-phenomenological perspective as well. American rehabilitation physician and scholar Gary Goldberg [2] explains how "brain injury deeply affect[s] the subjectivity of the person injured—that is, their existence as a human person—because of the potentially significant aspects of personhood impacted [...], it can also produce significant problematic impairment of self-awareness" (p. 397). Like neuropsychiatrist Kurt Goldstein [3] argued nearly a century earlier, Goldberg and others have called for a transformation of the philosophical paradigm that has traditionally been used to understand brain injury [4–9]. To this end, the present phenomenological analysis of PCS will be of interest to sport psychologists, clinical psychologists, and rehabilitation specialists working with acquired brain injury.

1.1 Medicalization and DSM

Since the third edition was published in 1980, *Diagnostic and Statistical Manual of Mental Disorders* (DSM) has used an increasingly biomedical model for explaining psychological disorders (1980). The biomedical model has replaced the psychoanalytic drive-theory model of explanation [10, 11].

The most recent iteration, *DSM-5* [1], continues down the pathway of biomedical explanation. The task-force explains: "The science of mental disorders continues to evolve. However, the last two decades since DSM-IV was released have seen real and durable progress in such areas as cognitive neuroscience, brain imagining, epidemiology, and genetics" (p. 5). They continue, "[s]uch an approach should permit a more accurate description of patient presentations and increase the validity of diagnosis (i.e., the degree to which diagnostic criteria reflect the comprehensive manifestation of an underlying psychopathological disorder)" (p. 5). Here we see that by "psychological disorder" the *DSM-5* task force has in mind an underlying pathogen, and diagnostic validity can be improved with advances in neuroscience, brain imaging, and so forth.

Medicalization, however, has its dissidents. *DSM-5* has been repeatedly criticized for its medicalization and somatization of psychological disorders. American philosopher of medicine Kevin Aho [12] has explained that this has led to a "growing dependence on biological explanations which tend to downplay socio-historical factors" (p. 3). Peter Kinderman, British psychologist and former president of the British Psychological Association's division for clinical psychology, recommends that a psychosocial model replace the medical model [13]. He suggests, for example, that "an effective way to reduce rates of mental health problems might be to reduce inequality in society" (p. 39). In an open letter to *DSM-5* task force, Division 32 of the American Psychological Association provides four specific examples of how the newer biomedically validated diagnostic criteria have actually lowered diagnostic thresholds, making it easier to receive a diagnosis [14]. In some cases, exclusionary criteria have been removed (such as the bereavement exclusion for depression of Major Depressive Disorder. In others, diagnostic requirements have been reduced (such as with the number of symptoms required for the diagnosis of adult attention-deficit hyperactivity disorder, ADHD).

Former director of the American National Institute of Mental Health, psychiatrist Tom Insel, has complained that the newest version of *DSM*, while *more* biomedical than previous editions, is still inadequately medicalized. On the NIMH website, he explained how "[i]n the rest of medicine, [psychological diagnoses] would be equivalent to creating diagnostic systems based on the nature of chest pain or the quality of fever" ([15]; in [16], p. 522). Indeed, the medicalization of psychological disorders is in presumed etiology only. ADHD, for example, is diagnosed based on patient symptoms which belong to the private world of the patient (e.g., "has trouble waiting his or her turn"). To this diagnosis a biomedical explanation is added. There are no biological tests for depression or ADHD, and the same can be said of a great majority of psychological disorders. It is uncertain what is gained by *explaining* them this way.

While there are many competing hypotheses about what causes depression (even among biomedical psychopathologists; [17]), depression is diagnosed based on behavioral signs and subjective symptoms. In an interview, Insel implores fellow psychiatrists to begin treating psychological disorders as brain disorders, e.g., relying exclusively on brain scans for depression diagnoses [18]. Until that day comes, depression will be diagnosed even in the absence of biomedical evidence.

Another troubling problem arises in addition to diagnostic validity. When biomedical factors are emphasized to the neglect of psychosocial, cultural, political, and historical factors, who benefits? The increasing medicalization of *DSM* has led to a suspicious partnership between the American Psychiatric Association and pharmaceutical companies [12, 19, 20].

2. Medicalization of PCS

PCS has not shared the fate of other psychological disorders. Like depression, PCS is diagnosed from behavioral and physiological signs (such as alcohol intolerance and problems shifting focus) and subjective symptoms (such as decreased music-listening pleasure). Also like depression, for PCS there is no neurological, biogenetic, or hormonal diagnostic procedure. However, depression remains in *DSM-5* and PCS does not. The *DSM-5* task force explains, "[s]ymptoms previously termed *postconcussive* (e.g., headaches, dizziness, sensitivity to light or sound, irritability, concentration deficits) can occur in brain-injured and non-brain injured populations, including individuals with acute stress disorder" ([1], p. 286). The argument is that the causal linkage between traumatic brain injury (TBI) and PCS breaks down because the symptoms of PCS can be attributed to additional causes (such as Acute Stress Disorder). As such, PCS is eliminated from *DSM-5*, and can be understood as either a variation of Acute Stress Disorder or TBI. An acquired brain injury rehabilitation specialist can be recommended for TBI; a clinical psychologist or psychiatrist can be recommended for

Acute Stress Disorder. The authors commend this reclassification because it recognizes that brain injuries are to be studied by neurologists and other medical specialists while transformations to one's existence are to be studied by psychologists.

While the present analysis aims at PCS in the latter psychological sense, it is worth mentioning that acquired brain injury (ABI) specialists have found it appropriate and even necessary to adopt an existential-phenomenological perspective as well. American rehabilitation physician and scholar Gary Goldberg [2] explains how "brain injury deeply affect[s] the subjectivity of the person injured—that is, their existence as a human person—because of the potentially significant aspects of personhood impacted..., it can also produce significant problematic impairment of self-awareness" (p. 397). Like neuropsychiatrist Kurt Goldstein [3] argued nearly a century earlier, Goldberg and others have called for a transformation of the philosophical paradigm that has traditionally been used to understand brain injury [4–9].

3. Using the phenomenological method to understand psychological disorders

The issues of diagnostic validity and medicalization emerge when the goal of scientific inquiry and treatment is law-governed explanation (*Erklären*). *DSM* reliance on neuroscience, brain imaging, and genetics is in service to explaining what constitutes a psychological disorder and, by extension, what causes each. Explaining phenomena is rooted in a Netwonian philosophy of science which views persons and things in their objectivity—that is, stripped of all qualities that cannot also be explained. Experimental procedures focus on identifying temporally and spatially proximal causes. This kind of knowledge is the goal of the natural sciences.

Erklären cannot reach human existence because existence is not divisible into objects. German philosopher Martin Heidegger [21] has argued that modern natural science has confused existence (i.e., *being*) with explanatory objects (i.e., beings). German philosopher Edmund Husserl, who inspired Heidegger, has also argued (1972) that modern natural science is incapable of understanding human experience. Husserl [22] has advocated for a humanistic science tasked with *understanding* human experience and proposed the phenomenological method for examining and describing the structure of human consciousness. This is in line with the methods of human science of 19th century German philosopher Wilhelm Dilthey (1833–1911) who emphasized *Verstehen* knowledge which focuses on meaning (*see* [23]).

Verstehen and *Erklären* are important for understanding psychological disorders because the latter are diagnosed through signs (objective behaviors) and symptoms (subjective experiences. Where *DSM-5* searches exclusively for physiological explanations for psychological disorders, it has either ignored the importance of understanding subjective experience (symptoms) or has confused symptoms with signs. To adequately address the breadth of psychological disorders, attention must be paid to understanding symptoms. This need has been identified for common psychological disorders [12] and advanced psychoses (*see* [24]). In the present article, the authors describe PCS with the goal of better understanding how it is experienced.

The descriptive phenomenological method begins, Giorgi explains, "by obtaining concrete descriptions of experiences from others who have lived through situations in which the phenomenon that the researcher is interested have taken place" [25]. These descriptions are the raw data of an empirical phenomenological analysis. This form of qualitative analysis follows three distinct steps: 1) Reading each protocol (that is, the raw data) for a sense of its whole. This means familiarizing oneself with the event as it has been described by each subject.

2) A determination of meaning units within the protocol. In this step of the analysis, the investigator tries to note any affective, experiential, or other shifts that occur within the protocol. 3) Transforming the natural attitude expressions into phenomenologically psychologically sensitive expressions. That is, the *psychological insights regarding the phenomenon* can be discussed without *reducing* the phenomenon to its psychological description.

4. Design

Authors obtained IRB approval before distributing a general call to university coaches and athletic trainers who supplied contact information for athletes interested in participating in a PCS study. Authors followed up with prospective participants and arranged interviews with three athletes. Participants 1 and 3 were males whose concussions had forced an early retirement from careers in football. Participant 2 was a female mountain climber. Interviews were recorded using a digital recording device and subsequently transcribed into text. Transcripts were analyzed using the descriptive phenomenological method [25]. Authors identified common themes across each interview and used free imaginative variation to describe the dimensions of the PCS experience.

5. Results

The participants who volunteered for this study had different experiences in recovery from TBI. Each participant succeeded in rehabilitating from injury but took very different paths in doing so. Common across each was a modification of personality and routine. Participant 3 had a complete recovery and full amelioration of symptoms in a relatively timely manner. He was able to do so with the least amount of adjustment. Participant 1, in comparison, had a long and turbulent recovery that involved the extension of symptoms over time and a severe and prolonged impairment in his psychosocial well-being. His recovery required a significant change to personality. Participant 2 made immediate adjustments in the wake of her injury and relied on social support to complete the readjustment and rehabilitation process.

As mentioned in the introduction and literature review, this examination of TBI and PCS focuses on the phenomenological dimensions of PCS—that is, how PCS is lived. Such examination requires we look closely at the meaning-centered aspects of recovery from head trauma, and examine how purpose, desire, and goal-orientation are adopted anew. Important themes during this process are identity formation, solidarity with others, and meaning. For our participants, psychosocial support proved to be the most significant factor affecting the severity of PCS and its rehabilitation.

The results are broken into two major subsections. The first is devoted to psychosocial factors which exacerbate PCS; the second to psychosocial factors which ameliorate PCS.

6. Impaired well-being

German hermeneutic philosopher Hans Georg Gadamer (1996) has found health a peculiar concept because it is not a good to be bought or sold. It is only when one is suffering that one comes to notice health at all. Illness and disease are impairments to health, but what is health itself but well-being? Each of our participants experienced an impairment to his or her well-being. Routines that marked ordinary life were upset by persistent concussion symptoms, impairing relationships and identity. Attempts to ignore or overcome the disruptions through willpower only increased the disruption.

6.1 Difficulties shifting identity

A significant problem of TBI is that the activity during which it occurs is itself one that brings a person fulfillment and pride. This was the case for our participants. Two were NCAA scholarship student-athletes, and the third was an amateur rock-climber. The injury threatened the continued enjoyment each participant could find in their chosen activity.

The participants who volunteered for this study had relatively different experiences in the recovery from a traumatic brain injury. Generally speaking, the three participants' experiences covered a wide swatch of the spectrum regarding the amelioration of symptoms, health, and life satisfaction in recovery. In terms of this spectrum of health and wellbeing, one participant (P3) had what we would describe as a full recovery and full amelioration of symptoms in a relatively timely manner. A second participant (P1) had what we would describe as a long and turbulent recovery that involved the extension of symptoms over time, as well as severe and prolonged impairment in his psychosocial wellbeing. Finally, the third participant (P2) had what we would term as a moderate recovery; one that involved significant challenges early in the process but, over time, turned to a full recovery after certain psychosocial factors came into place to support her through her PCS recovery.

Of the three participants in this study, P1 (whom the authors will call Roger) struggled the most as he faced the end of his career as a football player. Roger teared up as he described this realization: "It's like, I play football, I'm the alpha male and it's a scary feeling and it's like, 'what's going to happen?'"

Roger expresses clearly the difficulty that many athletes face when injured, deselected, or forced to retire. For Roger, the multiple concussions forced an abrupt retirement from football. Perhaps for the first time since late childhood when he realized his skill as an athlete, Roger is faced with the question of identity. Who is he if not alpha male?

During the interview, Roger vacillates between recognizing then ignoring the serious difficulty transitioning out of football. In a revealing statement, Roger admits that the loss of identity continues to be a source of anguish. "I can't just hop up and say, 'oh I'm going to be an athlete again.' That's something I worked forever to be. And that's not something that I can just wake up and be [...] again."

Like Roger, P3 (whom the authors will call Philip) was a division one NCAA football player. Philip must also face the loss of his identity as a football player, a consequence that occurred in the middle of his senior season. The depth of loss was exacerbated by a game where he would have played in front of 45,000 spectators. Philip explains;

That day was really, really tough for me emotionally. [...] Besides my family, football has been the one thing in my life that I have loved endlessly, and I'm never going to stop loving it, but you know I've been playing since elementary school and it's so tough to just immediately stop when I thought I was going to have 11 more games guaranteed. [...] And I think after this season I would have been content with stopping. At times I just felt like I was letting people down. I know I did not actually quit but it kind of felt that feeling of being like a quitter for the first time in my life.

Philip experiences a complicated blend of feelings about retiring from the sport and abandoning his team. Head injuries are less conspicuous than torn ligaments and broken bones, and this means the athletes have more responsibility in decisions to dis/continue. With a broken femur, suiting up for a game is out of the question. But with a lingering threat of another and possibly more severe concussion, the decision to play is left to the athlete, and Philip expressed guilt about his lack of commitment. To complicate this concern, upon returning to practice Philip had to wear a special uniform during practice indicating he was not to be hit. He explains, "It's like you've got this label on you that you're the kid that's injured that's no able to do the full practice. I don't want to say I felt weak but that's kind of how I felt." As a middle linebacker, Philip had a reputation of being tough. Vulnerability replaced toughness.

So too is it with the non-football player, P2 (whom the authors will call Maryann), who experienced a shift in identity following a rock-climbing head-injury. As a young college professor, Maryann prided herself in performing brilliantly and creatively in the classroom. Her brilliance was owed to endurance and focus during preparation, traits she lost after a concussion. She described the brilliant teacher as one who could roll into a classroom prepared to answer any question with ferocity and confidence. No longer able to rely on her cognitive agility, Maryann reports having to adjust to become "an economical teacher." As an economical teacher, Maryann has to ask for help in advance of, and leaned on her students during, her courses. However, she views this as a normal progression of becoming more mature as a professor. The concussion expedited this transition, but it was one towards which she found herself heading all along:

> *I am a little sad to lose the brilliance. I am a little sad to move out of that phase of my life. [However,] I almost wonder if it's not time to move into a different phase. And, so, this concussion just helped me to, like, stop, reconsider what's going on and then move in a different direction.*

All three participants experienced a loss of confidence in their identities where vulnerability supplanted strength. While the football players worry about how their weakness will be interpreted by others, Maryann sees the identity transformation as normal, even salutary. Her ease of transitioning to a post-injury life is owed to her willingness to experience vulnerability, and her openness to adopt a new professional identity. This may be compared to Roger and Philip who shared thoughts about transitioning to coaching, but who struggled to reconcile the new position on the football team with their alpha male identities (which they were unable to abandon).

6.2 Social isolation and support

Another significant factor working against participants during their recoveries was the absence of social support from peers, family, neighbors, and/or loved ones. When Roger had little to no social support for extended periods of time during his recovery, PCS symptoms were at their worst.

Roger was offered the least amount of social support across the three participants. He describes his experience of social isolation and perceived lack of social support from coaches after a serious concussion while playing for his university team:

> *I just felt as though they did not care. I was just like, they do not give a fuck about me. [...] They do not call me. The only time they called me is if I did something wrong. I got a concussion, you calling me about missing something called breakfast check (where players meet with coaches)? Like, I really did not care. I was just like, I'm not going to go to anything. I'm not going to do anything and they are going to have to find me if they want me.*

As a university athlete, Roger is away from his social support structure at home, and his new support structure is made entirely of teammates and coaches—people he believes do not value him outside of his contributions on the field. The athletic relationship between players and coaches is predominantly utilitarian. It is of deep value to consider the level of perceived isolation and dehumanization that is present in his social experience after high school.

It is difficult to separate actual from perceived social support. Roger seemed incapable of recognizing support when present. For example, he felt like his mother did not care about him even though she was regularly calling. "I'm like 'mom, I don't even want to be on Earth and you're not even asking me anything.' And she's like, 'but I am, I'm calling you everyday.' And I'm like, 'but you're not, you're not here.' It was never enough." The primary shortcoming of social support may not be from Roger's social environment at all, but his willingness to recognize support when present:

> *A second form of social isolation came with treatment itself. Roger explains:*
>
> *I went to the psychiatric facility for four days and I mean all they did was we would be in groups, we could be playing cards, we could be watching TV, and they say they were evaluating you but they were just writing is he walking or is he sitting. It wasn't that much of an evaluation, there wasn't that many people to evaluate 60 people in the place. There's no way everyone can be evaluated and keyed in on. They were just doing what they were supposed to be doing, writing little notes, writing little notes. [...] It can be a weekly visit with a psychologist or a counselor. I know that's what got me through, just talking to my friends and talking to my counselor. Because I can always talk to someone that has like a point of view because you go talk to that counselor, he does not know you really, so he's going to give you the raw of what's going on.*

The psychiatric facility is Roger's final place to turn for social support. However, just as he perceives apathy from coaches, loved ones, and family members throughout this process, the overworked and understaffed nature of the psychiatric facility is unable to meet his needs. It is the desire for interpersonal connection with and empathy and support from others that Roger seeks. The absence of such support is what stands out most significantly in Roger's experience with PCS.

Maryann's situation is similar. Her dependence on others reaches its peak following her injury. "In the aftermath," she explains, "I felt so lost. It was really, really astounding. Luckily I was able to stay with a friend for weeks, so I had somebody that I knew from before the accident." But then Maryann had to move, and she rented an apartment for a few weeks in a new town which was disorienting. "Nothing smelled like me. And I thought that I was losing my mind like, I really thought that I was going crazy because I had nothing, nothing that reminded me. [My partner at the time] took off, like didn't answer calls; just disappeared."

Knowledgeable about TBI, Maryann was looking for evidence that her personality had not changed. But her new environment and social isolation provided little in the way of homogeneity. Furthermore, she describes how the social nature of her life as an academic was not conducive to her recovery process:

> *I think the hardest part about academia for me is isolation. There's no question. I played team sports my whole life, I know teams. That's how I know how to function. Nobody here knows teams. Nobody here knows teams. I know like the idea of helping each other instead of getting ahead of each other. There is no doubt that my job made the recovery more difficult because of this.*

6.3 Resistance to personality change

Though each tried, all three participants were limited or unable to continue their pre-injury commitments and routines, leading to frustration and exhaustion. The longer the commitment lasted before the injury, the greater the severity of PCS.

It wasn't until he lost blocks of time and bits of memory during a phone conversation that Roger began to suspect he had suffered his fifth concussion. This occurred during a typical phone conversation when he had trouble remembering his previous day. He was also unable to read his notes without the words dancing around on the page. The impairments to his routine were considerable.

Philip was worried he would be unable to get through a workout without passing out. Even standing up too quickly resulted in light-headedness. This was a significant change. Philip reported being the strongest member of the football team during training. He had spent years of his life repeatedly training his muscles to engage in specific exercises. The fast-twitch anaerobic muscular strength upon which he relied was no longer there for him. His body was unfamiliar.

Maryann experienced trouble looking at the computer screen for long periods of time without getting dizzy, and this impaired nearly every aspect of her occupation as professor. Inability to concentrate affected normal daily activities like driving and grocery shopping. Indeed, it was her experience of dizziness while checking items off her grocery list that prompted her to see a physical therapist.

As with all illnesses [26], PCS is experienced through disruptions to routine. In the midst of routine, the body is taken for granted and absent to experience. It is only once these routines break down that the body is noticed at all. Attempts to continue the impaired routine results in disorientation and suffering—Roger studying for an exam, Philip finishing one more workout, and Maryann reviewing a course syllabus. It is only in the midst of such routines that one feels at home, and it is upon such routines that one builds one's identity and sense of life-satisfaction. To lose these routines is distressing, but it can also interrupt one's sense of time and space. It is as Maryann describes her routines: as "anchor[s] in the day to keep me moving from one point to the next. So that even if it's disorienting in between I know where I'm supposed to be when I'm supposed to be there and that's the foundation." Without routines one is adrift.

The desire to return to their pre-injury state is understandable, but impossible. It is only once the routine is adjusted that rehabilitation may begin. For Maryann, this started with adjustments in the classroom:

> *I was just honest with the students right up front and I said "you know I have a concussion. I can't use the computer and I need the lights to be off in the room because it's making me sick having the lights on." And they were really great about it, I mean, I got a lot of athletes in my class as well so hearing "concussion" they know what that means. Yeah, and then the other thing is I usually push too hard and with a concussion you cannot.*

Maryann recognized and accepted her newfound shortcomings which she was then able to strategically address. Strategies included being more patient with her work, taking breaks, and stopping to nap when necessary. These strategies are helpful not in recovering the pre-injury personality, but in developing a new one post-injury. To that end, Maryann was able to view these personality changes as important ones—changes the injury helped her make. Even before the injury, she recognized a needed help with work/life balance. The concussion helped her back off what she described as a tendency to be a "workaholic," and pay special attention to diet, nutrition, and social networks. "So one of the things that I've noticed is that

I have to make time for my hobbies and I have to make time for other people. [...] I needed to reexamine my sense of identity and commitment to priorities. I needed to make time away from work to be with others."

Finding meaning in injury and illness is an important part of what physician and philosopher of medicine Aaron Antonovsky has called sense of coherence (SOC). Patients that have a high SOC rehabilitate more quickly and live longer and more satisfying lives.

7. Social support and well-being

7.1 Solidarity and support

Participants credited social support for their ability to establish new forms of identity and purpose in their lives following TBI. Philip described the efforts of his teammates, family, peers, and coaches as beneficial for navigating the abrupt end of his football career. He describes a conversation with his father after Philip was sidelined with a concussion:

> *My Dad is like the hardest guy I've ever known, hardest worker. He's so supportive about football and he's played his entire life too. He loves the game and for him to be on the phone with me and to have him start crying and saying, "Alright, this is it, we got to hang it up." That's when I was like, "Alright, this is it." But, yes, I definitely felt supported by my parents throughout this process.*

Philip finds comfort in his father's empathy. He also found support from the team's linebacker coach who explained "if you were my son, I'd tell you to shut it down." Reflecting on his decision to retire from football, Philip explained that everybody around him was supportive:

> *And when it came down for me to actually say I was officially done, I sat down with my linebacker's [position-] coach and also the head coach and they were both like "this is the right decision for the long term and obviously we're going to miss you this year but your health is a lot more important".*

Support from coaches at an NCAA division I program, whose professional livelihoods are tied to young players like Philip, is difficult to overstate. With so much professional capital at stake, coaches can easily adopt a utilitarian relationship towards their players, squeezing every drop of performance from their players until there is nothing left. His position coach deliberately chooses to place himself in the position as Philip's mentor and caretaker, placing the personal well-being of his player above the productive value he might have had to the team as a starting linebacker. The whole coaching staff makes it clear that player health and well-being is more important than winning. Philip explains:

> *I have so much support from my friends, my family and no one's going to tell me that I did anything wrong in life or I was quitter or anything like that. I may have thought that but I think as I progress through my life, not doing contact sports is probably the better thing.*

Even with the family and coaching support, Philip still loses his typical in-season routines of training, practice, and competition. Though his coaches allow him to stay with the team in a quasi-coaching role, there's a noticeable hole left by physical training and performance.

Roger was also surprised by the support he received from university football coaches following his most serious concussion. After ignoring them for weeks for fear of being rejected, he finally told them what had happened. "It was just a big change. They checked in on me. They called to see if I was okay rather than getting on me about stuff I was doing wrong. [...] And that meant the world to me."

Roger took a break from school to adjust and began working in an athletic shoes store. This gave him an opportunity to build relationships outside of football while also maintaining continuity—from athletics to athletic equipment. "That was very good for me, being in a social, interactive environment helping people getting something that they need, which is shoes." Despite the lack of glamor, there are a series of factors in Roger's new job that support well-being: strong relationships with his new coworkers, a sense of purpose and identity in his work, and unique knowledge of the field.

7.2 Accepting personality change

Beyond strong relationships, empathy, and social support from peers and loved ones, another significant factor in building a sense of well-being for participants was their ability develop a new post-injury personality. We have seen the changes accepted by Maryann in the classroom. The loss for Roger and Philip was more significant, since the injury forced them into early retirement. Something new and significant had to replace football.

As mentioned, Roger's football career ended abruptly after a series of TBI's during the preseason of his senior year in college. He describes the process of refocusing his identity and relationships:

> *(Strong relationships are) what I did not think I was going to have. It was like even though I'm social, it was like okay I work with you, cool. But no, like we actually do things outside of work. We go to movies. We go out to eat and all that stuff. To find friends so fast was great for me. I felt like I would not find friends again. I thought that was going to be harder than what it was. To find another group of friends that I could talk to outside of sports was great. Usually all of my friends were from sports, playing on teams since I was younger. Most of my friends came from like, either, the travel team I played on, the school team I played on. And like, it was cool to have friends from different walks of life. One of the girls, she's gay and in the world we are in now just to have a friend that's gay is cool because the stuff that they go through may be totally different from what you go through. Just seeing a different perspective and talking to her or helping her for how she can handle situations when people are talking bad about her and all that stuff but, to see her, how she handles things is phenomenal. A lot of stuff just rolls right off her shoulder. It's great because if she can do that just because of her sexual preference, I can do that and nothing is really going on it's all up inside my head. So, those relationships at work really helped me just like, find myself again, to know that I was okay. Get back to being the regular me. So, this is about becoming the student I want to be again and that's probably the toughest part because my brain is not where it used to be. So, it takes me a little longer to do papers. And that's what's tough right now.*

Research shows that the shift in identity for athletes, especially after abrupt retirement due to injury, can be distressing and lead to psychosocial tension (Petitpas, et al., 2000). However, this line of research also speaks to the real benefits that retired athletes can receive from engaging in a flexible sense of identity. Roger continues, describing the process of refocusing his identity and relationships:

> *I felt like I would not find friends again. I thought that was going to be harder than what it was. To find another group of friends that I could talk to outside of sports was great. Usually all of my friends were from sports, playing on teams since I was younger. Most of my friends came from like, either, the travel team I played on, the school team I played on. And like, it was cool to have friends from different walks of life.*

Finally, Philip admits that nothing in life will match the feeling you get running out onto the football field but hopes to experience it in bits and pieces throughout life. "There's going to be aspects of my life later on where it's going to be those same emotions, those same strong feelings that I'm going to get while I'm playing football." Ultimately, Philip's combination of flexible identity and social solidarity offer a clear sense of career perspective for him, and allows him to be open, adaptable, and hopeful about the inevitable shift in life he faces.

7.3 Carving a novel path forward

Beyond strong relationships, empathy, and social support from peers and loved ones, another significant factor in building a sense of well-being for participants was their ability to carve out novel behaviors, goals, and routines in the aftermath of the TBI. For both participants Roger and Philip, their respective careers in sport were definitively ended after their final TBI. Therefore, moving forward into novel endeavors was essential for a myriad of professional, motivational and emotional reasons. Though she was not forced into definitive retirement, Maryann chose to step away from rock-climbing after her serious TBI as the presence of being in the arena caused psychological and somatic symptoms that were difficult to bear. Ultimately, all participants in this study were put in a position where carving out new behaviors, goals, and routines would be essential in moving forward in their professional and recreational lives.

Maryann expresses sentiments of needing to, in some ways, fundamentally restructure her habits, routines, and professional approach. She expresses how she experienced relief through streamlining her professional approach at work and establishing a sense of stoic efficiency:

> *I had to change my whole approach. You really have to because there's no time. All these students are really counting on you and relying on you, your department. There's no time for you to be sitting at home and crying that you are hurt. You just have to get up and do it, so what do you need to be able to get that done? It's like alright it happened, okay. Let us do what we have to, we have to run through to the end. No tears until you get home. And what do you need, like what do you need to be able to get it done? Like, to get through this day, what do you need today? And to finally ask yourself what do you need, not how much can I take from you but what do you need to be able to get through because we need to get this done. So, it's really developed a different relationship with myself.*

As mentioned throughout, Maryann feels a tremendous sense of accountability to her students and peers. Originally, this led to her decision to not take the proper amount of recovery time after her serious TBI. However, Maryann is able to find a novel way to move forward despite the limiting circumstances due to PCS. Her ability to adjust - to shift course and construct novel tendencies and behaviors in her day to day work - opens a space for her to overcome the immediate psychological and cognitive deficiencies in the aftermath of her TBI. As is the case with all three participants in this study, we argue that it is this ability to adapt after the TBI that supports wellbeing, psychosocial functionality, and the amelioration of symptoms for participants.

Though Philip still seems to be struggling with aspects of leaving sport - especially the emotional void that can come with leaving competition - he consistently describes how there a series of behaviors and outlets in his life that can replicate this emotional void. He expresses how he is optimistic about the possibility of his future career and its ability to fill any emotional void after football:

> *P: Being with all the guys; that's one thing that I'll definitely miss. But I think the work that you put into it just to win a football game, you realize that the entire work that you put into something made this product of a win. I know there's obviously other things in life where you put in so much time and you have a great outcome too but I think it's that one feeling when you run out onto the field and Sean Payton actually has a quote, he said, "You'll never get the same feeling when you run out onto a football field on a Friday night or a Saturday but you're going to get it in small pieces in your life" and that's like when you get married or have your first kid, you are going to get that same feeling. But it's just not going to come every single Saturday in the fall.*
>
> *I: Do you believe that? Do you believe that you will get tastes of it?*
>
> *P: Yeah, I think I definitely believe it. There's going to be aspects of my life later on where it's going to be those same emotions, those same strong feelings that I'm going to get while I'm playing football.*
>
> *I: Sure, but what about in your career? Do you think it will? Do you think in business, going into business it will replicate some of these, you said it well, strong emotions?*
>
> *P: I think so. Business is a competitive environment as well so I think the aspects that you need to be a collegiate athlete kind of transform into the business world too, so, I would say it would come here and there.*

Furthermore, he explains how deeper engagement in his academic work as a student and volunteer work outside of the classroom was deeply beneficial in the aftermath of TBI and, consequently, retirement:

> *I: What about as a student? Do you ever get it as a student?*
>
> *P: Yes. I think so.*
>
> *I: Does anything in academics or anything right now...is there anything that you do on a semi-regular basis that provides a similar kind of cathartic release to sports, or to football I should say?*
>
> *P: I do not know that's a tough one. I think I have not experienced the extent of some football emotions that you get while you are playing in the classroom but I think it's still a competitive environment obviously, you want to do better than some of the other students in the class.*
>
> *I: What about the solidarity thing? You said that you felt really connected to your teammates. Is there anything that you do outside of sports that makes you feel connected to the people around you? Even on a spectrum level? If it's not the same*

> *extent, is there anything that you do that falls on the spectrum of connection and solidarity?*
>
> *P: I do Big Brother Big Sisters so I've had a little brother over in the [College City] project for the past four years and I developed a really good relationship with him and just seeing him grow these past couple of years I think that's been a great experience as well. That's been something that I would say is pretty close to that team connection.*

Philip is fortunate enough to be at a college and in a social-professional culture that worked to promote a more holistic sense of identity beyond any exclusive notion of athletic identity. He describes how he feels like he can move between student-identity and service-identity after his athletic-identity is no longer available. These complementary forms of identity form a holistic sense of self and open space for him reconceptualize and broaden identity after sport. This allows him to experience how novel behaviors - intellectual engagement and service - can allow for a similar sense of satisfaction, solidarity, and competition after sport.

Finally, Philip expresses how he is relatively at peace with the end of his career and is anticipating the next chapter of life after football. He expresses how the combination of social support from his family, personal and team accomplishments have left him in a place where he is comfortable walking away:

> *I think I've definitely come to conclusions with my playing career. As I've thought about it, I'm like, okay, I got to play here at [College], I had a great experience, I had a really good career here. I played in high school. That was a great four years. I won a state championship in [State] with my best friends in high school and that was an unbelievable experience. I played my entire life with Pop Warner and as I've gone back and thought about my entire football career, I could not be more proud of myself. My parents could not be more proud of me so I think hearing that from them and I think look in the mirror at the end of the day and just actually being happy with myself and in my career I think it's made it a lot easier. I'm ready for the next chapter now.*

Philip's experience of PCS in the aftermath of a series of severe TBI and his consequent transition out of sport was undoubtedly the most expedited and successful in this study. This passage almost fully encapsulates the psychosocial factors that convalesce for P3 in order to navigate this transition so smoothly. The combination of both flexible identity and social solidarity, offer a clear sense of career perspective for him. Ultimately, this provides him a space to be open, adaptable, and hopeful about the inevitable shift that his life is undergoing.

7.4 Gaining a new sense of purpose

Participants experienced a higher level of life-satisfaction by gaining a new sense of purpose. TBI forces individuals to make significant alterations to their lives, routines, habits, and careers. This came more easily for Maryann and Philip than for Roger.

Roger's university playing career had only just begun, and his identity as a football player (which provided a full-tuition scholarship) was tied to his identity as a student, and he withdrew from school. After building relationships at his new job, Roger is able to look back with a heavy heart at those who suffer similarly from TBI, and has a compassion that only comes from having lived through it:

> *When I was talking to my psychologist, in his report, it says that I show signs of CTE. And it's like, wow, this is something I read about and saw it in a movie and I show signs of it, that's crazy. Now I want to help people and hopefully slow things down for future players or get better helmets or something because I feel like my last concussion was because the school did not have proper equipment. But, that's besides the fact, we just need to find the right combination for guys. It is something I want to be a part of.*

TBI's have fundamentally shifted the course of Roger's life and career. They have forced him to fully retire from football and withdraw from college. However, over time Roger describes how he begins to gain a sense of perspective on his own personal trauma. This leads to a deepening desire to offer solidarity and support to peers and former athletes who may have shared a similar experience of trauma. Roger continues, expressing a sense of compassion and desire to forward his support and care to other former contact-sport athletes who may also be suffering from the effects of head trauma:

> *I remember I was talking to my cousin and he works at a strip club and there was a guy who played for the Falcons. He's retired now but he's always there. I'm pretty sure he has CTE, but he's always drunk and he's fighting people and stuff like that. Him telling me that, while I was going through this is what made me step back from the situation and have a perspective on it. I do not want to be like that because that's the guy I did look up to when I was younger. (Player's name), I mean he played for the (NFL Team) and he was pretty good and to hear how he's doing in life now, after football, I do not want to be like that. I want to be able to still have intelligent conversations and talk to people just like this. Not "ah ugh you want to have a beer man?" No, that's not me. Of course, I can loosen up and have some fun but just to be yelling at people in the club because I'm drunk and mad for no reason? That's not me. I cannot do that and I hate that for him. And I told my cousin, if you can get in contact with him, I want to talk to him. Not on being a fan, I just want to talk to him just to help because he may have some insight for myself or I may have some insight for him. You never know. I do not care that he's an NFL player and played 16 years. I want to help because I feel as though in five years, we may be saying that (NFL Player) killed himself in a car accident or with a gun. Because that's crazy for him to really be having mood swings and drinking as much as he says he drinks, it's not good. It's not good at all. They're a person. We look at them like a piece of meat like, "Oh yeah, he made these plays or this play." But that's only inside of the helmet. He has a family. His purpose in life, in the world, may be bigger than just football to his family. That's what I look at it as. [...] Football is not, it does not define us, but it does get us to different places in life. It got me to college. And at times I did not think I was going to go to college, not coming from the neighborhood I came from. [...] So, seeing people from my same background doing things that I wanted to do and now he's going through that as far as being drunk all the time and being angry and all that stuff? That's not good. That's not good at all. I want to prevent that for someone maybe in my generation or the future generations, maybe even help people that are like him right now.*

Roger feels compelled to take up a greater sense of commitment to supporting individuals who, like himself, are possibly struggling in the aftermath of excessive TBI and career transition out of sport. He is able to recognize the stark reality that many face in the aftermath of their careers and the aftermath of head trauma. Though he did not make it to the NFL, he finds a shared sense of connection and experience with former NFL players who are facing a similar dark journey in the aftermath of TBI and their careers. He is clear here in recognizing that the difficulties of retirement are not merely limited to head trauma.

Finally, Roger mentions how symptoms of PCS are ameliorated when he is engaged in an activity that he is passionate about. He describes how his level of focus increases significantly when reading articles that are in the range of either his academic or personal interest:

> *I: And have you noticed any activities or even books or articles or movies that you do get really focused, that you can focus on?*
>
> *P: Sports. Anything with sports I can focus in good on. And it's frustrating because I was talking to my agent. She was like, normally what happens, because she's a psychology major, normally what happens is things that you get excited about, you are going to remember. I was just like, that sounds about right. But, I want to get excited about everything and remember everything. But that's just not how stuff is going to work. But it's just like, how do I get my brain to where I can retain what I used to retain? About things that are outside of sports?*
>
> *I: What about the research that you said that you did into the effects of marijuana on sleep? Were you able to focus on those things?*
>
> *P: Yeah because it was something that it was going to help me. Researching that it was more so reading what certain, what the certain strands did and the effects that it would have. And then if I was able to get my hands on it to see what it did to me, and most of the time if I got anything it was just I would get sleepy or I would get focused. And that was awesome to be able to focus in and do my work.*

Put simply, the presence of somatic and cognitive symptoms do not present universally for Roger. Instead, when he is engaged in an activity that finds personal passion and meaning in, many of the cognitive difficulties and symptoms are ameliorated. His description elucidates the role that meaning is likely to have on building focus and cognitive endurance even after a severe amount of TBI.

Maryann finds a sense of purpose in her recovery process and establishing a novel sense of purpose brings her to a greater position of well-being in the midst of her experience of PCS. She describes how getting back to the work she felt she owed her students was what drove her forward and helped her overcome the most difficult aspects of PCS:

> *I think part of the recovery was actually having something to do. You know, somewhere to be. Something to heal for because I did not want to let my students down. So that was really helpful in recovering and getting through the semester and being a bigger person for them.*

Similar to Roger, Maryann experiences a sense of cognitive endurance and the amelioration of symptoms when she is engaged in purpose-directed and meaningful activity. As mentioned throughout, she feels a sense of accountability to her peers and students and this drives her to return so quickly to work. Despite the difficulties of this early return, she gains a sense of cognitive strength through reorienting her own existential commitments through the trauma as a deep connection to her work and students.

As we have alluded to, compared to the other participants in this study (especially Roger), Philip was able to commit himself to a new sense of purpose with relative ease in the midst of experiencing PCS after the TBI that ended his career. He describes how he was able to establish a new purpose on the team after realizing his contributions on the field were no longer possible:

> *P: I would say so because obviously I'm not contributing on the field and it's tough for me to be like a coach and not try to overstep some boundaries here and there. At times I just felt like I was letting people down and I know I did not actually quit but it kind of felt that feeling of being like a quitter for the first time in my life.*
>
> *I: Did you feel that way?*
>
> *P: I did. At first it was really hard to kind of get over that fact that I had to stop because of my health but it was like was I kind of quitting almost?*
>
> *I: Were you able to find any ways to make contributions? Or anything that you felt was a contribution to the team? During those few weeks and months as you are going through this and you are not on the field, you are not playing, you are watching from the sidelines, was there anything you could've done there or is there anything that you did do during that time that made you feel like hey I am contributing something here to the team?*
>
> *P: Yeah, definitely. I helped. I went to every practice and helped out at all of those. So, I still felt that I was a part of the team even though I wasn't playing, you know? I got to go to all of the games.*
>
> *I: And you did feel like you were able to hold up with all of this work for the team?*
>
> *P: Yeah, I was able to chart plays for the defense and contribute as much as possible but I think not actually physically contributing to a win or loss kind of made me feel a little down on myself.*

Despite his inability to contribute to his team's success on the field, P3 is offered the opportunity to take up a pseudo-coaching and staff-support role for the team. Through this, he is able to bring some of his on the ground knowledge to his coaching staff while also offering an extra set of eyes and hands to the day-to-day work of practice and game day operations. Yet, he still expresses initial lament about not being able to physically contribute on the field to his team's efforts. P3 continues, explaining how he was able to establish a new sense of purpose and meaning through support from his coaches:

> *P: Yeah, I definitely felt supported. Even after the second concussion, I would always just talk to (Head Coach) on a Sunday. We'd talk about the game. He'd always ask me about my perspective. He would always ask me too, kind of like how the team was feeling. So, I was almost like the inside scoop for the coaching staff. Kind of the emotions of the team throughout the season.*
>
> *I: Are you grateful for that, looking back? That you were kind of able to act like this liaison between the players and coaches?*
>
> *P: Yeah I would say so. For him to trust my opinion and he asked me, "Alright, what do you think we need to do differently?" I think that was good too just to have him be supportive of my voice on the team.*

I: Did you still feel like you had some value and worth to the team by doing things like this?

P: Yeah I would say so. Definitely towards the end of the season, it got easier and easier that I wasn't playing and contributing, I think that obviously helped too just having my small role on the team.

I: I know it's hypothetical but if you did not have that what do you think it would be like? What do you think the season would have been like?

P: I think it would have been a lot harder. To be officially away from everything, that would have made it a lot lot tougher. And my parents said oh maybe you should just take some time off and not go to all of the practices and not go to the games ***but I felt it helped for me to actually still be a part of the team****. Because all of the guys in my senior class are my best friends for life. I know that's a relationship that I'm going to continue. Not being there with them in this final season of ours and how much we have gone through as a team and how many different coaches we have had, we are the first senior class of Coach Chesney obviously we have been through a lot, and if I wasn't able to be there with them, it obviously would have been a lot harder for me.*

P3 expresses, without equivocation, that the support of his coaching staff and the opportunity to reorient his identity and role on the team in the aftermath of a career ending TBI created a space for him to feel a novel sense of purpose for his life after football. His ability to take a role on the team and embrace these new behaviors, mindsets, and opportunities made him feel connected to his teammates and improved his sense of psychosocial wellbeing. This role allows him to feel that he is making a contribution to the team despite his inability to play. Ultimately, he does not stay stuck in a rigid sense of identity in the aftermath of the TBI. These new routines and behaviors are well within his acumen and ability after the TBI and build a sense of confidence and a novel concept of identity in his relationship to football. His embrace of this novel role is a new existential commitment that opens space for a reexamined life after football. This effort is aligned with both the amelioration of his symptoms and the increase in his psychosocial sense of wellbeing after the trauma.

8. Conclusion

The intention of this study was to demonstrate the need to deeply examine the psychosocial and existential realm present in individuals who are recovering from TBI. As mentioned throughout, each participant had a deeply singular experience of recovery from their major head injury. Participants who were able to conjure perspective, context, and a sustained sense of meaning around ending of their athletic career were able to recover a high level of psychosocial functioning, existential purpose, and, coincidentally or not, their symptoms were ameliorated.

Maryann and Philip were able to offer some unique perspective around the end of their career and the experience of no longer having the ability to participate in endeavors that caused their original TBI. Despite the myriad of trauma associated with her experience, Maryann continually described how she is grateful for rock climbing and how she can contextualize this experience with the longevity of her career. However, despite a traumatic ending and an injury that almost cost her health and life, she is able to put her career into perspective and expresses a sense of gratitude for her ability to engage in rock climbing. She knows that she cannot return to this arena of competition, however, she is cognizant of the sense of strength and confidence the sport offered her. The sport built her body and offered a consistent emotional release for her throughout the physical and somatic ailments she carried through her life. Even without the ability to return to this arena for the physical, emotional, and psychological strength it provides, she conceptualizes her career in sport as having deep and lasting meaning and is grateful for this experience despite any trauma incurred.

Similar to Maryann, Philip expresses a sense of gratitude and context around his full playing career despite experiencing a bevy of head injuries and abrupt ending to his career during his senior year. Though Philip acknowledges that sacrifices were made and injuries were incurred throughout his commitment to the sport, similar to Maryann, there is a sense of sustained meaning from and gratitude for his career and experiences in football. There is a similar sense of cognizance around what the sport offered despite what was taken from him through the trauma of his career ending injuries. The connection to his teammates, the emotional catharsis of competing and engaging in a contact sport, and the lessons learned and mindsets formed through discipline and commitment form a sense of sustained meaning for Philip. Ultimately, he is not blinding his awareness from the sacrifices made and asked. Instead, he is grateful for the game along with the trauma and struggles that were incurred in his career. Like Maryann, this sense of gratitude correlates with a sense of psychosocial wellbeing after the TBI and after his career has ended.

The aftermath of Roger's injury was undoubtedly the most physically, somatically, and psychosocially traumatizing. At least initially, he was offered little social support and struggled deeply to conjure a new identity without football. As he described, for some time, he felt like he was having a dissociative break from his identity, purpose, and experience of reality. However, in time, a novel sense of purpose and identity are conjured and the cognitive, somatic, and psychological symptoms of his TBI begin to subside.

Moving forward, more phenomenological research should be devoted to unearthing the lived experience of human beings who are recovering from traumatic brain injuries. Our argument is not that these psychosocial and existential factors have a causal effect on ameliorating somatic symptoms of TBI, however, it is possible that they play some significant role in aiding the holistic recovery of the traumatized person. The less we medicalize these injuries, the more we can build a holistic conceptualization of the traumatized human being. Ultimately, further phenomenological analysis of these lived experiences might be able to unravel the nuanced and complicated relationships between these systems.

Author details

Gary Senecal[1*] and Patrick Whitehead[2]

1 Assumption University, Worcester, MA, United States of America

2 Albany State University, Albany, GA, United States of America

*Address all correspondence to: gr.senecal@assumption.edu

References

[1] APA. (2013). *Diagnostic and statistical manual of mental disorders, fifth edition.* Washington:APA Press.

[2] Goldberg, G. (2017). Toward a postmodern pragmatic discourse semioethics for brain injury care: Empirically driven group inquiry as a dialogical practice in pursuit of the Peircean aesthetic ideal of 'reasonableness.' Physical Medicine and Rehabilitation Clinics of North America, *28*, 393-411.

[3] Goldstein, K. (2000). *The organism.* New York: ZONE Books. (Original work published in German in 1934)

[4] Fraas, M.R., & Calvert, M. The use of narrative to identify characteristics leading to a productive life following acquired brain injury. American Journal of Speech-Language Pathology, *18*, 315-328.

[5] Levack, W.M.M., Boland, P., Taylor, W.J., Siegert, R.J., Kayes, N.M., Fadyl, J.K., McPherson, K.M. (2014). Establishing a person-centred framework of self-identity after traumatic brain injury: a grounded theory study to inform measure development. Rehabilitation*Medicine, 4(5)*. doi: 10.1136/bmjopen-2013-004360.

[6] McGrath, J.C. (2007). The person at the centre of rehabilitation. In J.C. McGrath (Ed.). *Ethical practice in brain injury rehabilitation*. Oxford: Oxford University Press, 34-51.

[7] Morris, S.D. (2004). Rebuilding identity through narrative following traumatic brain injury. Journal of Cognitive Rehabilitation, *22*, 15-21.

[8] Muenchenberger, H., Kendall, E., & Neal, R. (2008). Identity transition following traumatic brain injury: A dynamic process of contraction, expansion, and tentative balance. Brain*Injury*, 22, 979-992

[9] Walsh, R. S., Muldoon, O. T., Gallagher, S., & Fortune, D. G. (2015). Affiliative and 'self-as-doer' identities: Relationships between social identity, social support, and emotional status amongst survivors of acquired brain injury. *Neuropsychological Rehabilitation, 25*, 555-573.

[10] APA. (1952). *Diagnostic and statistical manual of mental disorders, first edition.* Washington: APA Press.

[11] APA. (1968). *Diagnostic and statistical manual of mental disorders, second edition.* Washington: APA Press.

[12] Aho, K. (2019). *Contexts of suffering: A Heideggerian approach to psychopathology.* Lanham, MD: Rowman & Littlefield.

[13] Kinderman, P. (2014). *A prescription for psychiatry: Why we need a whole new approach to mental health and wellbeing.* New York: Palgrave Macmillan.

[14] Kamens, S.R., Elkins, D.N., & Robbins, B.D. (2017). Open letter to the DSM-5. Journal of Humanistic Psychology, 1-13.

[15] Insel, T.R. (2013). Transforming diagnosis. National Institute of Mental Health, April 13. [http://www.nimh.nih.gov/about/director/2013/transforming-diagnosis.shtml]

[16] Pickersgill, M.D. (2013). Debating DSM-5: Diagnosis and the sociology of critique. Journal of Medical Ethics, *0*, 1-5.

[17] Won Jeon, S., & Kim, Y. (2017). Molecular neurobiology and promising new treatment in depression. *International Journal of Molecular Sciences, 17*, 1-17.

[18] National Public Radio. (2019). Thomas Insel: Why are we afraid to discuss mental illness, if many struggle with it? *Erasing the Stigma, Part 3,* October 11.

[19] Frances, A. (2013). *Saving normal: An insider's revolt against out-of-control psychiatric diagnosis, DSM-5, big pharma, and the medicalization of ordinary life.* New York: William Morrow & Co.

[20] Lakeman, R. (2013). Review of A. Frances. *Saving normal: An insider's revolt against out-of-* control psychiatric diagnosis, DSM-5, big pharma, and the medicalization of ordinary *life,* 2013. New York: William Morrow. In *Psychosis: Psychological, Social, and Integrative Approaches*, September.

[21] Heidegger, M. (2008). *Being and time.* J. MacQuarrie & E. Robinson (Trans.). New York: Harper Perennial.

[22] Husserl, E. (2012). *Ideas: General introduction to pure phenomenology.* D. Moran (Trans.). New York: Routledge.

[23] Bransen, J. (2001). Philosophy of Verstehen and Erklären, in N.J. Smelser & P.B. Baltes (Eds.),*International encyclopedia of the social and behavioral sciences,* 16165-16170. New York: Oxford University Press.

[24] Sass, L., Parnas, J., & Zahavi, D. (2011). Phenomenological psychopathology and schizophrenia:Contemporary approaches and misunderstandings. *Philosophy, Psychiatry, and Psychology, 18(1),* 1-23.

[25] Giorgi, A. (2009). *The descriptive phenomenological method in psychology: A modified Husserlian approach.* Pittburgh, PA: Duquesne University Press.

[26] Whitehead, PM. (2019). *Existential health psychology: The blindspot in healthcare.* Cham: Palgrave Pivot.

Section 2

Brain Tumors

Chapter 3

Pre-Surgical and Surgical Planning in Neurosurgical Oncology - A Case-Based Approach to Maximal Safe Surgical Resection in Neurosurgery

Hanan Algethami, Fred C. Lam, Rafael Rojas and Ekkehard M. Kasper

Abstract

Use of functional neuroimaging capabilities such as fMRI, DTI, MRP, MRS, AS-PET-CT, SPECT, and TMS as noninvasive tools to visualize intrinsic brain and spine morphology in relation to function have developed over the past 30 years. Amongst these imaging modalities, functional magnetic resonance imaging (fMRI) is of particular interest since it follows the physiological coupling between neuronal electrical activity and metabolic structural (cellular) activity as it relates to tissue vascularity and perfusion states. This structure–function *synesis* (from the Greek noun, σύνεσις = being together), leads to three effects that contribute to the fMRI signal: an increase in the blood flow velocity, a change in the mean blood volume, and most importantly, alterations in the blood oxygenation level. The latter effect has lent to the development of blood-oxygenation-level-dependent or *BOLD* fMRI, which has been used in establishing the topographic relationship between eloquent cortex and neurosurgical planning. As an adjunct to this modality, MRI-based diffusion tensor imaging (DTI) allows further detailed radiographic assessment of fiber tracts in the brain in relationship to the surgical lesion of interest. Herein we review the roles of fMRI and DTI for presurgical mapping to allow for maximal safe resection procedures in neurosurgery with case-based illustrations.

Keywords: fMRI, DTI, neurosurgery, eloquent cortex, neuronavigation, neuromonitoring, tumor resection, neurosurgical oncology

1. Introduction

The goals of neurosurgical resection are best described by the statement: "*maximal safe resection with minimal morbidity*". In oncological neurosurgery, this often encompasses achieving a gross total resection (GTR), which can be challenging depending on the location (i.e. eloquent cortex), ease of accessibility (i.e. superficial *vs.* deep), and the presence of vital *en passant* fiber tracks. Pioneering work by Dr. Wilder Penfield at the Montreal Neurologic Institute by performing craniotomies and resections allowed for safe resection of epileptogenic foci in the brain, resulting in seizure control in his patients (superbly outlined in his recent biography) [1]. This concept was soon applied by Penfield and his team to other pathological entities affecting the cortex and subcortical areas and was subsequently adopted by many academic neurosurgical centers worldwide.

Penfield's pioneering brain mapping techniques have since laid the groundwork for the development of intraoperative cortical stimulation techniques to guide maximal safe extent of resection (EOR). However, we now understand the limitations of this technique, including the progressive decline in the spatial resolution of bipolar stimulation throughout the course of surgical resection; iatrogenic edema caused by tissue retraction and/or resection altering the resistance and conductance of brain tissue requiring adjusted increases in applied stimulus strength at the price of decreased spatial resolution; and finally, adjustment of stimulation parameters which could lead to spurious spread of excitation to areas not immediately next to the point of stimulation, which could introduce further uncertainty in determining the EOR. Another caveat is the fact that awake surgery also requires a larger craniotomy than the actual size of the lesion or area to be removed due to the fact that greater cortical access is often needed to place multiple electrodes over the hemispheric surface to localize both the lesional site as well as the topography of adjacent possibly eloquent brain areas.

Various emerging, invasive monitoring techniques have expanded the scope and utility of this approach such as: Extracellular cortical stimulation via implanted on-lay grids for epilepsy patients; Foramen ovale electrodes inserted via transbuccal access for patients with mesial temporal sclerosis; And/or intraoperative cortical surface stimulation with bipolar Ojemann-type electrodes. The latter is sometimes used in combination with monopolar fiber-track-stimulation via pointy tip electrodes for patients with deep seated intra-axial lesions, amongst other modalities. Another option is the application of transcranial (scalp) stimulation techniques for evoked motor or sensory potentials (MEPs or SEPs) to monitor the integrity of functional pathways. However, not all patients are suitable to undergo awake procedures or these invasive types of monitoring nor are all neurosurgeons trained to perform surgeries using these methods. Another disadvantage of these awake monitoring techniques is that a surgical procedure itself is required before valuable functional information can be obtained. As a result, important patient management decisions must be made upfront without complete knowledge of the anatomic relationships between the lesion borders and functionally eloquent cortex [2]. For these reasons, we consider it beneficial to obtain comprehensive preoperative imaging, in particular, fMRI and DTI, to identify eloquent cortex controlling movement, primary sensory perception, vision, and speech, and to understand the spatial relationships between critical *en passant* fiber tracts and these functionally eloquent cortical regions to allow for surgical planning and determining the EOR.

1.1 A historical perspective on functional magnetic resonance imaging

In 1890, Sir Charles Sherrington and Dr. Charles Roy at Cambridge University were amongst the first neuroscientists to experimentally demonstrate a link of brain function to cerebral blood flow [3]. In 1963, Drs. Linus Pauling and Charles Coryell reported differences in the magnetic properties of blood based on the oxygenation status of hemoglobin. Oxygen-carrying hemoglobin (oxy-Hgb) was weakly repelled by magnetic fields, whereas blood with de-oxygenated hemoglobin (deoxy-Hgb) was attracted by a magnetic field. However, it was not until the 1990's when two American researchers at Bell Laboratories in Murray Hill, New Jersey, recognized the utility of this phenomenon to study the oxygenation state of the brain using

MRI and clearly demonstrated that the metabolic effect of neuronal activation in brain tissue yielded distinct magnetic properties which correlated with deoxy-Hgb and oxy-Hgb concentrations. Ogawa and colleagues then demonstrated that blood oxygen level derived (BOLD) signals could be used to generate intrinsic MRI contrast which could be further augmented by gradient-echo techniques [4]. Kwong and colleagues then followed with the use of gradient-echo and inversion recovery echo planar imaging sequences to map signal changes within the human primary motor and visual cortices [5]. These studies laid the groundwork for the development of distinct protocols that are used in modern day fMRI studies.

1.2 The utilities of diffusion weighted and diffusion tensor imaging

Diffusion weighted imaging (DWI) assesses the restricted diffusion of intracellular water molecules in the brain and is routinely used for stroke assessment in hypoxic and metabolically compromised regions of the brain. Hypoxia-induced breakdown of the energy-dependent transmembrane potential can be demonstrated early on in the ischemic process by applying three gradient-directions to DWI sequences to estimate the "average diffusivity" allowing for very early radiographic detection (within minutes of the ischemic insult).

Diffusion tensor imaging (DTI) takes advantage of the fact that there is directionally restricted diffusion of molecules in certain tissues depending on the observer's viewing angle (i.e. along *vs.* perpendicular to nerve fibers) [6]. In DTI, each voxel has one or more pairs of parameters: a rate of diffusion and a preferred direction of diffusion, described in terms of three-dimensional space, for which that parameter is valid [7]. The properties of each voxel of a single DTI image are usually calculated by vector or tensor math from six or more different diffusion weighted acquisitions, each obtained with a different orientation (or viewing angle) of the diffusion sensitizing gradients [8]. The diffusion tensor model is a rather simple model of the diffusion process, assuming homogeneity and linearity of the diffusion within each image voxel. In order to measure the tissue's complete diffusion profile, one needs to repeat the MR scans and apply different directions (and possibly strengths) of the diffusion gradient for each scan. The high information which is contained by a DTI voxel makes it extremely sensitive to subtle pathologies in the brain. In addition, the directional information can be exploited at a higher level of structure to select and follow neural tracts through the brain — a process called *tractography*. The underlying molecular directional restriction is also called *anisotropic diffusion*. Such directionality can be color coded in three dimensions (anterior/posterior, superior/inferior, and lateral/medial) which is useful to visualize the axonal tract organizations of the brain. Fiber tractography is therefore an added three-dimensional reconstruction technique based on DTI data to assess axonal directions using the collected primary diffusion restriction data. DTI can therefore provide additional structural information about the organization of the white matter in and around primary and secondary brain lesions which is useful to the surgeon in procedural planning.

1.3 Current status of the field

Modern imaging technologies such as BOLD fMRI and DTI, as briefly outlined above, have allowed for significant improvements in the surgical team's ability to minimize perioperative neurosurgical morbidity. The complementary use of other non-invasive imaging modalities such as CT angiography or MR perfusion scans, MR spectroscopy, 3D single-molecule super-resolution microscopy, and more recently transcranial magnetic brain stimulation [9], further permits the surgical team to gain significant insight into the access and resectability of certain lesions and to reliably predict the maximally safe EOR. Furthermore, the ability to use these imaging modalities to engage patients is crucial in the obtained consent process.

One of the hindrances to such technology-driven and more transparent surgical disease management strategies remains the fact that not all these highly informative technologies are widely available. Hospital funding for subspecialty-trained MRI physicists and MRI technicians may be limited and there is hesitancy to implement these technologies due to several factors, including: 1) The absence of large scale randomized clinical trials to support the routine integration of fMRI and DTI for pre-operative surgical planning; 2) The problems encountered in some earlier fMRI studies with respect to precise spatial location of a lesion; 3) The inability to correlate imaging features to electrical activity surrounding the tumor in some earlier studies; 4) The inability to use fMRI for distinguishing brain regions that are considered not primary eloquent sites, yet appear to be essential areas for circuit functions *vs* those areas that may be sacrificed without causing a lasting major neurological deficit; and 5) High interobserver variability in fMRI threshold determinations and DTI segmentation algorithms, which require specialty training and experience. The situation is further complicated by the fact that many ancillary health care practitioners (including medical-, neuro-, and radiation oncologists) are not familiar enough with the potential that fMRI and DTI can bring to presurgical planning and the roles they can play for improving surgical outcomes.

2. fMRI and DTI methodology and limitations

Depiction of the classic surface anatomy of the brain has proven to be useful in native (non-lesional) cases, where anatomy is undistorted by pathological processes. High-resolution, thin-cut T2-weighted, FLAIR, and MPRAGE sequences provide a detailed morphological map to establish eloquent regions of the brain. Eloquent regions specifically refer to primary areas of the cerebral cortex which carry a distinct function which cannot be simply substituted by other areas or neuronal circuitry, including: a) Primary sensorimotor cortex; b) Primary auditory cortex; c) Primary visual cortex; and d) Primary expressive language area (Broca's Area). Distortion of these regions by space-occupying lesions can pose challenges for even the most skilled surgeon to safely navigate the resection safely based on gross anatomical landmarks alone. In these situations, presurgical fMRI superimposed on MPRAGE sequences can help the surgeon to achieve three goals:

1. To better assess determining the spatial relationship of a given lesion to the proximity of any eloquent area of concern and thus allow the surgeon to gauge the maximally safe EOR.

2. To better select patients who may benefit from intra-operative mapping in the situations where there may be considerable variability between anatomical loci and functional foci.

3. To provide a roadmap for the surgery itself by integrating fMRI with intraoperative neuro-navigation.

Limitations of BOLD fMRI are related to dependence of the technique to neurovascular coupling, hence any delays in hemodynamic response following neuronal activation leads to poor temporal resolution on fMRI with alterations of BOLD signal in regions of the brain with altered blood flow [10]. BOLD fMRI is task-related imaging and hence is subject to statistical rules and interpretation of data. Another use of BOLD signal application is resting-state fMRI (rs-fMRI), which does not require a stimulus or task and acquires spontaneous BOLD signal alterations [11]. Data acquisition occurs while the patient is at rest or by inferring resting-state data from periods of rest embedded within a series of tasks [12]. The lack of a need for a patient to perform tasks may overcome the limitations of BOLD fMRI in patients with neurologic, neurosurgical, and psychiatric conditions hence the growing popularity of the rs-fMRI for use in the clinical setting.

From early fMRI studies by Yetkin and colleagues, a now historic rule had been established that *the minimal safe distance between a lesion margin and the resection border should measure about 10 mm* [13]. This paradigm was established based on the observation that the rate of neurological deficits significantly increase when the distance between the margin and resection border falls below 10 mm [2]. It needs to be noted though, that this much quoted study result was significantly underpowered, thus not allowing to draw strong conclusions since these observations were obtained in a very small sized single center cohort with only a handful of patients entered in each group. Another criticism of the golden rule of a "must-respect minimal distance" comes from the fact that the observed BOLD signal in any given fMRI study represents the display of a **statistical threshold signal value** that can be arbitrarily set and adjusted by the fMRI analyst/investigator and that the underlying signal to noise ratio is profoundly dependent on a variety of technical factors as well as intraoperative scenarios (i.e., brain relaxation and progressive shift with resection). Vascular re-routing of blood by a lesion (commonly called "venous contamination") can also generate false signals that need to be accounted for. These can be assessed by a matching CTA/CTV scan.

One further aspect that was criticized in the past by fMRI skeptics is the lack of connectivity information in primary fMRI data which points to the fact that BOLD fMRI signal is a surface related signal of oxygen brain metabolism, not taking into account subcortical structures such as fiber tracts. As detailed above, the latter aspect can be remedied by simultaneous integration of modern DTI data. Once uploaded and fused on a single modern intraoperative neuronavigation platform (e.g., BrainLab; Stryker/Synaptiv) this adds the fiber tract component to the surgical planning step. This capability is especially valuable for deep seated intra-axial lesions such as gliomas which may be infiltrative to those tracts or in close topography to these essential structures. Another use of this imaging technology is the scenario, where surgical access to deep seated lesions is required and traversing the white matter is best accomplished via a route that minimizes damage to fibers running towards essential cortical regions.

A recent survey across American neurosurgical departments with a residency program assessing the surgeons' uses and experience with preoperative fMRI in surgical planning for neuro-oncology patients [14]. Indications and surgeons' preferences for using fMRI in pre-surgical planning were dominant hemisphere and functionally eloquent location of lesions, motor symptoms, and aphasia. Most common reasons for fMRI amongst surgeons surveyed included identifying language laterality (which yielded the highest interrater reliability), planning the extent of resection, and discussing surgical planning with patients. The majority of surgeons ordered fMRIs in patients with low- and high-grade gliomas (94% and 82%, respectively). However, 77% of surgeons resected an fMRI-positive functional site if it was "cleared" by cortical stimulation, and 98% of responders reported that if there was a discrepancy between fMRI and intraoperative mapping that they would rely on intraoperative mapping. There have been concerns about the sensitivity and specificity of fMRI, especially for language mapping, with sensitivity ranging from

59–100% and specificity ranging from 0–97% when compared across 9 published studies [15]. Tumors of oligodendroglioma subtype, tumor relative cerebral blood volume (CBV) > 1.5 on MR perfusion imaging, lower cortical CBV, and distance to tumor have also been shown to cause higher false-positive fMRI signals [16]. Southwell and colleagues presented another limitation of using pre-surgical fMRI planning in its inability to offer surgeons the ability to account for compensable areas that can be resected and critical areas that need to be preserved, leading to underselection of patients for surgery and increase the likelihood for achieving subtotal resections due to miscalculation of needing to preserve seeming critical areas [17]. They also achieved an average 90% resection with no new postoperative neurological deficits in a series of 58 glioma patient resections, further pointing out the limitations of fMRI [17].

Similarly, a study incorporating 96 individual surgical planning cases using DTI of ground-truth white matter tracts from 20 research groups found a high false-positive rate with many of the tractograms representing more invalid than valid bundles [18]. This was further corroborated by a study by Mandelli and colleagues demonstrating relatively poor performance in differentiating lateral vs. medial projections [19]. Leclercq and colleagues compared DTI to intraoperative subcortical language mapping and found that while 17 out of 21 positive cortical stimulation sites corresponded to DTI tractograms, negative tractograms did not rule out the presence of white matter tracts [20]. Another study reported intraoperative image distortion in over one-third of cases, negating the use of DTI whilst favoring the use of cortical stimulation as the superior intraoperative mapping modality [21]. Finally, a prospective study randomizing 328 glioma patients to either DTI, 3D MRI, or routine neuronavigation reported a higher rate of GTR in higher-grade glioma patients, however, the increase in GTR was only reported in high-grade tumors whilst the neuronavigation in the control arm did not utilize cortical stimulation and the authors only reported outcomes for motor function [22]. These above studies serve to indicate that functional imaging modalities such as fMRI and DTI are still in their infancy and should be used as an adjunct along with more established tools such as neuronavigation and cortical stimulation.

3. Case illustrations

3.1 Case 1: 36 year-old male with a recurrent atypical parasagittal meningioma

A 36 year-old male who had undergone a prior resection for a parasagittal meningioma 4 years ago at an outside institution was referred to our neurosurgical outpatient tumor clinic by radiation oncology with minimal gait abnormalities and a recurrent tumor in the same location. Pre-surgical post-contrast T1WI and CT demonstrated a large parasagittal contrast-enhancing lesion spanning the anterior to middle sections of the superior sagittal sinus (SSS, **Figure 1A–C**, yellow arrows). CT angiography reconstruction scans demonstrated significant occlusion of the SSS (**Figure 1D and E**, yellow arrows). fMRI scan localized the primary motor area (yellow) and the sensory area (green) just posterior to the lesion (**Figure 1F–I**), predicting likely success of resection as long as we remained anterior to these eloquent areas, only expecting a temporary supplementary motor area (SMA) syndrome. Surrounding venous anatomy was also taken into consideration during pre-surgical planning.

Thorough discussions with the patient regarding the spatial and anatomical relationships of his recurrent tumor to the functional eloquent regions of the brain, as shown on fMRI, were taken with an explanation of the risks of the surgery,

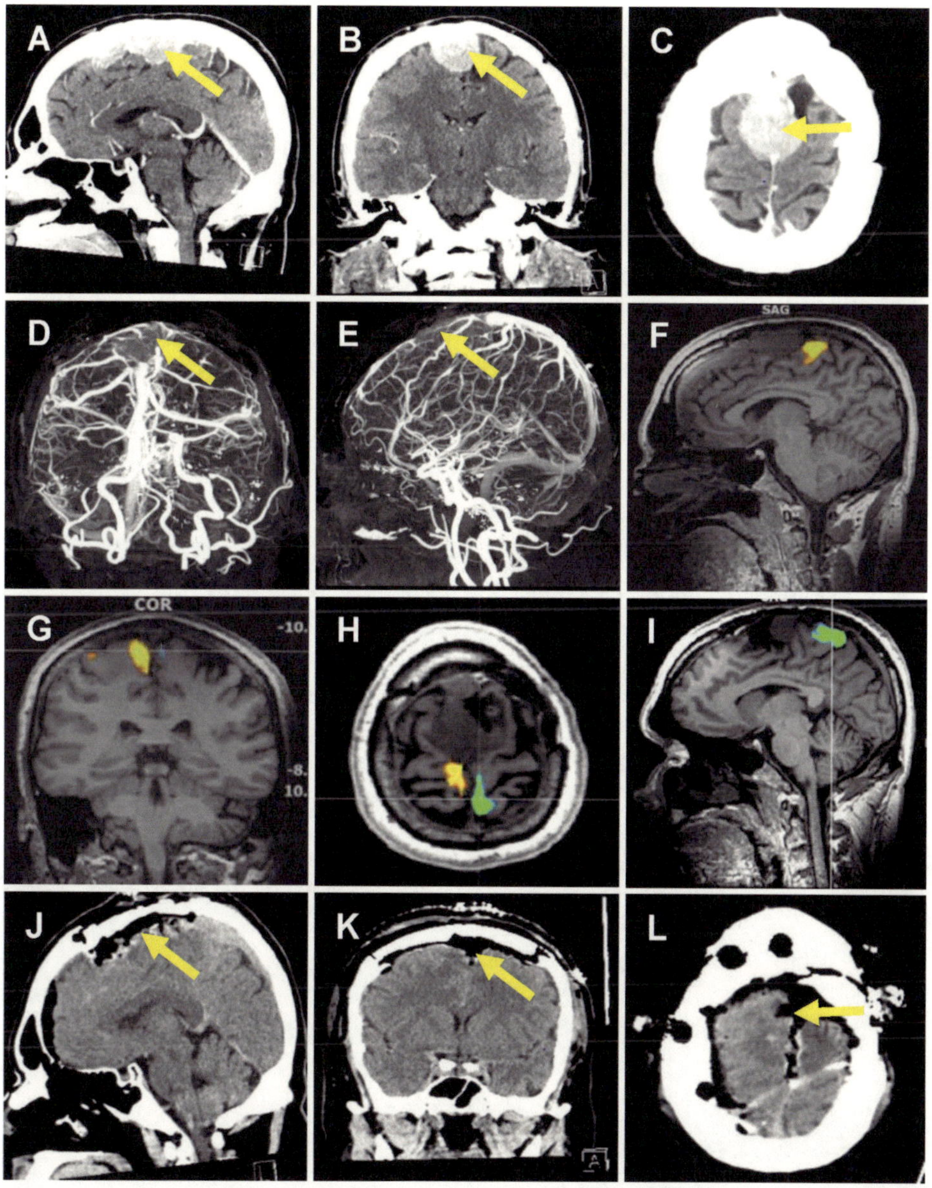

Figure 1.
Recurrent atypical meningioma. Pre-op MRI A) sagittal, B) coronal, and C) axial T1WI post-contrast scans showing a large, en plaque, recurrent parasagittal meningioma. Pre-op CTA D) coronal and E) sagittal views showing occlusion of the anterior third of the superior sagittal sinus. Pre-op fMRI showing F) sagittal, G) coronal views of the primary sensorimotor cortex (yellow) and H) axial, and I) sagittal views of the left primary motor cortex innervating the right leg (green). Post-op MRI J) sagittal, K) coronal, and L) axial TWI post-contrast scans showing resection of the meningioma.

including vascular injury to the sinus, and a post-operative SMA syndrome which would likely recover over the course of weeks. Surgery was recommended and the patient was taken to the operating room. A bilateral craniotomy was performed with intraoperative neuronavigation and the osseous midline bridge was dissected off. The SSS was tied off just anterior and posterior to the lesion, leaving the next surface draining veins intact. Surface mapping was used to confirm the motor strip location. A near gross total resection (GTR) was accomplished (**Figure 1J–L**) with a minimal 5 mm tumor cuff remaining which was encasing a draining vein in the posterior left SSS.

The patient woke up from surgery with a dense bilateral leg plegia, suggestive of a predicted SMA syndrome which recovered after 8 weeks requiring rehabilitation and physical therapy. He has since regained complete lower leg function and mobility at 6-months follow-up. Pathology came back WHO Grade II atypical meningioma. The patient was referred back to radiation oncology for post-operative stereotactic radiosurgery (SRS) to the tumor bed and the remaining cuff of tumor.

3.2 Case 2: 40 year-old male with a brainstem ependymoma

A 40 year-old male presented with cervical myelopathy (bilateral sensory loss in the hands, broad based gait, neck pain, and clonus). Imaging revealed a heterogeneously enhancing, intrinsic, intra-axial lesion at the craniocervical junction, with cystic and solid components (**Figure 2A** and **B**, yellow arrows). The index surgery was performed conventionally with intraoperative neuromonitoring (IOM) of somatosensory and motor evoked potentials (SSEPs and MEPs, respectively)

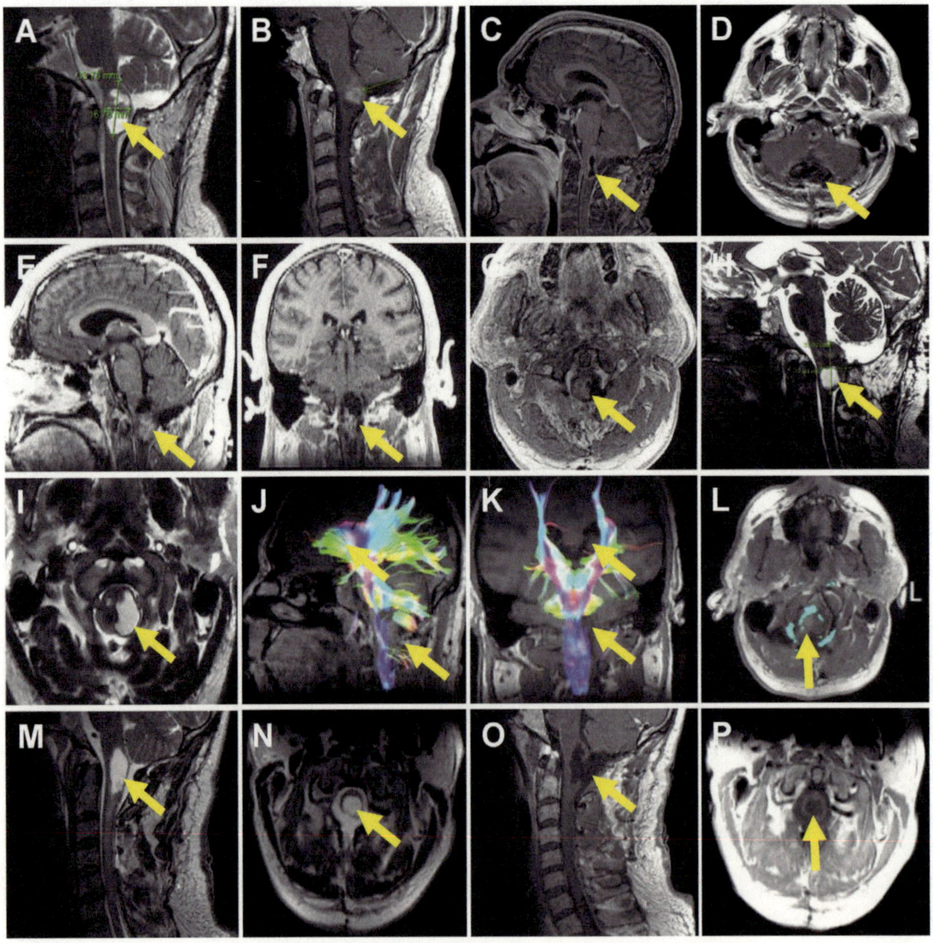

Figure 2.
Intra-axial cervico-medullary recurrent ependymoma. Pre-op MRI A) sagittal T2WI and B) sagittal T1WI post-contrast scan showing cystic partly enhancing lesion. Post-op MRI C) sagittal and D) axial T1WI post-contrast scans showing generous resection. Post-contrast E) sagittal, F) coronal, G) axial T1WI and H) sagittal, and I) axial T2WI showing tumor recurrence in the previous surgical bed. Pre-op fMRI showing J) sagittal, K) coronal, and L) axial views of the recurrent tumor completely displacing the motor fibers. Post-op MRI M) sagittal, N) axial T2WI and O) sagittal, P) axial T1WI post-contrast scans of the repeat resection cavity. Yellow arrows indicate location of the tumor.

via a posterior midline dorsal raphé approach with a myelotomy just inferior to the obex. Further resection was halted when the patient demonstrated prolonged drops in blood pressure and periods of asystole with ongoing dissection. Intra-operative frozen section pathology revealed a low-grade ependymoma. Post-operative imaging demonstrated a generous decompression (**Figure 2C** and **D**, yellow arrows). The patient had complete recovery of his myelopathy and he deferred adjuvant treatment, choosing to have follow-up surveillance with sequential imaging.

After 3 years of surveillance, the patient re-presented with recurrent symptoms and a recurrent tumor in the same location though significantly larger (**Figure 2E–I**). DTI images were acquired, clearly depicting that the pyramidal tract was displayed anterior and lateral to the lesion (**Figure 2J–L**, yellow arrows), allowing for a surgical window from posterior for resection. Resection for recurrent disease was again performed with IOM of SSEP, MEPs, monitoring of cranial nerves 5, 7, 9, and 12, as well as direct nerve stimulation. A suitable plane was established allowing for a gross total resection of what now was diagnosed as a tanycytic ependymoma. Only minimal amplitude drops in SSEPs were encountered during the surgery. Due to the manipulation of the recurrent surgical bed and delicate nature of the surgery, the patient was kept intubated following the surgery on high-dose steroids to prevent peri-operative edema of the surrounding brain stem tissues. He was successfully extubated on post-operative day 3 with no neurological deficits. Post-operative imaging showed no residual disease and a slim rim of cervical medullary parenchyma that carried all functional tracts with a large access window posteriorly positioned exactly between the posterior funiculus (**Figure 2M–P**, yellow arrows).

3.3 Case 3: 68 year-old female with a left subfrontal glioma

A 68 year-old female patient presented to our emergency department with new onset speech arrest episodes interpreted as seizures and secondary manifestation as Grand Mal. She had an unremarkable past medical history and no systemic signs of infection. The patient was started on antiepileptic drugs with an MRI scan revealing multiple ring enhancing lesions in the left frontal lobe (**Figure 3A–C**, yellow arrows). Differential diagnosis included primary CNS malignancies (e.g. malignant glioma), secondary malignancy (e.g. metastasis or lymphoma), or abscess. fMRI scan showed localization just adjacent to Broca's area but without infiltration of the frontal operculum (**Figure 3D–F**). A frontotemporal image-guided craniotomy was performed with intraoperative frozen pathology indicative of malignant glioma. Post-operative imaging demonstrated a generous resection (**Figure 3G–I**, yellow arrows). The patient went on to receive post-operative concurrent chemo-radiation as per the Stupp protocol.

3.4 Case 4: 38 year-old male with a fourth ventricular ganglioglioma

A 38 year-old male presented with episodes of headaches and nausea with no neurological deficit. MRI scan revealed a 1.5 cm ring enhancing lesion in the inferior 4th ventricle that was considered to be a neoplasm or infection (**Figure 4A–C**, yellow arrows). It was difficult to ascertain from the MRI scans whether the lesion was intra-axial or intraventricular. CTA showed low vascularity of the lesion (**Figure 4D–F**, yellow arrows). DTI showed displaced corticospinal fibers with a suitable access corridor from posterior using a planned unilateral telovelar approach (**Figure 4G–I**, yellow arrows). Surgery was performed with IOM, SSEP, MEP and cranial nerves 5, 7, 8, 9, and 10 monitoring. A small remnant of tumor was left laterally in situ since attempts for a complete resection caused cranial nerves 9 and 10 signal changes. Successful

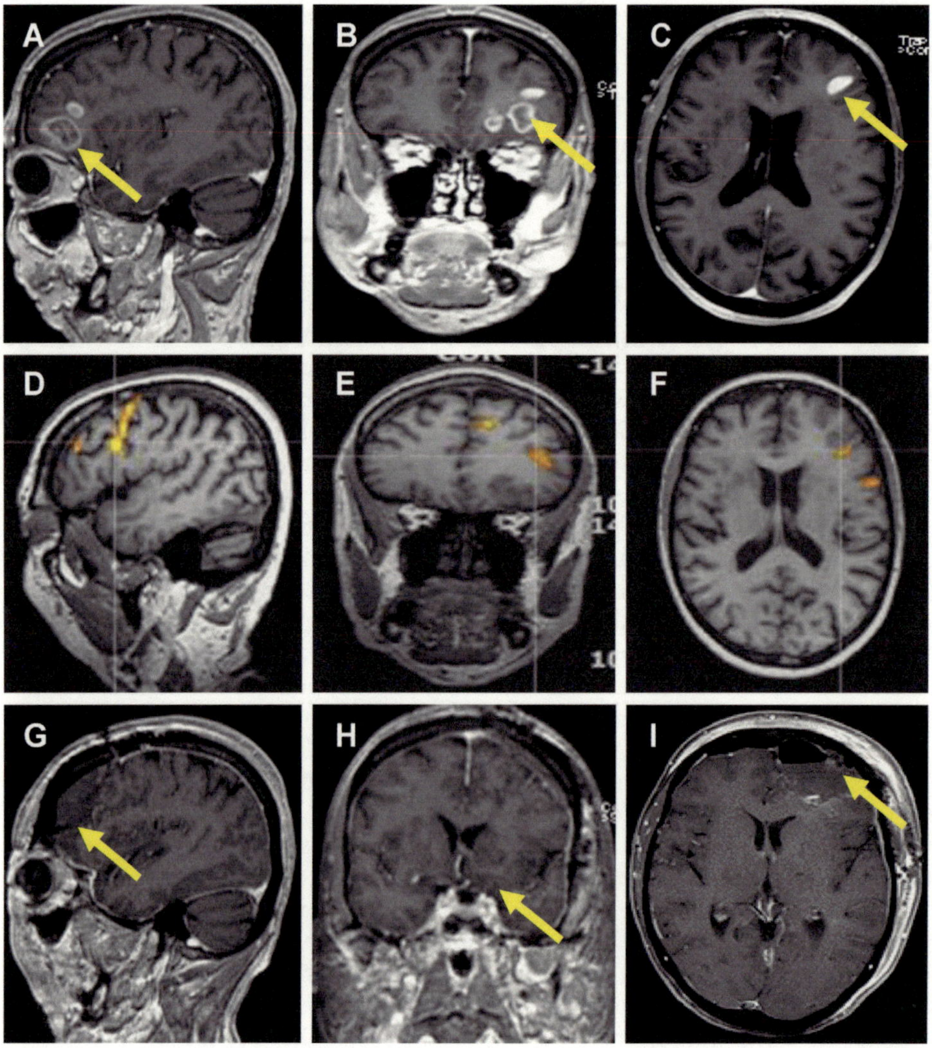

Figure 3.
Left sub-frontal glioma. Pre-op MRI A) sagittal, B) coronal, and C) axial T1WI post-contrast scans showing solid-cystic, multi-focal, enhancing lesions in the left subfrontal cortex. Pre-op fMRI scans showing D) sagittal, E) coronal, and F) axial anterior inferior frontal gyrus, Broca's area, and composite language map. Post-op MRI showing G) sagittal, H) coronal, and I) axial T1WI post-contrast scans of the frontal resection cavity.

subtotal resection was accomplished with pathology revealing a benign WHO Grade I ganglioglioma (**Figure 4J–L**, yellow arrows). The patient did not suffer any surgical morbidity and is being followed with surveillance imaging. Should there be further progression of disease, SRS *vs* a second repeat resection could be contemplated.

3.5 Case 5: 53 year-old female with a recurrent left temporal lobe glioma

A 53 year-old female had a previous subtotal resection of a small left temporal lobe GBM followed by concurrent chemo-radiation as per the Stupp protocol. She presented 2 years later to our institution's multidisciplinary tumor board, neurologically intact, with a left recurrent temporal lobe lesion (**Figure 5A–C**, yellow arrows). The differential diagnosis was recurrent disease *vs* radiation necrosis or pseudo-progression.

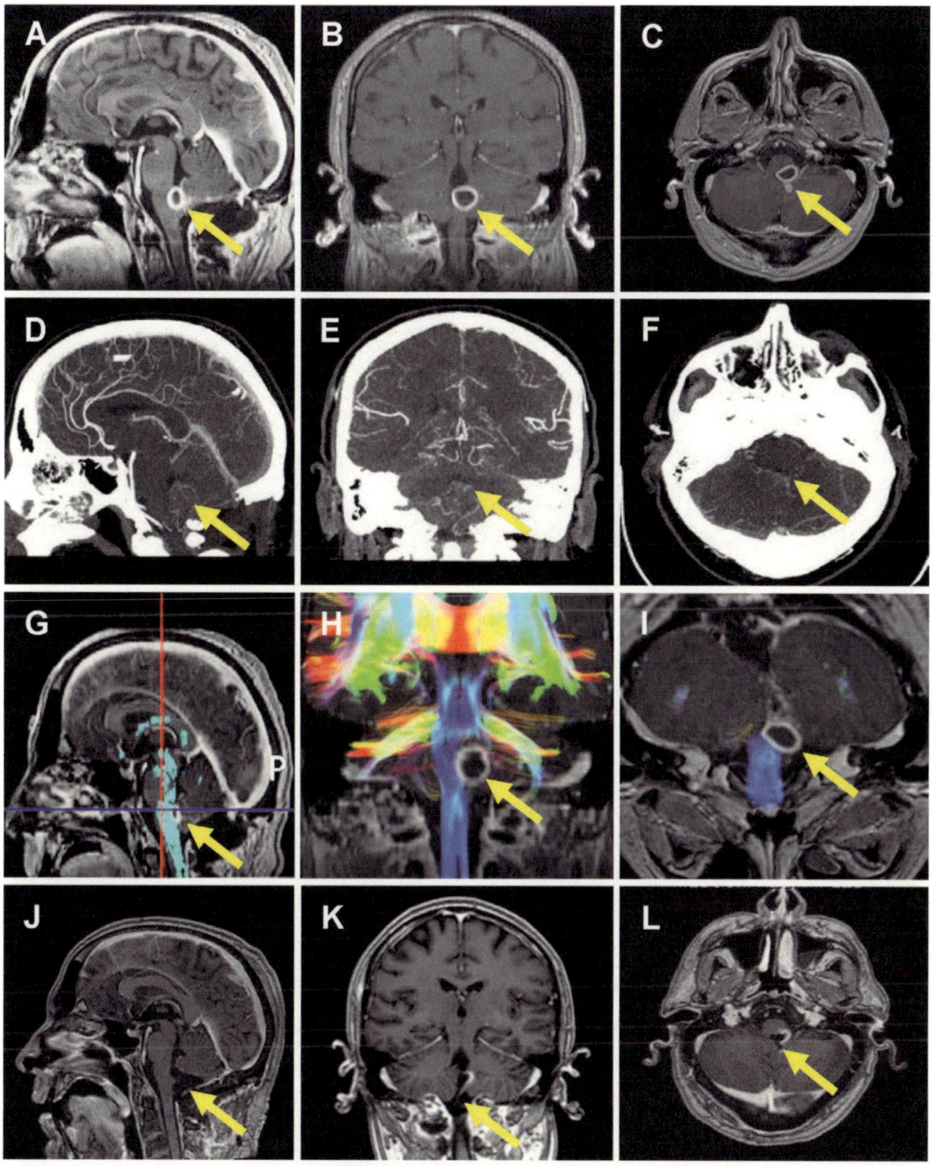

Figure 4.
Fourth ventricular ganglioglioma. Pre-op MRI A) sagittal, B) coronal, and C) axial T1WI post-contrast scans showing ring-enhancing cystic lesion originating from the floor of the 4th ventricle. Pre-op CTA D) sagittal, E) coronal, and F) axial views to assess vascularity of the lesion. Pre-op fMRI G) sagittal, H) coronal, and I) axial images showing clear anteromedial displacement of the pyramidal tracts by the lesion. Post-op MRI J) sagittal, K) coronal, and L) axial T1WI post-contrast scans assessing near total resection of the tumor. Yellow arrows depict location of the lesion.

MR perfusion (MRP) scan confirmed a hyper-perfused area in the left middle temporal fossa corresponding to the area of enhancement on MRI (**Figure 5D**, yellow arrow). Given the location of the recurrence (anterior to the 6 cm line measured from the temporal tip) with predominantly mesial extension with no proximity to the superior temporal gyrus and sparing anatomical language areas, we decided to perform a conventional asleep temporal lobe resection without the need for awake surgery with language mapping. The patient did not have any post-operative neurological deficits with good radiographic evidence of resection of contrast-enhancing disease (**Figure 5E** and **F**, yellow arrows) and a generous anterior mesio-temporal

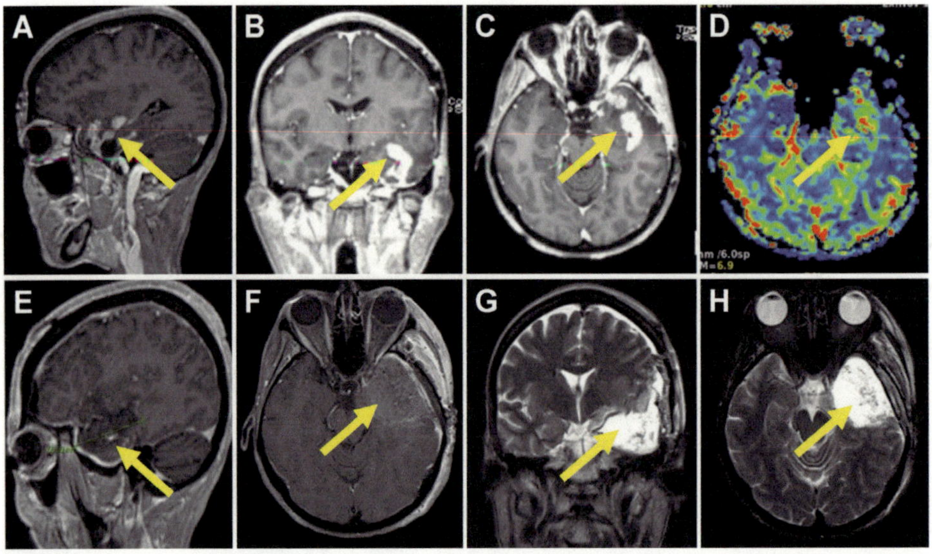

Figure 5.
Left mesiotemporal recurrent glioma. Pre-op MRI A) sagittal, B) coronal, and C) axial T1WI post-contrast scans of a left intra-axial anterior temporal lobe recurrent glioma. D) MR perfusion scan showing relative increased cerebral blood velocity in the left anterior temporal lobe corresponding to the area of increased enhancement on MRI. Post-op MRI E) sagittal, F) axial T1WI post-contrast, and G) coronal, and H) axial T2WI scans of the resection cavity. Yellow arrows define tumor bed.

resection cavity (**Figure 5G** and **H**). This case demonstrates the ability to do a safe maximal surgical resection in the absence of DTI or fMRI as long as there is strong correlation with other imaging modalities such as MRP delineating areas of suspected disease recurrence and an adequate anatomical distance between the resection margins and eloquent areas of the brain.

4. Conclusion

In summary, the combination of non-invasive functional and metabolic neuroimaging modalities such as fMRI and MRP in conjunction with anatomical mapping modalities such as DTI can help inform neurosurgical planning for lesions associated with eloquent cortex or in challenging anatomical locations such as the brainstem. Collaboration with a multidisciplinary team including neurosurgeons, neuro-oncologists, neuroradiologists, radiation oncologists, medical imaging physicists, and neurorehabilitation specialists, will help offer patients a comprehensive treatment plan which will achieve maximal surgical resection, disease control, and improved quality of life and survival.

Acknowledgements

The authors would like to thank Dr. Amy Harrison, a very talented and dedicated neuroimaging scientist in Diagnostic Services of Hamilton Health Sciences, for her tireless effort, diligence, and willingness to perform fMRI studies on many of our patients, including those presented in this book chapter. This work would not have been possible without Dr. Harrison's expertise and contributions to the team.

Author details

Hanan Algethami[1†], Fred C. Lam[2†*], Rafael Rojas[3] and Ekkehard M. Kasper[1*]

1 Division of Neurosurgery, McMaster University Faculty of Health Sciences, Hamilton General Hospital, Hamilton, Ontario, Canada

2 Department of Neurosurgery, Northwell Health, Donald and Barbara Zucker School of Medicine at Hofstra/Northwell, Manhasset, New York, USA

3 Division of Neuroradiology, Department of Radiology, Beth Israel Deaconess Medical Center, Harvard Medical School, Boston, Massachusetts, USA

*Address all correspondence to: flam1@northwell.edu and kaspere@mcmaster.ca

† These authors have contributed equally.

References

[1] Leblanc, R., *Radical Treatment*. 2020: McGill-Queen's University Press. 288.

[2] Sunaert, S., *Presurgical planning for tumor resectioning*. J Magn Reson Imaging, 2006. 23(6): p. 887-905.

[3] Raichle, M.E., *A brief history of human brain mapping*. Trends Neurosci, 2009. 32(2): p. 118-126.

[4] Ogawa, S., et al., *Brain magnetic resonance imaging with contrast dependent on blood oxygenation*. Proc Natl Acad Sci U S A, 1990. 87(24): p. 9868-9872.

[5] Kwong, K.K., et al., *Dynamic magnetic resonance imaging of human brain activity during primary sensory stimulation*. Proc Natl Acad Sci U S A, 1992. 89(12): p. 5675-5679.

[6] Alexander, A.L., et al., *Diffusion tensor imaging of the brain*. Neurotherapeutics, 2007. 4(3): p. 316-329.

[7] O'Donnell, L.J. and C.F. Westin, *An introduction to diffusion tensor image analysis*. Neurosurg Clin N Am, 2011. 22(2): p. 185-196, viii.

[8] Soares, J.M., et al., *A hitchhiker's guide to diffusion tensor imaging*. Front Neurosci, 2013. 7: p. 31.

[9] Sollmann, N., et al., *Intra- and interobserver variability of language mapping by navigated transcranial magnetic brain stimulation*. BMC Neurosci, 2013. 14: p. 150.

[10] Hermes, D., M. Nguyen, and J. Winawer, *Neuronal synchrony and the relation between the blood-oxygen-level dependent response and the local field potential*. PLoS Biol, 2017. 15(7): p. e2001461.

[11] Lv, H., et al., *Resting-State Functional MRI: Everything That Nonexperts Have Always Wanted to Know*. AJNR Am J Neuroradiol, 2018. 39(8): p. 1390-1399.

[12] Korgaonkar, M.S., et al., *Establishing the resting state default mode network derived from functional magnetic resonance imaging tasks as an endophenotype: A twins study*. Hum Brain Mapp, 2014. 35(8): p. 3893-3902.

[13] Yetkin, F.Z., et al., *Functional magnetic resonance imaging assessment of the risk of postoperative hemiparesis after excision of cerebral tumors*. Int J Neuroradiol, 1998. 4: p. 253-257.

[14] Stopa, B.M., et al., *Preoperative functional MRI use in neurooncology patients: a clinician survey*. Neurosurg Focus, 2020. 48(2): p. E11.

[15] Giussani, C., et al., *Is preoperative functional magnetic resonance imaging reliable for language areas mapping in brain tumor surgery? Review of language functional magnetic resonance imaging and direct cortical stimulation correlation studies*. Neurosurgery, 2010. 66(1): p. 113-120.

[16] Kuchcinski, G., et al., *Three-tesla functional MR language mapping: comparison with direct cortical stimulation in gliomas*. Neurology, 2015. 84(6): p. 560-568.

[17] Southwell, D.G., et al., *Resection of gliomas deemed inoperable by neurosurgeons based on preoperative imaging studies*. J Neurosurg, 2018. 129(3): p. 567-575.

[18] Maier-Hein, K.H., et al., *The challenge of mapping the human connectome based on diffusion tractography*. Nat Commun, 2017. 8(1): p. 1349.

[19] Mandelli, M.L., et al., *Quantifying accuracy and precision of diffusion MR tractography of the corticospinal tract in*

brain tumors. J Neurosurg, 2014. 121(2): p. 349-358.

[20] Leclercq, D., et al., *Comparison of diffusion tensor imaging tractography of language tracts and intraoperative subcortical stimulations.* J Neurosurg, 2010. 112(3): p. 503-511.

[21] Ostry, S., et al., *Is intraoperative diffusion tensor imaging at 3.0T comparable to subcortical corticospinal tract mapping?* Neurosurgery, 2013. 73(5): p. 797-807; discussion 806-7.

[22] Wu, J.S., et al., *Clinical evaluation and follow-up outcome of diffusion tensor imaging-based functional neuronavigation: a prospective, controlled study in patients with gliomas involving pyramidal tracts.* Neurosurgery, 2007. 61(5): p. 935-48; discussion 948-9.

Chapter 4

Intraoperative MRI in Brain Tumor Surgeries

G. Krishna Kumar, Anandh Balasubramaniam, K. Pradeep and Nitin Manohar

Abstract

Intraoperative MRI (ioMRI) has evolved since it used in 1991. ioMRI has been effective tool not only in glioma surgeries but also in other neurosurgical procedures. It provides real time information with high quality resolution and it is not affected by brain shift. ioMRI images can be uploaded in the navigation which helps in further resection of residual tumors. ioMRI can be used for confirmation of complete excision of tumor or location of microelectrode catheter tip DBS/sterotatic biopsy. It provides valuable information like location and amount of residue which guides surgeon for further resection safely as possible. ioMRI requires specialized operation theater with MRI compatible instruments which makes this setup expensive and it is available in only few centers across the globe.

Keywords: Intraop MRI, glioma surgery, MRI guided resection

1. Introduction

In 1991 at the Brigham and Women's hospital first intraoperative MRI (ioMRI) was used. Since then, its use and techniques have evolved. It is the most accurate imaging in intraoperative setting as it provides the real time information of tumor residue and guides further resections even if anatomy is distorted by brain shift [1]. The extent of resection is a prognostic factor in most tumor surgeries, like surgery for gliomas. These patients will benefit from ioMRI. The role of ioMRI is not only restricted to gliomas but other tumors/procedures as well. Designated operation theaters, operative instruments and MRI-compatible monitoring devices were required for ioMRI which has made this an expensive modality, with only few centers in the world able to afford such a facility. In this chapter we will discuss about types of ioMRI, anesthesia considerations and its role in different types of neurosurgical procedures.

2. Evolution and types of ioMRI

The first intraoperative MRI for neurosurgical operations, was developed in 1991 by the combined efforts of the Departments of Neurosurgery and Radiology of the Brigham & Woman's Hospital of the Harvard Medical School in Boston and the General Electric Medical Systems [2]. It was 0.5 T open type. Low field open type with Horizantal gap MRI was used for interventional procedures by Gronemeyer and colleagues [2, 3] which provided access to patients. Later Vertical gap MRI was developed which increased patient access and was used for various interventional, endoscopic and open surgeries. Many MRI compatible equipment had been developed since then along with ioMRI, with all ferromagnetic instruments replaced with titanium. The main drawback for open type configuration has been low field strength of magnet which does not yield good image resolution. Both vertical and horizontal systems had double doughnut magnets. The IMRIS system was developed later by a neurosurgeon, Dr. Garnette Sutherland of Calgary, Alberta, Canada. This system offered a uniquerail-mounted MRI system in which the scanner could be mobilized to the patient. It was closed type 1.5 T ceiling mounted rail system, which was moved between two rooms [4].

ioMRI scanner can be open or closed type. Open type (with horizontal gap or vertical gap) has better access to patient while compromising on image quality. Closed type (small bore or long bore) has better quality of images with no access to the patient.

Based on field strength ioMRI are classified as low field (0.2 T), mid field (0.5 T) and high field (1.5 T & 3 T). Low-field systems are the GE Signa, the Hitachi 0.3 tesla system, and the Polestar0.15 tesla system. SIGNA SP 0.5 T is a midfield ioMRI system. High-field systems are Siemens Brain Suite, IMRIS system, and the Philips systems. High field ioMRI provides good quality of images with better spatial and contrast resolution with precision and some of the studies like perfusion, DTI and fMRI are possible compared to low or mid field ioMRI [5, 6].

The imaging in ioMRI can be truly intraoperative or interoperative in nature. Intraoperative imaging is done while surgery is ongoing in the scanner without any interruption of procedure. Horizontal and vertical donut models were used for it. These are mid field ioMRIs. These are the actual real time imaging which were performed during the surgery similar to fluoroscopy. The draw backs of this system were poor image quality, need of MRI compatible instruments including microscope, navigation which were very expensive and space constrains for movement. In interoperative imaging, surgery is stopped temporarily and either patient or gantry mobilized to acquire images. This type has been developed more commercially as there is no need for continuous intraoperative imaging and imaging is required only for certain periods like, to confirm extent of resection, location of residue or guiding further resection. This type allows installation of high field strength MRI in the area near the operating room or within the same room with operating table outside of the 5 gauss line. This allows surgeon to use non-MRI compatible instruments during surgery. Patient transportation is the main drawback which takes 20–40 minutes and requires proper trained staff [4].

High field ioMRI operative rooms (OR) are of different types. First type was IMRIS. In this type MRI was rail mounted and placed between two operating rooms and mobilized into the OR when required. During imaging instruments moved beyond the 5 gauss line. The operating rooms had to be RF shielded to acquire good images. Second type was RF shielded OR in which MRI and operating table are in the same room, when imaging is required, patient is moved into gantry to require images. This type has a rotating table, during surgery head end of the table is beyond 5 gauss line. When imaging is planned table is rotated so that head goes into the gantry. This was developed by Siemens and BrainLab companies combined. BRAIN SUITE is an integrated operative area away from the magnet in which interventional procedures can be done. MRI compatible instruments are not required.

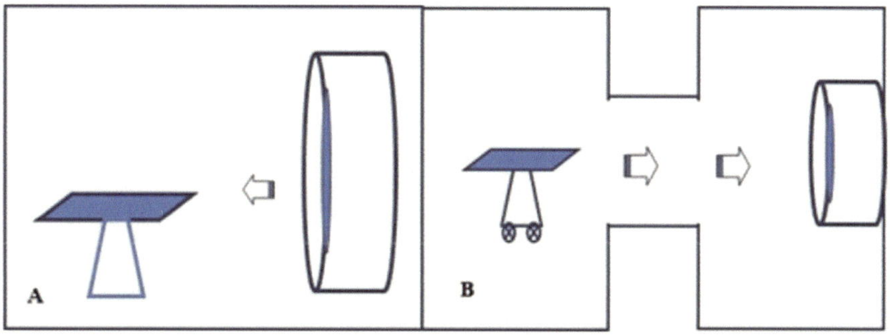

Figure 1.
Representational images. A. RF shielded ioMRI OT in which MRI moved towards operating table B. Nearby OT model, in this model patient shifted on mobile MRI compatible table top.

It also has incorporated Neuronavigation with auto registration. All of these systems are possible in high volume centers or in institutes with research interest, as the cost is prohibitive [4]. Other more commercially viable concept is "nearby OT type" –in which MRI machine is fixed in separate room adjacent to OR and operating table is transferred into MRI suite. In nearby OT type, the MRI can be used for imaging other patients through separate entry to access the MRI which can be cost effective. Whenever ioMRI is planned the MRI is room is cleaned and sterilized, the outside entry is closed and OR entry is opened to receive the patient in operative position draped, under anesthesia. All these require special protocols, trained staff, and proper communication between MRI technician, surgeon, anesthesiologist and OT staff.

Authors are using "Nearby OT model" – Siemens 3 T ioMRI and have found to be cost effective. Initially it took around 85.6 minutes for shifting in and out ioMRI and restart surgery which latter reduced to 37.4 minutes by multiple mock drills and continuous training of involved staffs [7, 8] (**Figure 1**).

3. Anesthesia considerations

The main challenge during ioMRI anesthesia is to have uninterrupted access to the patient while allowing high-quality real-time MRI images with minimal electrical noise interference. All standard monitors, equipment and anesthesia workstation should have minimal electrical noise interference and MRI compatible. Monitors can be classified as MRI unsafe (prohibited inside suite), MRI conditional (permitted not beyond 5 Gauss line inside the MRI suite), MRI safe (can be allowed freely inside the suite) [9].

Anesthetist should be aware of ECG changes like ST segment changes, P wave abnormalities, AF, Ventricular fibrillation can happen due to static magnetic field, pulse gradient and high frequency field. If these changes occur along with hemodynamic instability then it should be managed accordingly.

All patients should be screened for any metallic objects, piercings, tattoos (lead), metallic implants, pacemakers, deep brain stimulators, implantable defibrillator, vagal stimulator, aneurysmal clips during pre-operative assessment to know the MRI compatibility.

During ioMRI patient access is limited and so all IV lines and tubings should be long, tightly fixed and secured. Proper checklist has to be followed to avoid mishaps and accidents. Anesthesia depth has to be maintained throughout the procedure either with intravenous or inhalational anesthesia. Nitin et al. [10] reported thermal injuries due to radio frequency energy. It can be avoided with skin to skin packing, avoiding looping of wires, lines and tubing. Noncompatible equipment (Temperature probe and depth monitors and flexometallic tubes) are removed. Nitin Manohar et al. [11] also reported that IONM electrodes can interfere with the signals and produce artifacts affecting the image quality. Patient positioning for ioMRI requires additional attention. Position should be tailored so that head fixed to the head clamp moves freely within the ioMRI bore. ioMRI compatible Mayfield clamps are used for positioning and final position should be confirmed with bore gauge that is provided along with ioMRI compatible operative table, to avoid possible collision with the gantry. During awake procedure or surgery, preoperative counseling regarding the MRI sound, use of ear plugs and sedation should be done.

Emergency drugs should be ready in case of contrast induced reactions or hemodynamic instability during the scan. Mock drills to cope up with emergency situations for all OT and MR staff should be done with everyone knowing all steps and well versed in their roles with even quenching of MRIif needed (**Figures 2** and **3**) (Box 1).

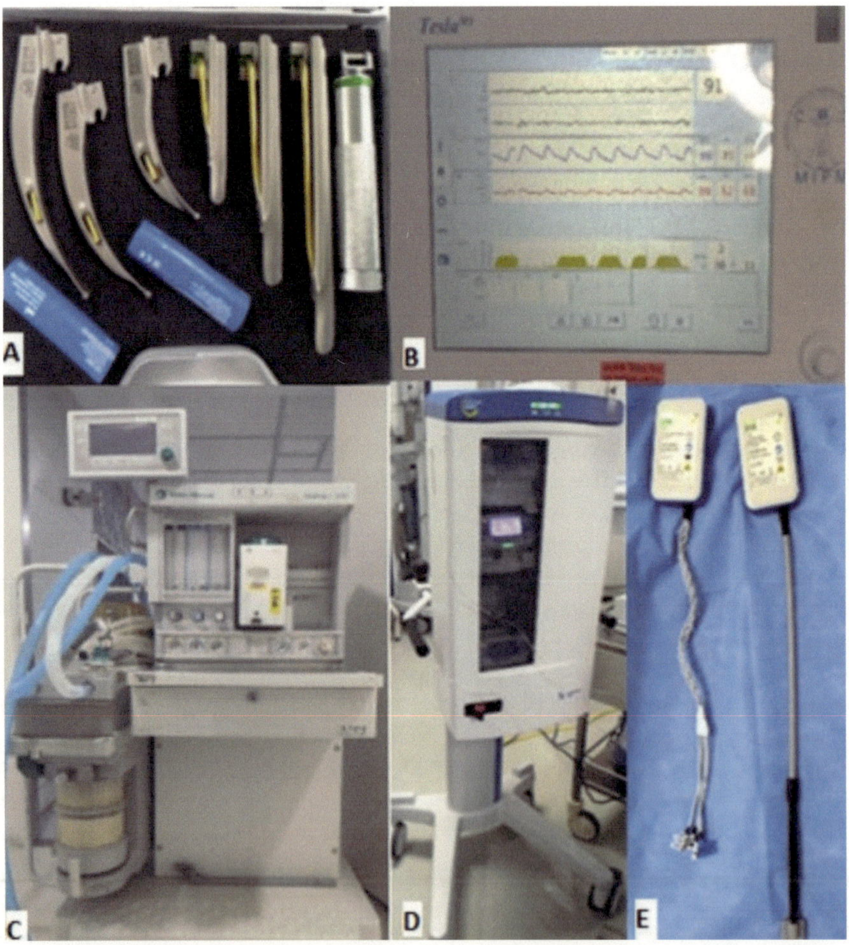

Figure 2.
MRI compatible instruments A. Laryngoscopes, B. Monitor, C. Ventilator, D. Infusion pump and E. ECG electrodes.

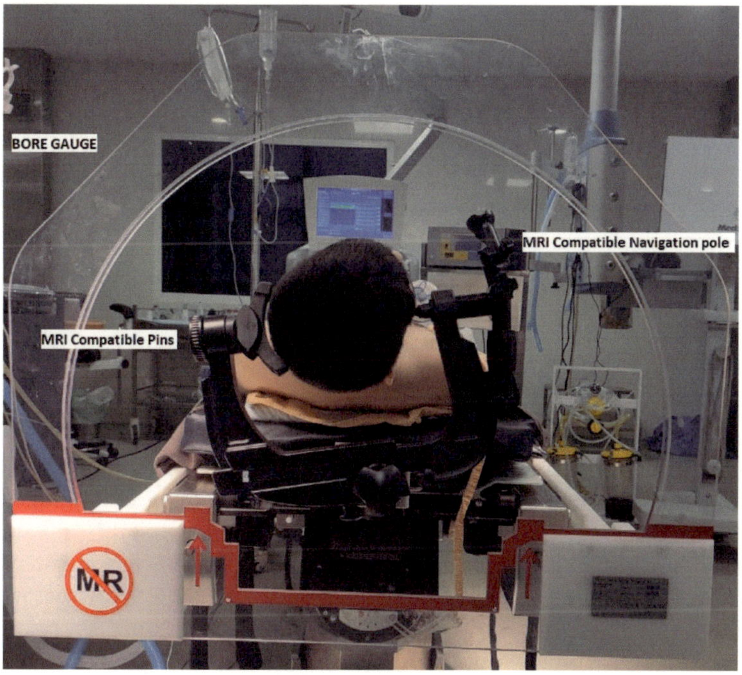

Figure 3.
Positioning of patient in operative table with MRI compatible Mayfield clamps and navigation probe. Final position is confirmed using bore gauge so that patient moves in and out of MRI machine freely.

CHECKLIST FOR INTRA-OP MRI:

(To be Completed mandatorily prior to Wheeling-1a; Please Tick on the boxes on checklist completion)

- MRI Compatible ECG electrodes: ☐
- No metallic ornaments: ☐
- No metallic Implants, Heart valves, Pacemakers in patient: ☐
- Arms insulated from body: ☐
- Padding from skin to skin: ☐
- No staplers, sand bags, metal objects in sheets, sisters check done: ☐
- OT table sheets tucked under to help sliding: ☐
- Temp probe removed: ☐
- Bag free: ☐
- Warmer disconnected: ☐
- Antibiotic repeated: ☐
- Inform MRI Technician: ☐
- Cautery pad removed: ☐
- Emergency drugs box sent in: ☐
- OT personnel moving into the MRI Suite screened for metallic objects: ☐
- MRI Compatible Monitor Ready: ☐
- MRI Anaesthesia Machine SWITCHED "ON" CHECKED: ☐
- OT Table & MRI Table ALIGNED & LEVELLED ☐
- Infusion pump casing: ☐
- Long breathing circuit (Double): ☐
- Long IV line extension (200 ml): ☐
- Long infusion extension (200 ml): ☐
- AMBU, Bains circuit ready ☐
- Compatible Laryngoscope Ready: ☐
- Relaxant bolus ☐

Box 1.
ioMRI checklist.

4. Role of ioMRI in neurosurgery

It is useful in both intra and extra axial tumors. Depending upon the situation ioMRI can be used as completion study, residue seeking or guidance for further resection. It is also used in epilepsy surgery, deep brain stimulation (DBS), sterotactic biopsies. Apart from extent of resection and location of residue, ioMRI also gives us information like hematoma in and around operative cavity, ischemia (diffusion restriction), hydrocephalus, location of electrode tips in DBS, proximity to neurovascular bundles which guides surgeon for further planning and proceeding in the same sitting of surgery.

4.1 Intraaxial tumors

Gliomas are the most common primary brain tumors. These are infiltrating tumors along the subcortical white fibers. In low grade gliomas it is difficult to differentiate from adjacent normal tissue. During surgery extended resection can cause neurological deficits or inadequate resection may leave significant residue which can progress, decreasing overall survival of the patient. Preoperatively MRI is usually done in patients with glioma which gives us valuable information about the nature of the lesion. Important sequences being FLAIR, contrast study, perfusion study, DTI, functional MRI (fMRI)and spectroscopy. Information from these sequences are compared with the ioMRI providing the valuable information for improving the safety and efficacy of the resection [12–14].

ioMRI is an ideal tool for the resection of low grade gliomas (LGGs) because of their superior resolution in differentiating tumor from the surrounding brain, it allows accurate localization of residual tumor. It allows near-real-time assessment of extent of resection and also allows correcting for the brain shift, a disadvantage for Neuronavigation, which happens as surgery progresses. In LGGs, ioMRI flair sequence compared with preoperative image shows the residual tumor. Perfusion study will demonstrate the hyperperfusing area around the surgical cavity and thereby increase the extent of resection. In high grade gliomas (HGGs) usually the lesions are contrast enhancing, post-contrast study in ioMRI will show us the extent of resection of contrast enhancing tumor. Perfusion study helps us to identify the hyperperfusing areas in the non-enhancing part of HGGs which can be resected. Resecting hyperperfusing areas in HGGs will definitively increase the extent of resection and thereby increasing progression free survival [12–14] (**Figures 4** and 5).

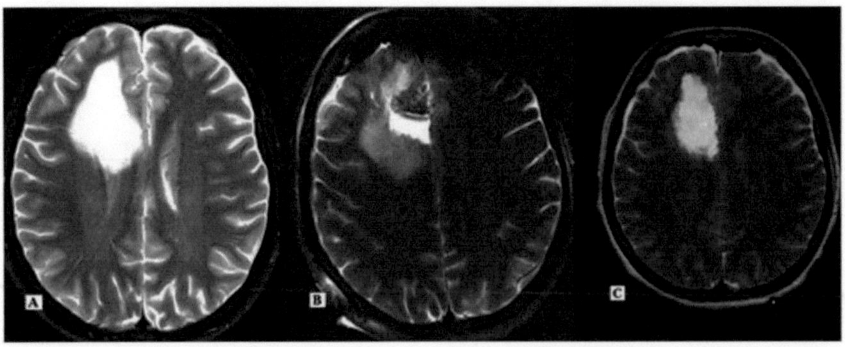

Figure 4.
A. Preoperative MRI of a patient showing T2 hyperintense LGG involving right medial frontal lobe B. ioMRI showing residue around the surgical cavity which was excised in the same sitting. C. Post-op MRI showing.

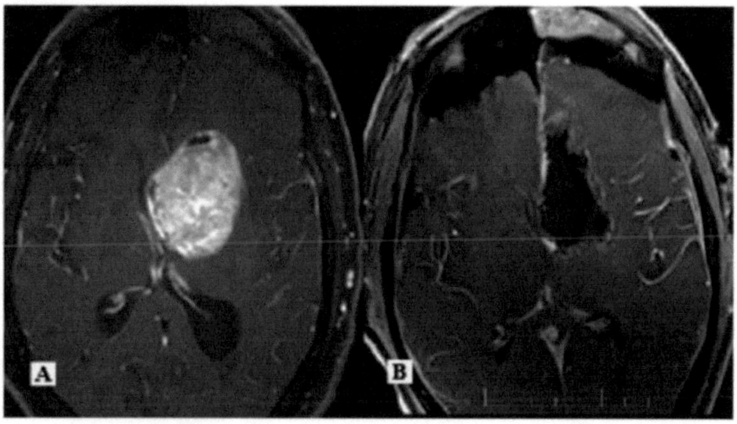

Figure 5.
A. Preoperative MRI of patient with high grade lesion which was contrast enhancing, involving left caudate and periventricular region. B. ioMRI shows no residue of the contrast enhancing lesion.

ioMRI is a valuable tool in awake craniotomy. ioMRI shows the location of residual tumor and one can perform fMRI to correlate its position with eloquent areas. If the residue is in the region of BOLD signals of fMRI then one can leave behind the residue without causing any permanent neurological deficits. Intraoperative neuromonitoring will guide us the intactness of long fiber tracts. ioMRI in intra-axial tumors involving or in proximity with these tracts will tell us the extent of residue as well as the intactness of tract using DTI imaging. During resection of the intraaxial tumors, sometimes the wall of cavity collapses and blinds a part of tumor. Deep seated tumor or tumorat difficult angles/corners may be left behind. These tumor residues can be located and resected with ioMRI guidance with additional navigation support from the newly acquired images [12–14].

In the prospective studies done by Senft and colleagues [15] and Hatiboglu and colleagues [16] with ioMRI guidance, it was established that the MRI group had a complete resection of their enhancing tumor compared with the control group [4, 16]. Also in nonenhancing tumors Hatiboglu and colleagues showed increased complete resection from 63–80% with the help of ioMRI [16]. Pamir MN et al. studied 56 patients of LGG who underwent resection with ioMRI. They found that the use of ioMRI increased the number gross total resection of from 31 to 41, up by 32.3% [17]. Coburger and colleagues in their multicenter retrospective assessment of LGGs surgery under ioMRI guidance showed that high-field ioMRI was significantly associated with gross total resection (GTR). WithGTR in 85% of cases compared with 57% with a low-field ioMRI [18]. Similarly ioMRI also used in other intraaxialtumorsandintraventicular tumors, which guides the extent of resection and location of residue.

With ioMRI we had achieved significant reduction in residual tumor volume. The mean residual tumor volume improved from 22.5 cm^3 to 11.7 cm^3 after ioMRI in 29 patients of LGGs. Also the overall extent of resection improved from 72.9% to 88.4% with ioMRI.

4.2 Extraaxial tumors

4.2.1 Sella-suprasellar tumors

ioMRI role is well established in the pituitary tumors. It is important for both functional and nonfunctional pituitary adenomas. With the advent of endoscopic

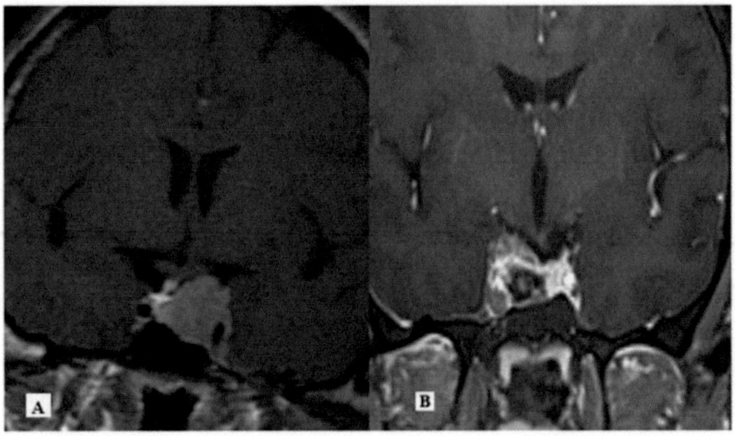

Figure 6.
A. Pre-operative MRI showing pituitary macroadenoma B. ioMRI showing residue (arrow) in left side which was removed in the same sitting after ioMRI.

pituitary excision the extent of resection has significantly increased compared to that of the microscopic approach, though the complete excision is still around 50–60%. The residual disease is strongly associated with complications like postoperative hemorrhage, need for adjuvant radiotherapy or hormonal therapy, significant higher risk of adenoma regrowth and possibly reduced life expectancy. Thus Gross total resection is recommended for both NFPAs and FPAs. With ioMRI one can locate the residue and chase it. In functional adenomas complete resection is mandatory to achieve cure, with ioMRI it is achievable. With ioMRI normal pituitary can be identified and preserved so that we can avoid post-operative hypopituitarism [19–21].

In various large series involving non-iMRI-guided transsphenoidal endoscopic resection of pituitary tumors, Dehdashti AR et al. [22] reported gross total resection of 79% and Serra C et al. [23] reported between 44–88%, while on analysis of studies that involved iMRI guided eTSS for PAs, average initial gross total resection rates at iMRI was only 51% which was increased to 73% help of ioMRI guided resection [24]. Berkmann et al. [25] observed new onset hypopituitarism of any one of the axes in 29% patients in iMRI guided resection group versus 45% in control group operated without iMRI guidance. They also observed that post-operatively RT was required in 3 patients in group without ioMRI compared to that none of the patients in ioMRI group.

ioMRI also used in craniopharyngiomas, one can assess whether adequate decompression has been achieved like decompression of optic chiasm. It also gives us information about contrast enhancing residue if any that is accessable for resection.

In our centre with ioMRI, we achieved gross total resection rate from 52–80% (p value <0.05) in 57 patients of pituitary macroadenoma (**Figure 6**).

4.2.2 Other extra axial lesions

Large extra axial lesions in the CP angle and skull base are difficult to excise completely due to its relations with cranial nerves, blood vessels and vital neural structures like brainstem. Due to its complexitysometimes surgeons lose the direction or leave behind large residues. In such cases ioMRI gives valuable information about volume and location of the residual lesion. When gross total resection of skull base lesions is not feasible then ioMRI can be a used for tailored tumor resection.

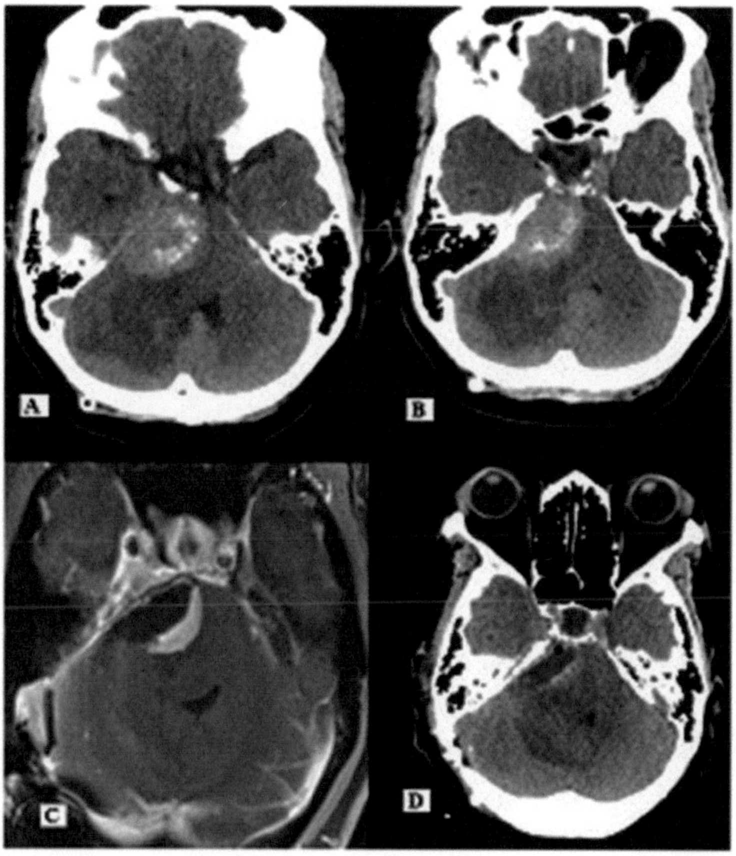

Figure 7.
A&B preoperative CT image showing CP angle meningioma, C. ioMRI showing the residue along the brainstem which was difficult to mobilize hence it was left behind and size was less than 2 cm which was subjected for SRT, D post-operative CT showing residue without any operative site hematoma. In this patient ioMRI helped to guide the surgeon to stop further resection and safely subjected for SRT without causing any neurological deficits.*

With ioMRI one can achieve maximum safe resection and decrease the size of residue so that it can become suitable for sterotactic radiosurgery [26] (**Figure 7**).

Mario Giordano et al. [27] recruited 19 patients of para-sellar meningiomas includes clinoidal, tuberculum sellae, and cavernous sinus who underwent surgical resection using intraoperative MRI. In 7(37%) of 19 patients, further tumor resection was performed based on information from the ioMRI. 56% of patients with cavernous sinus meningioma benefited by ioMRI by further safe resection of tumor. Dr. Chakraborty et al. [28] conducted a retrospective review of 70 operations performed on 66 patients with intracranial meningiomas. Among them 30 were skull base meningiomas. 9(12.8%) patients required additional tumor resection based on ioMRI findings, and in 4 patients (6%), ioMRI imaging allowed for the avoidance of further dissection near-critical neurovascular structures (**Figure 8**).

Hussam Metwali et al. [29] performed a retrospective analysis of 15 patients with skull base chordomas with ioMRI. 8 patients had complete resection confirmed by ioMRI. Out of 7 patients 3 hadtumor residual requiring further resection was located in the clivus and in 4 patients in the intradural space. All the intradural residue patients had significant improvement in preoperative deficits which was possible with ioMRI guidance for locating the residue. Joseph C. Dort et al. [30] did a prospective, non-randomized, cohort study on 31 patients with skull base lesions.

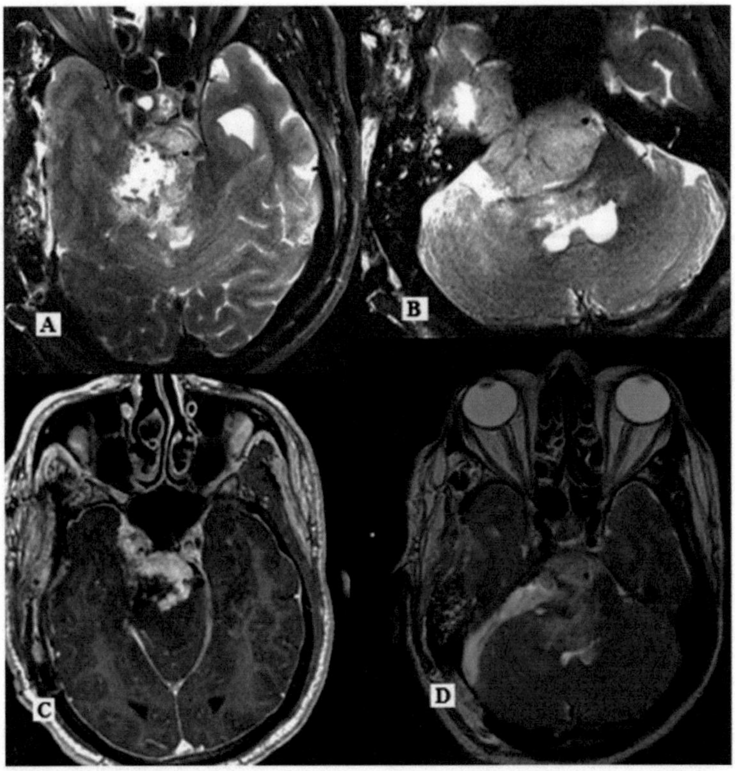

Figure 8.
A&B ioMRI images of sphenopetroclival meningioma, initially tumor was decompressed by subtemporal approach but due to intra operative bleeding and hard calcified which was unable to mobilize. In this case ioMRI helped surgeon to approach by retromastoid craniotomy and achieve further resection of tumor as safely as possible in the same sitting. C&D. post-operative MRI images showing residual tumor. Volume of the residue is significantly reduced compared to that of in ioMRI.

All these patients underwent surgery in a 1.5-Tesla ioMRI suite. 11 out of 31 patients surgical course altered with the help of ioMRI and maximum safe resection was achieved. ioMRI is a valuable adjunct to skull base surgery.

In our center we did ioMRI in 30 skull base meningiomas. 16 patients had residual lesion, of which 12 patients had subjected for further resection in same sitting. They had significant reduction in volume of residual lesion. we achieved Simpson grade 2 excision in 6 out of 12 patients. Other 4 patients, residual lesion was not chased due to its proximity to neurovascular structures.

5. Other neurosurgical procedures

Epilepsy surgery has evolved over the past few decades. ioMRIisalso a valuable tool to achieve complete resection of abnormal areas especially those with lesions. Nilesh S. Kurwale et al. [31] studied on role of ioMRI in achieving seizure control in 39 pharmacoresistant epilepsy patients. This study included tumor (31%), focal cortical dysplasia (28%), mesial temporal lobe surgeries (18%), and disconnectionsurgeries (23%). In lesionalgroupioMRI helped infurtherresections about 21% (5/23) patients. Complete resection was achieved in 87% of patients. ioMRI increases the extent of resection especially in lesionalepilepsy surgeries and thereby good seizure outcomes. Kaibara et al. [32] reported about50% patients had residual hippocampus in ioMRI aiding further resection resulting in 93% seizure freedom at 17 months. Michael Buchfelderet al. [33] assessed 61 patients with pharmacoresistant epilepsy. In this study 32 nonlesional cases underwent surgery using ioMRI, the extent of the tailored 28 temporal resection and 4 callosotomy was well documented. Out of 29 lesional cases the complete resection was done in 23 patients. In three patients lesion was extending into eloquent areas and further resection was not done. In other 3 patients ioMRI enabled to achieve complete resection. ioMRI evaluates the extent of resection or disconnection in epilepsy surgery.

ioMRI during DBS surgery provides real time confirmation of lead placement and other complications. Commonly the microelectrode placement in DBS is done with intraoperative microelectrode recording (MER) in awake conditions. With evolution of ioMRI now a days DBS is being done with ioMRI alone or along with MER. Zhiqiang Cui et al. [34] have done microelectrode placement for movement disorder patients under local anesthesia with MER and ioMRI. 56 (27%) of 206 DBS electrodes were adjusted after initial ioMRI. Another 6 times repositioned after 2 and 3 ioMRI in the same sitting. ioMRI revealed intraparenchymal hemorrhages in 2 patients. Martin Jakobs et al. [35] performed 86 surgeries in 81 patients with Parkinson's disease, essential tremor and dystonia with intraoperative stereotactic MRI-only DBS electrode implantation. A total of 167 electrodes were implanted. In 96.5% of cases the surgeries could be finished as planned. Both length of surgery and the time spent in the stereotactic frame could be significantly reduced. Caio M. Matias et al. [34, 36] evaluated placement accuracy and clinical outcomes in patients with frame-based stereotaxy and ioMRI without MER after induction under general anesthesia in DBS patients. 33 patients underwent implantation, 64 leads in total. MR images were acquired immediately after the procedure and fused to the preoperative plan to verify accuracy. At the last follow-up there was significant improvement ($p < 0.001$) in symptoms compared to preoperative state. Placement of microelectrodes in DBS with ioMRI reduces the operative time as well as the time in frame. Microelectrode tip location can be confirmed and also any intraoperative complications can be diagnosed. ioMRI is not affected by brain shift due to csf leak or intracranial air, but one has to be aware of the artifacts created by these electrodes. Role ioMRI in DBS is certainly promising and needs further validation in future.

6. Future directions in ioMRI

AMIGO (Advanced Multimodality Image Guided Operating Suite) is a three-room configuration involving the PET-CT room, operating room, and MRI room. It involves multidisciplinary teams to guide treatment before, during, and after surgery in the operating room. PET provides functional and metabolic information with molecular biomarkers. The combination of MRI and CT with PET gives anatomical, functional, and metabolic combined information to surgeons intraoperatively for further decision-making [37].

MRI-guided focused ultrasound (MRgFUS) is a noninvasive thermal ablation method.IT uses MRI for target identification, planning, and energy deposition. It allows to ablate targeted tissue without damaging normal structures. MRgFUS has been approved for the treatment of uterine fibroids. It is also evaluated for targeted drug delivery and gene therapy, which can temporarily change vascular or cell membrane permeability and release or activate various compounds. High field strength of MRI (3 T) aids better quality of images it helps both diagnosis and surgical ablation. 3 T MRI also has improved sensitivity to temperature measurements which enables multi-slice or three-dimensional thermometry. Trails are being conducted for its use in brain tumors [38].

The Smart Cyber Operating Theater (SCOT), the next generation operating room has been developed by Japan Agency for Medical Research and Development with AMED. It has a treatment room communication interface called "OPeLiNK" which projects all the information like patient data, navigation, IONM, anesthesia monitoring, operative field, ioMRI, etc. in a 70 inch screen. Approximately 20 types of equipment are connected to the system. Surgical information from these sources are sent through an application and displayed to the surgeon and it enables precision in surgery with low risk and high therapeutic effect [39].

7. Conclusion

ioMRI is a valuable tool which not only locates the residue but also guides further resections with enhanced safety. Its importance has been well documented in pituitary surgeries and gliomas. The drawbacks of ioMRI are the cost and time involved. But it is certainly beneficial for the patients in terms of improved functional outcomes and survivals.

Author details

G. Krishna Kumar, Anandh Balasubramaniam*, K. Pradeep and Nitin Manohar
Yashoda Hospital, Secunderabad, Hyderabad, India

*Address all correspondence to: anandhbala@gmail.com

References

[1] Mislow JM, Golby AJ, Black PMJMRIC. Origins of intraoperative MRI. 2010;18(1):1-10.

[2] Grönemeyer D, Seibel R, Erbel R, Schmidt A, Melzer A, et al. Equipment configuration and procedures: preferences for interventional micro therapy. 1996;9(2):81.

[3] Grönemeyer D, Seibel R, Schmidt A, Melzer A, Dell MJSiHT, et al. Two- and three-dimensional imaging for interventional MRI and CT guidance. 1996;29:62-76.

[4] Seifert VJNI. Intraoperative MRI in neurosurgery: technical overkill or the future of brain surgery? 2003;51(3):329.

[5] Zhuang D-X, Wu J-S, Yao C-J, Qiu T-M, Lu J-F, et al. Intraoperative multi-information-guided resection of dominant-sided insular gliomas in a 3-T intraoperative magnetic resonance imaging integrated neurosurgical suite. 2016;89:84-92.

[6] Ginat DT, Swearingen B, Curry W, Cahill D, Madsen J, et al. 3 Tesla intraoperative MRI for brain tumor surgery. 2014;39(6):1357-65.

[7] Manohar N, Mohapatra D, Balasubramaniam A, Rao K, Srinivas D, et al. Setting Up Workflow of an Intraoperative MRI Unit: A Single-Centre Experience of First 53 Cases. Journal of Neuroanaesthesiology and Critical Care. 2018;5(03):177-183.

[8] Multani KM, Balasubramaniam A, Rajesh BJ, Kumar MS, Manohara N, et al. Utility and pitfalls of high field 3 tesla intraoperative MRI in neurosurgery: A single centre experience of 100 cases. Neurology India. 2020;68(2):413.

[9] Gandhe RU, Bhave CPJIJoA. Intraoperative magnetic resonance imaging for neurosurgery–An anaesthesiologist's challenge. 2018;62(6):411.

[10] Manohar N, Palan A, Deora H, Rajesh BJ, Balasubramanium A, et al. Thermal injuries during intraoperative magnetic resonance imaging: Mechanisms and prevention. Journal of Neuroanaesthesiology and Critical Care. 2019.

[11] Manohar N, Palan A, Mohapatra D, Rao K, Srinivas D, et al. Intraoperative Magnetic Resonance Imaging with Evoked Potential Monitoring: Tailored Method of Scalp Corkscrew Electrode Placement to Reduce Image Artifacts. Journal of Neuroanaesthesiology and Critical Care. 2019;6(1).

[12] Yrjänä S, Tuominen J, KoivukangasJJAR.Intraoperativemagnetic resonance imaging in neurosurgery. 2007;48(5):540-549.

[13] Mohammadi AM, Sullivan TB, Barnett GH, Recinos V, Angelov L, et al. Use of high-field intraoperative magnetic resonance imaging to enhance the extent of resection of enhancing and nonenhancing gliomas. 2014;74(4):339-350.

[14] Brown TJ, Brennan MC, Li M, Church EW, Brandmeir NJ, et al. Association of the extent of resection with survival in glioblastoma: a systematic review and meta-analysis. 2016;2(11):1460-1469.

[15] Senft C, Bink A, Franz K, Vatter H, Gasser T, et al. Intraoperative MRI guidance and extent of resection in glioma surgery: a randomised, controlled trial. 2011;12(11):997-1003.

[16] Hatiboglu MA, Weinberg JS, Suki D, Rao G, Prabhu SS, et al. Impact of intraoperative high-field magnetic resonance imaging guidance on glioma surgery: A prospective volumetric analysis. 2009;64(6):1073-1081.

[17] Pamir MN, Özduman K, Dinçer A, Yildiz E, Peker S, et al. First intraoperative, shared-resource, ultrahigh-field 3-Tesla magnetic resonance imaging system and its application in low-grade glioma resection. 2010;112(1):57-69.

[18] Coburger J, Merkel A, Scherer M, Schwartz F, Gessler F, et al. Low-grade glioma surgery in intraoperative magnetic resonance imaging: results of a multicenter retrospective assessment of the German Study Group for Intraoperative Magnetic Resonance Imaging. 2016;78(6):775-786.

[19] Bodhinayake I, Ottenhausen M, Mooney MA, Kesavabhotla K, Christos P, et al. Results and risk factors for recurrence following endoscopic endonasal transsphenoidal surgery for pituitary adenoma. 2014;119:75-79.

[20] Raverot G, Vasiljevic A, Jouanneau EJP. Prognostic factors of regrowth in nonfunctioning pituitary tumors. 2018;21(2):176-182.

[21] Brochier S, Galland F, Kujas M, Parker F, Gaillard S, et al. Factors predicting relapse of nonfunctioning pituitary macroadenomas after neurosurgery: a study of 142 patients. 2010;163(2):193.

[22] DeKlotz TR, Chia SH, Lu W, Makambi KH, Aulisi E, et al. Meta-analysis of endoscopic versus sublabial pituitary surgery. 2012;122(3):511-518.

[23] Dehdashti AR, Ganna A, Karabatsou K, Gentili FJN. Pure endoscopic endonasal approach for pituitary adenomas: early surgical results in 200 patients and comparison with previous microsurgical series. 2008;62(5):1006-17.

[24] Serra C, Burkhardt J-K, Esposito G, Bozinov O, Pangalu A, et al. Pituitary surgery and volumetric assessment of extent of resection: a paradigm shift in the use of intraoperative magnetic resonance imaging. 2016;40(3):E17.

[25] Berkmann S, Fandino J, Muller B, Remonda L, Landolt H. Intraoperative MRI and endocrinological outcome of transsphenoidal surgery for non-functioning pituitary adenoma. Acta Neurochir (Wien). 2012;154(4):639-647.

[26] Adeolu A, Sutherland GJWAjom. Intraoperative magnetic resonance imaging and meningioma surgery. 2006;25(3):174-178.

[27] Giordano M, Gallieni M, Metwali H, Fahlbusch R, Samii M, et al. Can Intraoperative Magnetic Resonance Imaging Be Helpful in the Surgical Resection of Parasellar Meningiomas? A Case Series. 2019;132:e577-ee84.

[28] Chakraborty S, Zavarella S, Salas S, Schulder MJJoET, Oncology. Intraoperative MRI for resection of intracranial meningiomas. 2017;12(2).

[29] Metwali H, Samii A, Gerganov V, Giordano M, Fahlbusch R, et al. The Significance of Intraoperative Magnetic Resonance Imaging in Resection of Skull Base Chordomas. 2019;128:e185-ee94.

[30] Dort JC, Sutherland GRJTL. Intraoperative magnetic resonance imaging for skull base surgery. 2001;111(9):1570-1575.

[31] Kurwale NS, Chandra SP, Chouksey P, Arora A, Garg A, et al. Impact of intraoperative MRI on outcomes in epilepsy surgery: preliminary experience of two years. 2015;29(3):380-385.

[32] Kaibara T, Myles ST, Lee MA, Sutherland GRJE. Optimizing epilepsy surgery with intraoperative MR imaging. 2002;43(4):425-429.

[33] Buchfelder M, Fahlbusch R, Ganslandt O, Stefan H, Nimsky CJE. Use of intraoperative magnetic resonance

imaging in tailored temporal lobe surgeries for epilepsy. 2002;43(8):864-873.

[34] Cui Z, Pan L, Song H, Xu X, Xu B, et al. Intraoperative MRI for optimizing electrode placement for deep brain stimulation of the subthalamic nucleus in Parkinson disease. 2016;124(1):62-69.

[35] Jakobs M, Krasniqi E, Kloß M, Neumann J-O, Campos B, et al. Intraoperative Stereotactic magnetic resonance imaging for deep brain stimulation electrode planning in patients with movement disorders. 2018;119:e801-e8e8.

[36] Matias CM, Frizon LA, Nagel SJ, Lobel DA, Machado AGJJoN. Deep brain stimulation outcomes in patients implanted under general anesthesia with frame-based stereotaxy and intraoperative MRI. 2018;129(6):1572-1578.

[37] Wang G, Zhang J, Gao H, Weir V, Yu H, et al. Towards omni-tomography—Grand fusion of multiple modalities for simultaneous interior tomography. 2012;7(6):e39700.

[38] Jung NY, Chang JWJJoKms. Magnetic resonance-guided focused ultrasound in neurosurgery: taking lessons from the past to inform the future. 2018;33(44).

[39] Iseki H, Muragaki Y, Tamura M, Suzuki T, Yoshimitsu K, et al., editors. SCOT (Smart Cyber Operating Theater) project: advanced medical information analyzer for guidance of the surgical procedures. Proceedings of the international display workshops; 2012.

Chapter 5

Management of Brain Tumors in Eloquent Areas with Awake Patient

José Luis Navarro-Olvera, Gustavo Parra-Romero, Stephani Dalila Heres-Becerril, David Trejo-Martínez, José D. Carrillo Ruiz, Kleber Gonzalez Echeverría and Gustavo Aguado-Carrillo

Abstract

This chapter aims to provide an overview of the transdisciplinary work of the Neurosurgeon, Neuroanesthesiologist and Neuropsychologist before, during and after the resection of a neoplasm in eloquent areas with the patient conscious under the 3A anesthesia modality (asleep, awake, asleep). The diagnostic approach and the logistics to carry out this procedure and achieve better results will be shown. At present there is growing evidence regarding the benefits of surgery in awake patients, with application in the treatment of epilepsy, abnormal movements and oncological surgery. The benefits of awake craniotomy are increased lesion removal, with improved survival benefit, whilst minimizing damage to eloquent cortex and resulting postoperative neurological dysfunction. Other advantages include a shorter hospitalization time, hence reduced cost of care, and a decreased incidence of postoperative complications. This approach has allowed to achieve a higher degree of resection with less morbidity and a higher quality of life.

Keywords: brain tumors, eloquent areas, neurosurgery, awake craniotomy

1. Introduction

This chapter aims to provide an overview of the transdisciplinary work of the Neurosurgeon, Neuroanesthesiologist and Neuropsychologist before, during and after the resection of a neoplasm in eloquent areas with the patient conscious under the 3A anesthesia modality (asleep, awake, asleep). The diagnostic approach and the logistics to carry out this procedure and achieve better results will be shown.

At present there is growing evidence regarding the benefits of surgery in awake patients, with application in the treatment of epilepsy, abnormal movements and neurooncological surgery [1]. The benefits of awake craniotomy are increased lesion removal, with improved survival benefit, whilst minimizing damage to eloquent cortex and resulting postoperative neurological dysfunction. Other advantages include a shorter hospitalization time, hence reduced cost of care, and a decreased incidence of postoperative complications [2, 3]. This approach has allowed to achieve a higher degree of resection with less morbidity and a higher quality of life [2, 3].

1.1 History of brain surgery with awake patient

Throughout the history of neurosurgery it is known from archeological findings that therapeutic trepanation has existed since the Neolithic period between 8,000–500 BC, this type of treatment was performed for headaches, fractures, localized cranial deformity, mental changes, infections or seizures [4].

The earliest descriptions in the modern era of neurosurgery date back to descriptions in the treatment of epilepsy in the 17th century. However, the most identifiable antecedent dates back to the beginning of the last century with Penfield's descriptions in the 1920s of intractable epilepsy surgery in awake patients and later in 1937 with the exposure of the intraoperative electrical stimulation technique used for the treatment of epileptogenic foci close to the language area [5, 6].

It was not until 1970 that the intraoperative cortical mapping technique began to be used for the resection of neoplastic lesions by Whitaker and Ojemann, who perfected the technique and published the first series that demonstrated the usefulness of this technique, describing it as safe, simple and adequately tolerated by most patients [5–7]. Later, in the last decade of the 20th century, Berger began to treat infiltrating neoplasms in eloquent cortical areas, improving the cortical mapping technique with the posterior publication of his experience [5, 8, 9]. Finally, in recent decades, new neuroanatomical studies and the popularization of the cortical mapping technique have led to a better understanding of the cortical and subcortical anatomy, improving the technique and prognosis of patients with infiltrating CNS lesions [10, 11].

For centuries there has been an incessant search to associate specific neurological functions with specific areas of the nervous system. At the beginning of the 19th century, explanatory models of functional neuroanatomy were built. The first to develop a model was Franz Joseph Gall (1776–1832) and his disciple Spurzheim. Dr. Gall is the founder of phrenology, based on the interpretation of the different neurological functions, on the basis that the greater development of a certain function resulted in hypertrophy of a specific brain region and that this hypertrophy conditioned a variation in the external configuration of the skull. This ability of the nervous system to "hypertrophy", erroneously in the past, is now one of the main properties of the central nervous system used by modern radiology, such as the BOLD effect (increased blood supply to an area that is developing functional activity) or PET (increased glucose metabolism) [12, 13].

Walter Moxon (1836–1886) published the first cases that exposed the principle of hemispheric lateralization, associating the right hemiplegia with aphasia and, therefore, breaking the principle of hemispheric symmetry and locating language in the dominant left hemisphere. Later, Paul Broca presented the case of Monsieur Leborgne a patient suffering from septic gangrene in the lower limb. He was admitted to the Salpetriere hospital in Paris with a clinical presentation described by Broca as "expressive aphemia", that is, he did not present facial motor deficit or comprehension problems, but the patient was unable to articulate words. An autopsy study identified the lesion in the posterior part of the lower left frontal gyrus. Pierre Marie (1853–1940), reexamined the brain of M. Leborgne, despite confirming the anatomical - functional association made by Broca 50 years earlier, he also concluded that the lesion was not limited to Broca's area only, but it extended subcortically to the striatum and posterior to the angular gyrus [12–14].

Carl Wernicke in 1874 gave name and anatomical location to sensory aphasia that he located in the primary auditory cortex, in the posterior part of the superior left temporal gyrus. Decades later Theodore Meynert (1833–1892) was the first to associate auditory aphasia with the posterior part of the superior left temporal gyrus. Wernicke not only correlated the types of aphasia with different areas, but also established the term conduction aphasia (inability to repeat words) for those syndromes of disconnection between the sensory and motor areas of language, associated with the lesion of the arcuate fascicle (AF) [13, 15].

Geschwind succeeded in introducing one more level into the theory of language: the fundamental idea of networking and interconnection of the central nervous system. There are some basic Broca - Wernicke nodes and their main connection, which is the arcuate fascicle, but they do not work in isolation [16].

Damasio published the implication of the associative areas of the left medial frontal gyrus and the premotor area when performing tasks of understand words when related to animals, tools, or people. Also the implication of the inferotemporal cortex in the assimilation of the semantic concept of language, regardless of the stimulus pathway through which the word, visual (reading) or auditory information arrives, the precise implication of the dominant temporal pole in the memory-language association with the name of famous faces or places. He also characterized the difference between the pure primary auditory cortex in the transverse gyrus of Heschl and the posterior temporal area in T1 proper language, establishing the high regional cortical specialization for language understanding and he introduced the participation of the right hemisphere in the assimilation of concepts [17, 18].

1.2 Anatomy of brain eloquent areas

Once the historical review of the intraoperative cortical mapping has been carried out, it is important to emphasize that it is an evolving paradigm. Nowadays the vision of functions dependent on a specific anatomical cortical site has given way to a new dynamic and integrative paradigm with structural and functional connectivity and reciprocal influence, in this manner a lesion in a given site does not affect only one function, but the system as a whole [19, 20]. For this reason, pre-surgical functional studies are not superior to intraoperative mapping.

Although it is accepted that the mapping should be directed towards the area where the lesion is located, the wide anatomical and functional variability between individuals, limitations in presurgical neuroimaging, and functional modifications caused by the tumor must be considered [21, 22]. Usually, the evaluation of 8 main domains is accepted, which are adapted to the location of the lesion, activity of each patient and the evaluation of the benefit of a broad resection against the loss of functionality/neuroplasticity [20, 22]:

1. Movement.
2. Somatosensory function.
3. Visual Function.
4. Vestibular/auditory function.
5. Language (spontaneous, nominate, understand, repeat, read, write).
6. Higher functions (calculation, memory, attention, cognitive control, judgment).
7. Spatial orientation.
8. State of consciousness **(Table 1)**.

Function	Cortical Areas	Subcortical pathways
Motor function	Central region, SMA, premotor cortex	Pyramidal pathways (corona radiata, internal capsule, mesencephalic peduncles)
Somatosensory	Central region (primary and secondary somatosensory areas), insula	Thalamocortical pathways
Oral language		
Ventral semantic stream	Posterior temporal regions, orbitofrontal and dorsolateral prefrontal areas (dorsal and ventral)	Inferior occipital fasciculus
Dorsal phonological stream	Posterosuperior temporal cortex, inferior frontal gyrus	Direct SLF (arcuate fasciculus)
Articulatory loop	Supramarginalis gyrus, ventral premotor cortex	Indirect SLF III (lateral, anterior)
Speech production	Dominant anterior insula (articulatory planning), ventral premotor cortex, primary sensorimotor area of the mouth	Operculo-insular fibers, descending pathways from the ventral premotor cortex, pyramidal tract and lentiform nucleus.
Writing	Inferior and superior parietal lobules, insula, second and third frontal convolutions, SMA	SLF
Reading	Visual cortex, visual object (word) form area	Inferior longitudinal fasciculus
Visuospatial cognition		
Visual	Temporo-parieto-occipital junction, visual cortex	Optic radiations
Spatial awareness	Right supramarginal gyrus, right superior temporal cortex	Right SLF
Vestibular	Right inferior parietal cortex, posterior insula, superior temporal cortex	Right SLF
Higher cognitive / executive functions		
Language switching	Left inferior frontal gyrus, posterosuperior temporal area	SLF
Working memory	Inferior frontal gyrus, dorsal premotor cortex, supramarginal gyrus	SLF
Syntactic processing	Left inferior frontal gyrus, left inferior temporal gyrus	SLF
Judgment, decision making, understanding	Left dominant prefrontal cortex, Left posterior temporal cortex.	Inferior occipitofrontal fasciculus
Selection, inhibition, attention	SMA, cingulum, frontal eye fields.	Subcallosal medialis fasciculus, head of the caudate nucleus

SLF: superior longitudinal fasciculus.
SMA: supplementary motor area.
From: De Benedictis A, Duffau H. Brain hodotopy: From esoteric concept to practical surgical applications. Neurosurgery 2011;68:1709–23.

Table 1.
Cortical and subcortical structures involved in major brain functions as detected by direct cerebral stimulation.

The cortical mapping must be adapted in each patient, according to location of the lesion. The following paragraphs review the main tasks and effects of cortical stimulation.

1.2.1 Frontal lobe

The main functions to evaluate correspond to the motor paradigm, which traditionally has an anatomical correlate in the primary motor cortex in the precentral gyrus, and surrounding subcortical regions, therefore it is necessary to map this area to avoid contralateral paresis or plegia. Corona radiata is considered the posterior subcortical limit of a frontal lesion resection. Cortical mapping is performed by asking the patient to perform movements while stimulating the specific area with respect to the Penfield homunculus, which will lead to its inhibition, or in a patient at rest the stimulation will cause involuntary movement [21, 22] **(Vignette 1).**

Vignette 1. Intraoperative cortical electrical stimulation

It is the most widely used technique in awake patient surgery to delimit essential brain regions for some functions such as movement and language. It consists of the administration of an electric current in milli-amperes directly on the cerebral cortex (authors recommend bipolar stimulation, short train, 1 ms duration and 200 Hz frequency, with 5-20 mA intensity) in order to cause depolarization of a group of neurons belonging to a cerebral system to produce a positive symptom (such as a muscle contraction) or negative (such as the arrest during number counting).

Thanks to this technique, the organization of the representation of the body in the cerebral cortex was described by the eminent neurosurgeon Wilder Penfield in the 1950s and later important contributions were made on the organization of language in the brain by George Ojemann.

Among the most important advantages is the speed with which a wide region of the cerebral cortex can be mapped, in cases where the neoplasm delimited in the cortex can be observed, the edges of the lesion can be delimited. In the same way, it is possible to stimulate subcortically in the white matter.

Among the most important limitations is the little time available to carry out a cognitive task. For example, it is ideal to explore the denomination since the electrical stimulus can be administered immediately after asking the patient for the name of an object represented in a slide (several seconds), however it would not be possible to administer an electrical stimulus during the elaboration of a narration (**Figures 1–3**).

The supplementary motor cortex (SMA) is responsible for preparation, initiation, and monitoring movement, and it is located anterior to the cortical representation of the lower limb of precentral circumvolution. In the dominant hemisphere it exerts a function in the articulation of language, so its stimulation can cause alterations in the fluency of language when asking to name pictures. [22, 23].

The frontal premotor cortex (PMC) has a ventrolateral division responsible for the articulation of language, which when stimulated can cause anarthria; while the dorsolateral division is involved in the naming network, causing anomia when stimulated, this mainly in the dominant hemisphere. This location is where the intensity values of the stimulation are determined to obtain responses in the rest of the areas to explore [22, 23].

The cortex of the inferior and middle frontal gyri, when stimulated, causes impairment in writing.

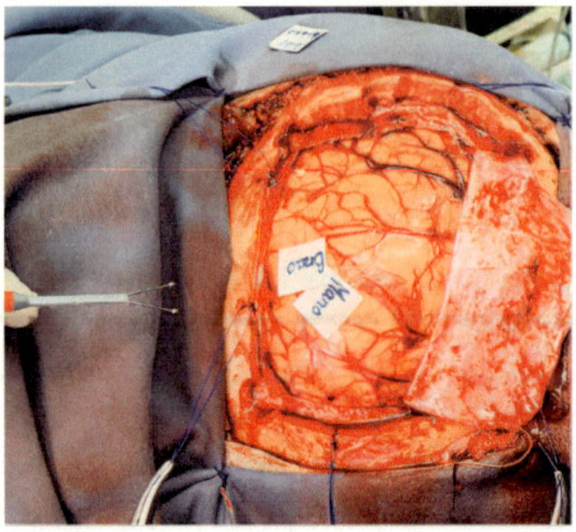

Figure 1.
Cortical stimulation with bipolar.

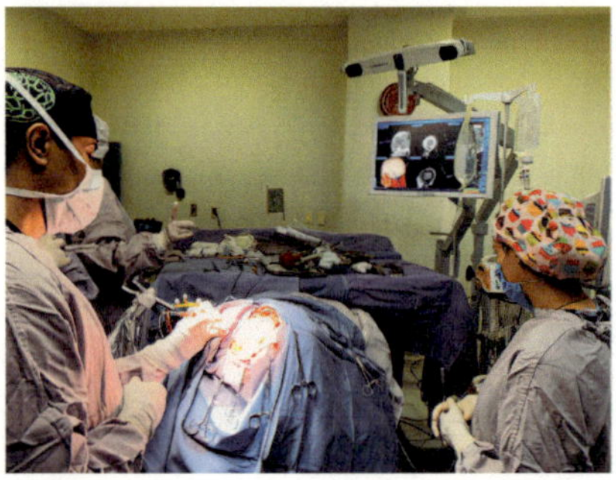

Figure 2.
Use of cortical stimulation guided by navigation.

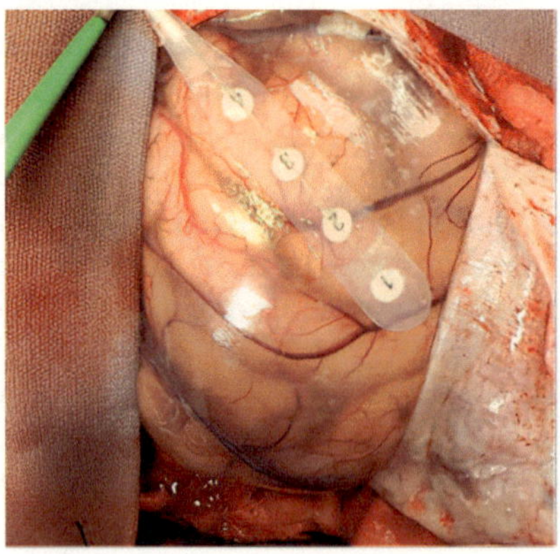

Figure 3.
Cortical stimulation using various contacts.

Regarding the frontal subcortical mapping, these fasciculi are evaluated by counting, naming, and reading tasks, the main tracts to evaluate in this area are:

a. *Superior Longitudinal Fasciculus (SLF):* it has the cortical projections of the frontal, temporal and inferior parietal lobe. SLF stimulation through the arcuate fasciculus (AF), can cause problems in the production of language, memory alterations and phonemic paraphasia.

b. *Subcallosal fasciculus*: it links the frontomesial structures with the striatum, so its stimulation causes a decrease in fluency or difficulty in initiating language.

c. *Anterior part of Inferior Frontooccipital fascicle (aIFOF):* projects the orbitofrontal and dorsolateral prefrontal cortex with the temporooccipital cortex. aIFOF stimulation causes semantic paraphasia and failures in facial recognition. aIFOF represents the lower limit of resection of frontoorbital lesions [22–24].

Executive functions, working memory, attention, control, judgment and decision-making, functions related to perisylvian and prefrontal areas are also evaluated.

1.2.2 Parietal lobe

The primary somatosensory cortex is located posterior to the primary motor cortex and, if necessary, it is possible to resect it without significant alterations in the sensory function, since other association areas can supply its function. However, the thalamocortical radiation must be preserved, representing the anterior limit of resection of parietal lesions [22–24].

The cortical region of the inferior parietal lobe, the supramarginal and angular gyrus, affect language in the dominant hemisphere and spatial awareness in the non-dominant hemisphere. Writing and calculation tests should be done to avoid iatrogenic Gertsman's syndrome. In the subcortical region of the dominant inferior parietal lobe (Geschwind territory), there are continuity of the pathways that communicate Broca's area (inferior frontal cortex) with Wernicke's area (posterior temporal cortex), the AF and SLF, therefore the stimulation of these areas can cause paraphasia and alteration in the production of language [22, 25].

1.2.3 Temporal lobe

In the temporal cortex, the main function to identify is language, especially in lesions of the dominant hemisphere. The posterior limit of a temporal pole resection is the arcuate fasciculus, which when stimulated causes paraphasia. Other temporal cortical and subcortical functions are visual recognition and dependent language, which is assessed with picture recognition. Likewise, temporary optic radiation should be evaluated in periventricular lesions in this region, in order to avoid postsurgical hemianopia [23].

1.2.4 Occipital lobe

The primary visual cortex is the main area to be explored, which when stimulated can produce phosphenes, blurred vision, visual hallucinations, and scotomas. Regarding the subcortical mapping, the final portion of the IFOF can produce alteration in the recognition and conceptualization of objects, so semantic paraphasia can be found [22, 23].

1.2.5 Insular lobe

The insular cortex and its corresponding subcortical tracts are considered unresectable, since they represent an important anatomical seat of essential functions of sensory, motor, limbic, vestibular and language integration. It is explored using a picture naming test [22, 26].

In a report, Ius et al., were able to identify sites considered unresectable after cortical mapping and resection of the lesion; in the dominant hemisphere the primary sensory and motor areas for the upper and lower extremities, the ventral premotor cortex, Wernicke's area in the posterior part of the superior temporal gyrus, and the supramarginal and angular gyrus; while in the non-dominant hemisphere the primary motor and sensory cortex and the angular gyrus. In certain cases it was possible to excise the rest of the association areas under the principle of maximum resection without greatly affecting the function [20–22]. Likewise, regarding the tracts, the following were considered unresectable: the cortico-spinal tract, posterior limit in patients with frontal lesion; thalamic-cortical radiations, anterior limit in patients with parietal lesions; the stratum sagittale, medial border of temporo-parietal lesions; anterior part of IFOF and perisylvian network [21, 22].

1.3 Brain lesions affecting the eloquent areas and surgical criteria

In general, neoplastic intracranial lesions can displace or invade brain structures. The first group of lesions are not usually candidates for awake resection, since the symptoms are produced by the effect of mass on the cortex and tracts, but their resection does not involve functional areas. Unlike the second group of neoplasms that can infiltrate or even originate in functional areas, and whose resection without the appropriate quality of life approach, can have unacceptable consequences for the functioning of patients. Also, since the patient should be comfortable as much as possible for resection of the lesions, the awake and cortical mapping approaches usually involve convexity or superficial, intra-axial, supratentorial lesions [1, 27].

In a review of several reported series of awake cortical mapping, gliomas are the neoplasms that are most frequently approached by this technique, up to 60%. High-grade astrocytomas such as OMS GIV glioblastoma is the most frequent glioma reported, followed by oligodendrogliomas, oligoastrocytomas, and low-grade astrocytomas [2, 28, 29]. The second group in frequency are brain metastases, mainly pulmonary and mammary origin. Finally, non-neoplastic lesions such as cavernous angiomas are usually reported as accessible lesions using this technique [30].

Although it is true that all the lesions described in the previous paragraph benefit from a wide resection, at present special emphasis has been placed in low-grade gliomas since these are lesions that usually occur in young adults, and it migrates through white matter tracts at an average rate of 4 mm/year [23, 31]. This raises new paradigms in which a supramarginal resection has been proposed even at the cost of function, hoping that brain plasticity in young patients improves the prognosis and quality of life in the long term [32].

1.3.1 Surgical criteria

The main criteria that are considered in neurosurgery to determine that a patient is considered for this type of procedure can be consulted in **Figure 4** in the form of a flow chart. Some of the most important criteria will be mentioned below according to the purpose of this chapter:

a. The lesion should be located intra-axial (typical of the brain parenchyma), in a brain region that implies a high risk of post-surgical neurological and/or cognitive alterations. Generally, cortical and/or subcortical sensorimotor and periinsular regions of the dominant hemisphere. However, other "highly specialized areas" should be considered according to the profession of each patient.

b. In relation to the radiological characteristics of the tumor, ideally with little cerebral edema, without significant midline deviation.

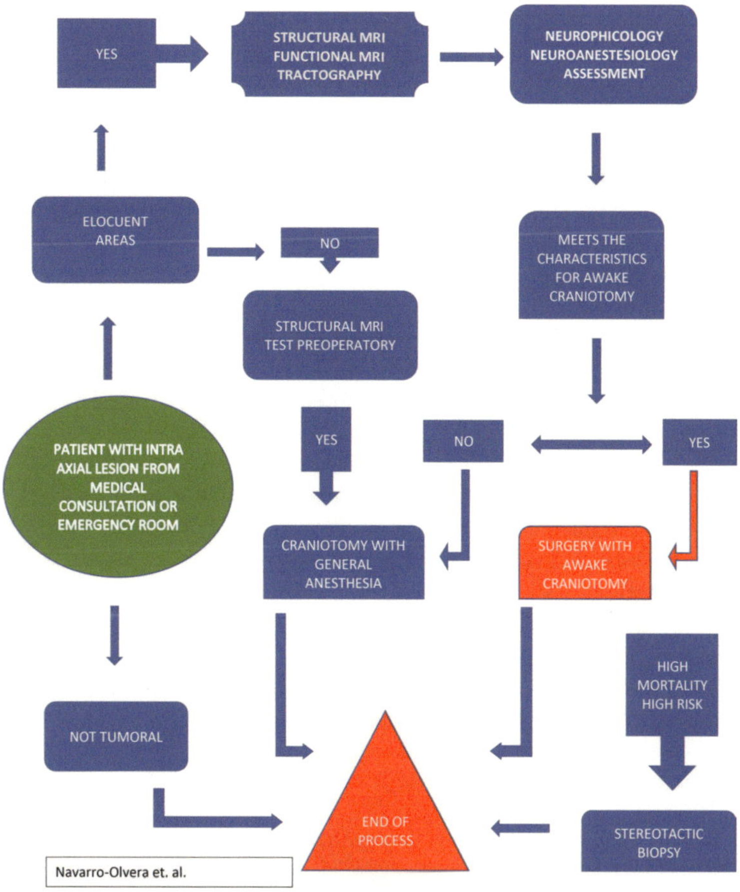

Figure 4.
Diagram showing the flow of neurosurgical conditions that must be considered to determine that a patient is a candidate for awake surgery (red line). Patient admitted to neurosurgery, from the outpatient or emergency department with an intra-axial lesion, located in a highly specialized area. Candidate for structural, functional and tractography MRI. Neuropsychological assessment confirmed the possibility of surgery with a conscious patient. Surgery is scheduled with a navigation method for resection of the lesion.

c. Degree of malignancy. Previously it was considered that the tumor should be low grade (histologically) since having a good survival prognosis, the benefit of keeping it neurologically intact was essential However, nowadays it is currently considered that it should also for patients with a high-grade, to promote quality of life.

d. Patient can decide to accept the procedure and agree to collaborate once he knows the type of surgery that is proposed.

e. Patient with no history of anxiety or impulsivity disorder because these may be exacerbated during surgery (e.g. refusing to cooperate or presenting psychogenic symptoms that make evaluation difficult) (**Table 2**).

1.4 Pre-operative evaluation

Once the patient has been selected for resection of the lesion with cortical mapping, extension studies should be carried out to bring us more evidence regarding the patient and their environment through neuropsychological and neuro-anesthesiology assessment. In addition, to plan the intraoperative mapping, it is advisable to perform:

a. Diffusion tensor tractography (DTI): identifies the main tracts of white fibers (corticospinal, superior longitudinal fasciculus, arcuate fasciculus, uncinate fasciculus, inferior orbitofrontal fasciculus, optic pathways) their location and infiltration or displace. However, the variability between imaging and the effect of medical treatment on the injury and associated vasogenic edema must be taken into consideration.

b. Functional MRI: it helps to locate functional cortical areas through dependent sequences of blood oxygenation, which detects the increase in cerebral perfusion to certain areas when specific tasks are performed. The most studied paradigms are motor, sensory and speech **(Vignette 2)**.

Vignette 2. Functional Magnetic Resonance (fMRI)
The functional Magnetic Resonance images are based on the changes in the oxygen levels in the blood related to an activity by the subject. It is an indirect measure of brain functionality since the equipment detects changes in signal intensity caused by vascular changes (demand for oxygen supply through the blood). Since the construction of the images depends on the use of complex mathematical algorithms, it is not possible to completely eliminate the noise sources that may occur, causing false positives, that is, activations in some brain region that are not real.

Prior Concerns	Current Solutions
Significant mass effect (>2-cm midline shift) despite preoperative diuretics & steroid	Staged internal debulking (asleep) using functional imaging (MEG/MSI) followed by reoperation w/ awake mapping or LMA
Obese patient (BMI >30)/obstructive apnea	LMA before & after mapping (limits subcortical mapping during resection if LMA is used)
Psychiatric history/emotional instability	Treated mood disorders no longer a contraindication
Age (yrs)	
>10	Awake
<10	2-stage procedure w/ implanted grid
Intraop seizures	Iced Ringers solution, propofol IV 6 inches from vein
Smoker	Cough suppressants w/ or w/o light sedation
Intraop nausea	Preop medication w/ antiemetic drugs (ondansetron hydrochloride, scopolamine) & high-dose dexamethasone (10 mg)
Reop (dural scar)	Focused craniotomy w/ negative mapping is acceptable
Severely impaired preoperative function*	Attempt to improve function w/ up to 5 days of preoperative high-dose steroids w/ or w/o diuretics
Tumor location presumed to be w/in functional cortical or subcortical pathways on preop imaging	The decision to offer surgery is not made based on preop anatomical or functional imaging (attempt is always made to map, identify, & preserve functional sites).

*BMI = body mass index; IV = intravenous; MEG = magnetoencephalography; MSI = magnetic source imaging. *Motor function <2/5 or baseline naming/reading errors.*
From: Hervey-Jumper SL, Li J, Lau D, Molinaro AM, Perry DW, Meng L, et al. Awake craniotomy to maximize glioma resection: Methods and technical nuances over a 27-year period. J Neurosurg 2015;123:325–39.

Table 2.
Relative contraindications and solutions for awake craniotomy patients.

In the same way, false positives can occur due to the pathology of the brain tissue itself due to the pathological vasculature.

It is currently one of the most common methods in cognitive neurosciences due to its safety in healthy subjects.

Figure 5 shows motor paradigm during evaluation of a patient with a supratentorial glioma.

Other functional extension studies such as positron emission tomography (PET) or magnetoencephalography allow planning the procedure but none of them is superior to intraoperative cortical mapping, which is considered the gold standard.

1.5 Anesthetic management

1.5.1 Neuroanesthetic perioperative management

Benefits of awake craniotomy are greater resection of the lesion, with improvement in survival, while the damage to the eloquent cortex, which generates postoperative neurological dysfunction, is minimized. Other advantages include shorter hospitalization times, hence a reduction in care costs, and a decrease in the incidence of postoperative complications.

The term "awake craniotomy" is misleading as the patient is not fully awake during the entire procedure. The most painful moments of surgery require different levels of sedation or anesthesia, nonetheless, patient is fully awake while mapping or during resection [33].

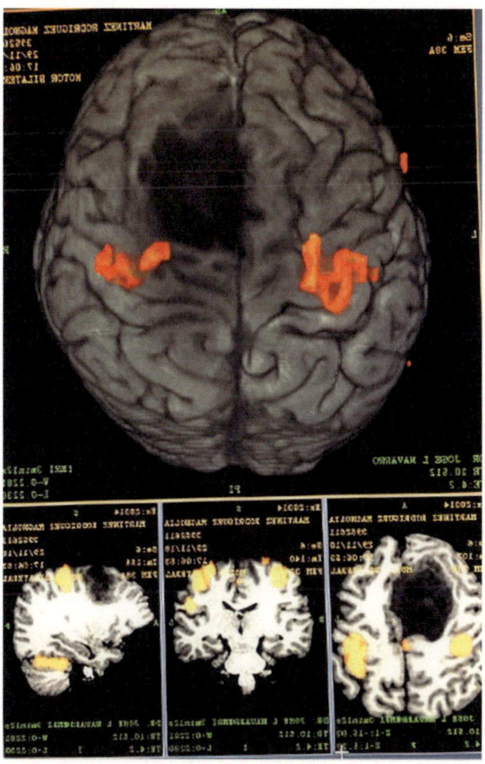

Figure 5.
Functional MRI with motor paradigm.

1.5.2 Preoperative evaluation

A very important aspect in an awake craniotomy is the adequate selection and full preparation of the patient by a multidisciplinary team in order to avoid intraoperative failures [34].

All patients should have consultations with the neurosurgeon and neuroanesthesiologist to assess whether the patient is a good candidate for this technique **(see Table 3)** and to prepare the patient for the procedure. This includes a complete evaluation of patient's comorbidities, which must be optimized before surgery, in or Patients in whom a difficult airway is anticipated may have problems during the intraoperative period that possess the neuroanesthesiologist to a very difficult airway scenario. Children are not psychologically fit to undergo this procedure although individual development of each child must be considered.

Preoperative evaluation includes getting detailed information from the patient, in turn the patient must know what to expect and know the risks inherent to anesthesia. Usually this includes verbal and written informed consent [34, 35].

Pre-operative consultations provide an invaluable opportunity for the multidisciplinary team to create a rapport with the patient and therefore encourage trust.

1.5.3 Operating room preparation

The layout of the operating room and the position of the patient must be taken into account. The ability to communicate with the patient must be maintained at all times and access to the patient during adverse events is of equal importance.

As in every surgery, the operating table should be as comfortable as possible, since the patient is going to be lying in the same position for several hours. The operating room temperature should be comfortable for the patient, and the number of people should be minimized to reduce unnecessary noise and reduce patient anxiety [36].

The position of the patient is determined by the location of the lesion. **(Figure 6)** This is usually a lateral or supine position, in the case of occipital lesions and evaluation of the visual cortex, a sitting position may be used. In either position, it's important that when patient is fully awake during mapping, he can see and communicate with the neuroanesthesiologist or neuropsychologist. Sterile drapes used should not invade the patient's face, as this may cause claustrophobia and difficulty in communicating [37].

Absolute
Patient refusal
Inability to lay still for any length of time
Inability to co-operate, for example confusion
Mental retardation
Anticipated difficult intubation
Obstructive sleep apnea
Children <10 years
Relative
Patient cough
Learning difficulties
Inability to lay flat
Patient anxiety
Language barriers
Obese patients

Table 3.
Anesthetic contraindications.

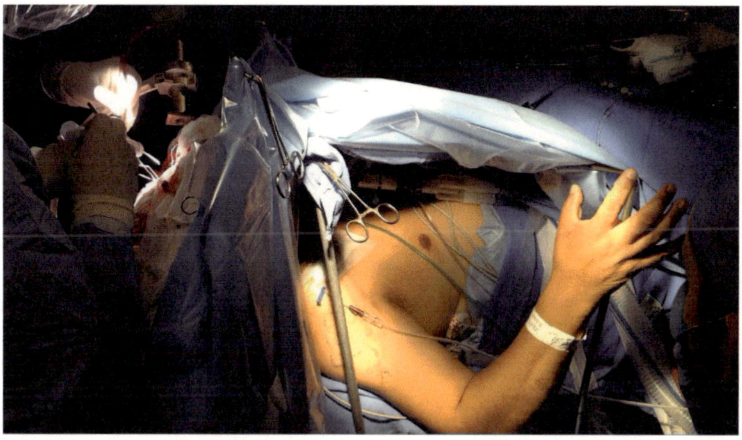

Figure 6.
Position of the patient and the evaluator during the surgical procedure to carry out the neuropsychological and movement evaluation.

1.5.4 Anesthetic generalities

The choice of the anesthetic agent even within a preferred anesthetic technique varies, but the general principles are common to all of them; the need to maximize patient comfort, prevention of nausea and vomiting that may increase intracranial pressure, the need for hemodynamic stability, and the use of short-acting drugs that allow acute control of the patient's level of consciousness.

Premedication is not common, but reflux prophylaxis should be considered, patients should continue their prescribed medication such as steroids, antiepileptic drugs, or antihypertensives. Prophylactic antibiotics and usually one or more antiemetics are administered in every patient before the incision. The most common options are ondansetron and dexamethasone. Dexamethasone can also be used to diminish brain edema during the operation.

Standard anesthetic monitoring is used. Depth of anesthesia monitors, for example Bispectral Index Monitoring (BIS™), are sometimes used to reduce the dose of anesthetic agents administered and thus time required for patient emergence and cortical mapping cooperation [37, 38].

Capnography under general anesthesia is considered basic monitoring, but carbon dioxide monitoring for sedated or awake patients during mapping is also a common practice. Although carbon dioxide levels may be inaccurate, it is used to confirm ventilation [39].

A large-bore intravenous access is obtained and most neuroanesthesiologist place also an arterial line, usually sedated or asleep. The use of other forms of monitoring is variable.

1.5.5 Anesthetic techniques

There is not a recognized consensus on the best anesthetic approach for awake craniotomy. This is because neuroanesthesiologists vary the technique depending on neurosurgeon's preferences, pathology, duration of the surgery and patient's factors.

There are two dominant anesthetic approaches to solving this problem: monitored anesthetic care (MAC) and asleep-awake-asleep (AAA).

The goal of the MAC approach is to decrease the sedative dose to avoid an abrupt transition from sleep to awakening, which can lead to hypoactive or hyperactive delirium upon emergence and to decrease the reliability of mapping.

MAC technique for awake craniotomy involves spontaneous ventilation and low doses of sedative drugs [38].

The AAA technique involves induction of general anesthesia and control of the airway with a supraglottic device such as laryngeal mask airway (LMA) or intubation. When neurocognitive testing and intraoperative mapping need to be started, anesthetic drugs are reduced or stopped, and the device is removed from the airway. Once resection of the lesion is complete, return to general anesthesia and reintroduction of the airway device is done. Advantages of this technique include the ability to control ventilation and thus control carbon dioxide concentrations and prevent airway obstruction and hypoventilation. It also facilitates a greater anesthetic depth during the most painful moments of surgery. Anesthetic drugs used for this technique are varied, but propofol and remifentanil TCI are the most common, followed by the use of a volatile anesthetic and remifentanil infusion. The use of dexmedetomidine has also been reported with this technique, and it's generally used during the awake stage of surgery and closure [39].

1.5.6 Scalp block

The cornerstone of awake craniotomy analgesia is regional scalp block along with infiltration of the incision line. A scalp block also provides hemodynamic stability and decreases the stress response to painful stimuli [40].

The scalp block technique includes infiltration of local anesthetic into seven nerves on each side. This is an anatomical block and not just a ring block. A ring block will require large volumes of local anesthetic, increase the risk of toxicity, and will not provide deep anesthesia to the temporal fascia.

Most neuroanesthesiologist place a bilateral scalp block before pinning of the head with Mayfield skull clamp. Occasionally, a scalp blocker is not applied and relies on local anesthetic infiltration by the surgeon.

The total dose of local anesthetic with and without epinephrine must be calculated individually for each patient. Studies have shown that the rise in plasma concentration of levobupivacaine and ropivacaine is faster compared to other local anesthetics and similar in all patients. Despite the quick rise in plasma levels, there were no signs of cardiovascular or central nervous system toxicity. The use of bupivacaine, levobupivacaine, and ropivacaine in varying concentrations with and without epinephrine has been described for use in a blockage of the scalp. The addition of epinephrine, usually 1: 200,000, increases the total amount of local anesthetic that can be used, decreases localized bleeding, and maximizes duration. However, systemic absorption may cause tachycardia and hypertension, and intraarterial injection into the superficial temporal artery is possible when the auriculotemporal nerve is blocked [37].

1.5.7 Adverse events

Awake craniotomy is generally a well-tolerated procedure with a low conversion rate to general anesthesia and a low complication rate. One of the most common complications is intolerance of the patient to the procedure, often due to urinary catheter or prolonged positioning and intraoperative seizures.

Seizures, focal or generalized, are more likely to occur during cortical mapping. The frequency of seizures during awake craniotomy ranges widely from 2.9–54%. These are treated by irrigating the brain tissue with ice-cold saline, they usually stop with this treatment, but sometimes benzodiazepines, antiepileptic drugs or re-sedation with airway control are required [41].

The efficacy of prevention of intraoperative seizures with anticonvulsants remains doubtful. The latest systematic review on this topic revealed no benefit of prophylaxis. However, it should be noted that most of seizure prevention trials are based on the use of phenytoin or valproate. On the other hand, there are new data that support the superiority of levetiracetam in the prophylaxis of seizures. However, there are insufficient data to recommend its routine use in awake craniotomy.

An emergency plan for airway control must be in place at all times and this can be challenging as the patient's head is fixed on the clamp and often away from the ventilator. Options include insertion of an LMA which may be easier than endotracheal intubation.

1.5.8 Closure and postoperative

Once resection is complete, patient may be re-sedated or re-anesthetized with reattachment of the airway device, even if in the lateral position. Dura, bone flap, and scalp are then closed, pins are removed, and patient is awakened.

If remifentanil has been used, it can be given at low infusion rates to aid for a "soft" awakening and prevent coughing.

It is imperative that close neurological monitoring continues as postoperative hematomas may develop, especially in the first 6 h after operating. This may require an urgent evacuation of the clot.

After scalp block has worn off, systemic pain relief is used. The use of postoperative pain relief can be decreased in patients who have received a scalp block. Regular paracetamol and opioids are used.

1.6 Neuropsychological management

Some generalities of intraoperative neuropsychological evaluation will be mentioned in the light of new neurocognitive technological and theoretical tools that allow us to carry out current forms of evaluation, always outlined based on the objectives of the surgical plan of the transdisciplinary group of the treating physician, as well as the type of tumor, location and extension.

The selection of the methodology for the intraoperative neuropsychological evaluation is described in detail in accordance with the current literature on a recent vision of Functional Neurosurgery in brain tumors called hodology [19], which implies a radical change to the classical view on a rigid and exclusively cortical cerebral organization of brain functions. **(Vignette 3)** The advances that have occurred in recent decades on neurocognitive aspects in patients with brain tumors allow the more specific evaluation of some aspects of language, for example the name by visual confrontation has been a very important way of assessing an aspect of language in the operating room [9] but until recently attention has been paid to the type of stimuli that are presented and how to do it, that is, we currently know that the findings may be different if they are presented for the naming, an image or drawing in black and white compared to a color image with three-dimensional properties, in addition to the control of psycholinguistic variables of the words [13]. The same can be mentioned in other cognitive domains, for example the advance in the knowledge of the participation of subcortical structures in cognition, the participation of the right hemisphere in language at the narrative level, social cognition, brain reorganization in the recovery process, participation of the insula in cognitive aspects, to name a few [41].

Vignette 3 - Brain Hodotopy

This term refers to a current vision in functional neurosurgery in which the classic trend of localize functions in the cerebral cortex is changed by a concept called hodological mechanism (from the Greek hodos, path or path) related to the cognitive alteration caused by affection in anatomical connectivity rather than a lesion in the cerebral cortex.

This approach conceives the Central Nervous System as a comprehensive system integrated by a plastic network made up of functional cortical epicenters connected by short and long fibers of white matter. Thus, brain functions are the result of the confluence of parallel information pathways, dynamically modulated in a widely distributed, interactive and multimodal circuit.

This view is of great relevance, especially in brain tumor neurosurgery due to the brain plasticity that is induced by the neoplasm itself. This phenomenon makes the dissociation between anatomy and functional delimitation especially valid, that is, to determine anatomically an area (for example the precentral gyrus) does not guarantee that it functionally corresponds to motor regions. This new perspective opens the possibility of contemplating the performance of surgical procedures in regions that were previously considered inoperable. Broca's area is an example of this new vision, since if it is considered inoperable, different brain mapping techniques such as cortical electrical stimulation can currently be used to functionally delimit this region through naming tasks. Broca's area is also a good example to show the brain plasticity that the hodological approach considers, since we frequently observe neoplasms in these regions with a patient without deficit (dynamic, not rigid system), and it is well known that in order to presents an alteration compatible with Broca's aphasia, the lesion must include cortical and subcortical regions (cortical epicenters and connectome), since a lesion limited only to the cerebral cortex corresponding to Brodmann's area 44 and 45 is associated with a transitory alteration less severe.

Transoperatively evaluating a cognitive domain with all the theoretical complexity that we currently have can take a long time, bringing an apparent contradiction, since on the one hand we require time to assess details of the domains, however, during surgical procedures with the patient awake, only they have several seconds and in some cases minutes. This leads to apparently unrelated cognitive areas that will be evident in the postoperative period. To exemplify this, we can take the case of the famous patient HM, one of the best known cases in the history of modern neurosciences who was operated awake during the bilateral resection of hippocampal structures in 1953. At that time, it was only considered important to explore the understanding and expression of language, without considering the exploration of other cognitive domains, resulting in the tragic history of memory loss that we all know. Without devaluing the merit of surgery in the context of the time, this story teaches us that it is essential to carry out a broader neuropsychological evaluation in terms of cognitive domains, apparently little related to the intervened brain region, so that the consideration of the activities to perform during the intraoperative is essential in order to optimize the time and tasks to be performed.

Among the most important neuropsychological criteria is that the patient wishes to cooperate and his neurological and psychological condition allows it, that is, the patient must understand why the suggestion of this surgery modality so that he openly expresses that he wants awake modality, knowing that it can be stressful to a certain extent and that your participation is essential. A second important criterion is not to present alterations that may obstruct the intraoperative neuropsychological evaluation. In this sense, the patient could find conditions that allow him to have a functional daily life, however, it may be that for the surgical procedure it is not suitable, for example a tumor in prefrontal regions that could affect uninhibited behavior. This could be dangerous because the integrity of the patient could be compromised by refusing to participate during surgery. Another example could be the difficulty in understanding long sentences or marked slowness when carrying out the instructions. These examples show that, even though the patient understands the importance of the procedure and shows the willingness to cooperate, it should be considered, since in the last example it could be determined that it would be enough to be able to carry out the monitoring of gross motor aspects, so it could be done.

An important aspect is to know, through anxiety, depression and impulsivity scales, the degree that the patient can manifest in the face of stress, since the procedure can facilitate the appearance of behaviors that could hardly be observed in daily life.

In our experience, awake surgery involves a series of stages prior to the intraoperative that the patient must undergo to guarantee a greater chance of success. That is, if it is true that success depends largely on what happens in the operating room, it is also true that a lot has to do with the preparation of the patient, the collection of neuropsychological and psychological data, and in some cases the family dynamics before the surgery, as it must be remembered that patient participation is essential, so that an inadequate preparation (eg, lack of understanding of the purpose of the procedure) could turn into limited cooperation and vulnerable to fatigue due to the small discomforts that could present.

In the same way, follow-up is important to guide the family and the patient about neuropsychological or personality changes that may occur, some of them may require neuropsychological intervention or orientation to primary caregivers.

The entire conventional neuropsychological clinical interview is conducted paying attention to traits or probable personality disorders, how to manage stress in the daily life and impulse management. It should be remembered that surgery can represent a time of stress in which the patient can behave differently from the way they do it in their daily life (explain with appropriate psychological terms that it can be psychologically unstructured), in addition to the use of medications that they could contribute for that moment. (If you are in stress, you can request to be put to sleep or decide not to cooperate, making the procedure considerably more difficult).

A conventional neuropsychological evaluation is performed. In brain tumors, large batteries are used in terms of functions, e.g. The Comprehensive Neuropsychological Exploration Program Test Barcelona completes and complementary tests.

One of the purposes is to detect qualitatively and quantitatively. All this to detect obvious or subtle alterations that the neoplasm is already causing and think about the possibility that these alterations are highlighted.

Psychological approach in which the patient's real expectations and fantasies must be detected. Anxiety and depression must be identified. Follow-up is encouraged for the next stages, gives an overview of what might happen if the tumor is malignant or non-malignant. This stage is mixed with the Psychological intervention and the intervention plan must begin here.

Other aspects that influence this stage are:

the carving explanation of the procedure, beginning, end, when waking up, when sleeping, when to sedate it, activities to perform, activities to perform, possible discomfort, procedure simulation, stereotactic frame simulation. As far as possible, visit the operating room from the outside, explanation of a video of a patient with a similar tumor.

1.6.1 Family involvement

This gives you a lot of neuropsychological material to ask questions during surgery, e.g. If so, a description of the coffee harvest can already be requested (since he is involved in the process in his place of origin). This constitutes a great deal of material to use in assessing spontaneous language.

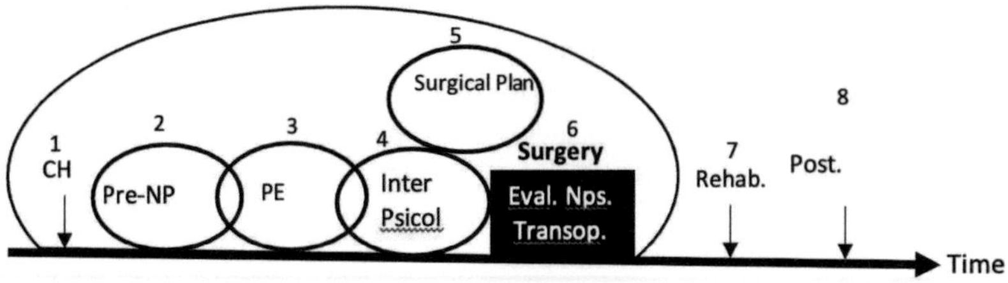

Figure 7.
General diagram (timeline) of the transdisciplinary treatment and location of the intraoperative neuropsychological evaluation. The steps prior to the neuropsychological assessment represented by interconnected circles represent the independence of each step, but the close relationship between them. CH: Clinical History, Pre-NP: Preoperative Neuropsychological Evaluation, PE: Psychoeducation, Inter Psicol - Psychological Intervention, Post: Postoperative neuropsychological follow-up, Rehab: Neuropsychological rehabilitation.

Activities are designed according to the neuropsychological profile and the surgical plan. This stage can be better understood in the section on the intraoperative neuropsychological evaluation plan.

Ecological evaluation plan, what the patient requires for her daily life.

Neuropsychological rehabilitation and orientation to the family on apparently permanent and transitory alterations, including personality changes.

Follow-up at 6 months and 1 year. **Figure** 7.

2. Conclusions

The most important objective of this surgical modality is the cognitive preservation and neurological function of the patient and at the same time achieving the greatest amount of tumor resection, that is, the removal of the greatest amount of brain tumor with the least amount of sequelae. This is especially valid for those patients who have a low-grade tumor with an adequate prognosis for life, recently also for those with a tumor with a higher grade of malignancy that will limit survival to several months. In both cases, the amount of pathological tissue that can be removed is of vital importance since the success of the rest of the complementary postsurgical treatments such as radio or chemotherapy depends largely on this.

The most serious intra-surgical complications include seizures, respiratory depression, air embolism, cerebral edema, and the cardiac trigeminal reflex. The total reported complication rate is about 16.5%, and in 6.4% of patients it is not possible to complete the mapping procedure.

The main causes of failure are the appearance of seizures and the loss of cooperation of the patient due to severe drowsiness, agitation, or the development of mixed dysphasia. Failed craniotomies are associated with a lower incidence of gross total resections, greater speech impairment after the procedure, and a longer hospital stay.

The application of awake craniotomy has continually evolved. The key to the success of this procedure is to pay attention to each of the components, such as careful patient selection, prior psychological preparation, building a solid relationship, ensuring the solid position of the patient, optimal regional anesthesia, the correct selection of agents and anesthetic technique, preparation and timely management of crises, and constant communication between group members.

Author details

José Luis Navarro-Olvera[1]*, Gustavo Parra-Romero[1],
Stephani Dalila Heres-Becerril[3], David Trejo-Martínez[2], José D. Carrillo Ruiz[1],
Kleber Gonzalez Echeverría[1] and Gustavo Aguado-Carrillo[1]

1 Functional Neurosurgery, Stereotactic and Radiosurgery Department, Mexico General Hospital "Dr. Eduardo Liceaga", Mexico

2 Neuropsychology Department, Mexico General Hospital "Dr. Eduardo Liceaga", Mexico

3 Neuroanesthesiology Department, Mexico General Hospital "Dr. Eduardo Liceaga", Mexico

*Address all correspondence to: luiginavarro97@hotmail.com

References

[1] Ibrahim GM, Bernstein M. Awake craniotomy for supratentorial gliomas: why, when and how? CNS Oncol 2012;1:71-83. https://doi.org/10.2217/cns.12.1.

[2] Sacko O, Lauwers-Cances V, Brauge D, Sesay M, Brenner A, Roux FE. Awake craniotomy vs surgery under general anesthesia for resection of supratentorial lesions. Neurosurgery 2011;68:1192-8. https://doi.org/10.1227/NEU.0b013e31820c02a3.

[3] Lu VM, Phan K, Rovin RA. Comparison of operative outcomes of eloquent glioma resection performed under awake versus general anesthesia: A systematic review and meta-analysis. Clin Neurol Neurosurg 2018;169:121-7. https://doi.org/10.1016/j.clineuro.2018.04.011.

[4] Bulsara KR, Johnson J, Villavicencio AT. Improvements in brain tumor surgery: the modern history of awake craniotomies. Neurosurg Focus 2005;18:5-7. https://doi.org/10.3171/foc.2005.18.4.6.

[5] Kobyakov GL, Lubnin AY, Kulikov AS, Gavrilov AG, Goryaynov SA, Poddubskiy AA, et al. Awake craniotomy. Zh Vopr Neirokhir Im N N Burdenko 2016;80:107-16. https://doi.org/10.17116/engneiro201680188-96.

[6] July J, Manninen P, Lai J, Yao Z, Bernstein M. The history of awake craniotomy for brain tumor and its spread into Asia. Surg Neurol 2009;71:621-4. https://doi.org/10.1016/j.surneu.2007.12.022.

[7] Surbeck W, Hildebrandt G, Duffau H. The evolution of brain surgery on awake patients. Acta Neurochir (Wien) 2015;157:77-84. https://doi.org/10.1007/s00701-014-2249-8.

[8] De Witt Hamer PC, Robles SG, Zwinderman AH, Duffau H, Berger MS. Impact of intraoperative stimulation brain mapping on glioma surgery outcome: A meta-analysis. J Clin Oncol 2012;30:2559-65. https://doi.org/10.1200/JCO.2011.38.4818.

[9] Haglund M, Berger MS, Shamseldin M, Lettich E, Ojemann G. Cortical Localization of Temporal Lobe Language Sites in Patients with Gliomas. Clinical Study. Neurosurgery 1994;34:1689-99.

[10] Duffau H. Contribution of cortical and subcortical electrostimulation in brain glioma surgery: Methodological and functional considerations. Neurophysiol Clin 2007;37:373-82. https://doi.org/10.1016/j.neucli.2007.09.003.

[11] Duffau H. Stimulation Mapping of Myelinated Tracts in Awake Patients. Brain Plast 2016;2:99-113. https://doi.org/10.3233/bpl-160027.

[12] Buckingham HW. The Marc Dax (1770-1837)/Paul Broca (1824-1880) controversy over priority in science: Left hemisphere specificity for seat of articulate language and for lesions that cause aphemia. Clin Linguist Phonetics 2006;20:613-9. https://doi.org/10.1080/02699200500266703.

[13] Tate MC, Herbet G, Moritz-Gasser S, Tate JE, Duffau H. Probabilistic map of critical functional regions of the human cerebral cortex: Broca's area revisited. Brain 2014;137:2773-82. https://doi.org/10.1093/brain/awu168.

[14] Iwata M. Anatomical Error of Pierre Marie's "zone Lenticulaire." Front Neurol Neurosci 2019;44:23-9. https://doi.org/10.1159/000494948.

[15] Rahimpour S, Haglund MM, Friedman AH, Duffau H. History

of awake mapping and speech and language localization: From modules to networks. Neurosurg Focus 2019;47:7-12. https://doi.org/10.3171/2019.7.FOCUS19347.

[16] Nasios G, Dardiotis E, Messinis L. From Broca and Wernicke to the Neuromodulation Era: Insights of Brain Language Networks for Neurorehabilitation. Behav Neurol 2019:1-10. https://doi.org/10.1155/2019/9894571.

[17] Damasio AR. Brain and language: what a difference a decade makes. Curr Opin Neurol 1997;10:177-8.

[18] Damasio H, Grabowski TJ, Tranel D, Ponto LLB, Hichwa RD, Damasio AR. Neural correlates of naming actions and of naming spatial relations. Neuroimage 2001;13:1053-64. https://doi.org/10.1006/nimg.2001.0775.

[19] De Benedictis A, Duffau H. Brain hodotopy: From esoteric concept to practical surgical applications. Neurosurgery 2011;68:1709-23. https://doi.org/10.1227/NEU.0b013e3182124690.

[20] Duffau H. Hodotopy, neuroplasticity and diffuse gliomas. Neurochirurgie 2017;63:259-65. https://doi.org/10.1016/j.neuchi.2016.12.001.

[21] Ius T, Angelini E, Thiebaut de Schotten M, Mandonnet E, Duffau H. Evidence for potentials and limitations of brain plasticity using an atlas of functional resectability of WHO grade II gliomas: Towards a "minimal common brain." Neuroimage 2011;56:992-1000. https://doi.org/10.1016/j.neuroimage.2011.03.022.

[22] Coello AF, Moritz-Gasser S, Martino J, Martinoni M, Matsuda R, Duffau H. Selection of intraoperative tasks for awake mapping based on relationships between tumor location and functional networks: A review. J Neurosurg 2013;119:1380-94. https://doi.org/10.3171/2013.6.JNS122470.

[23] Duffau H. New concepts in surgery of WHO grade II gliomas: Functional brain mapping, connectionism and plasticity - A review. J Neurooncol 2006;79:77-115. https://doi.org/10.1007/s11060-005-9109-6.

[24] Duffau H. Stimulation mapping of white matter tracts to study brain functional connectivity. Nat Rev Neurol 2015;11:255-65. https://doi.org/10.1038/nrneurol.2015.51.

[25] Vanacôr CN, Isolan GR, Yu YH, Telles JPM, Oberman DZ, Rabelo NN, et al. Microsurgical anatomy of language. Clin Anat 2020:1-15. https://doi.org/10.1002/ca.23681.

[26] Duffau H, Capelle L, Lopes M, Faillot T, Sichez JP, Fohanno D. The insular lobe: Physiopathological and surgical considerations. Neurosurgery 2000;47:801-11. https://doi.org/10.1097/00006123-200010000-00001.

[27] Dziedzic T, Bernstein M. Awake craniotomy for brain tumor: Indications, technique and benefits. Expert Rev Neurother 2014;14:1405-15. https://doi.org/10.1586/14737175.2014.979793.

[28] Brown T, Shah AH, Bregy A, Shah NH, Thambuswamy M, Barbarite E, et al. Awake Craniotomy for Brain Tumor Resection. J Neurosurg Anesthesiol 2013;25:240-7. https://doi.org/10.1097/ana.0b013e318290c230.

[29] Hervey-Jumper SL, Li J, Lau D, Molinaro AM, Perry DW, Meng L, et al. Awake craniotomy to maximize glioma resection: Methods and technical nuances over a 27-year period. J Neurosurg 2015;123:325-39. https://doi.org/10.3171/2014.10.JNS141520.

[30] Chua TH, See AAQ, Ang BT, King NKK. Awake Craniotomy for

Resection of Brain Metastases: A Systematic Review. World Neurosurg 2018;120:e1128-35. https://doi.org/10.1016/j.wneu.2018.08.243.

[31] Duffau H. Diffuse low-grade glioma, oncological outcome and quality of life: A surgical perspective. Curr Opin Oncol 2018;30:383-9. https://doi.org/10.1097/CCO.0000000000000483.

[32] Duffau H. Higher-Order Surgical Questions for Diffuse Low-Grade Gliomas: Supramaximal Resection, Neuroplasticity, and Screening. Neurosurg Clin N Am 2019;30:119-28. https://doi.org/10.1016/j.nec.2018.08.009.

[33] Akay A, Islekel S. Awake craniotomy procedure: Its effects on neurological morbidity and recommendations. Turk Neurosurg 2018;28:186-92. https://doi.org/10.5137/1019-5149.JTN.19391-16.1.

[34] Kulikov A, Lubnin A. Anesthesia for awake craniotomy. Curr Opin Anaesthesiol 2018;31:506-10. https://doi.org/10.1097/ACO.0000000000000625.

[35] Eseonu CI, ReFaey K, Garcia O, John A, Quiñones-Hinojosa A, Tripathi P. Awake Craniotomy Anesthesia: A Comparison of the Monitored Anesthesia Care and Asleep-Awake-Asleep Techniques. World Neurosurg 2017;104:679-86. https://doi.org/10.1016/j.wneu.2017.05.053.

[36] Osborn I, Sebeo J. "Scalp block" during craniotomy: A classic technique revisited. J Neurosurg Anesthesiol 2010;22:187-94. https://doi.org/10.1097/ANA.0b013e3181d48846.

[37] Özlü O. Anaesthesiologist's approach to awake craniotomy. Turk Anesteziyoloji ve Reanimasyon Dern Derg 2018;46:250-6. https://doi.org/10.5152/TJAR.2018.56255.

[38] Stevanovic A, Rossaint R, Veldeman M, Bilotta F, Coburn M. Anaesthesia management for awake craniotomy: Systematic review and meta-analysis. PLoS One 2016;11:12-23. https://doi.org/10.1371/journal.pone.0156448.

[39] Jones H, Smith M. Awake craniotomy. Contin Educ Anaesthesia, Crit Care Pain 2004;4:189-92. https://doi.org/10.1093/bjaceaccp/mkh051.

[40] Hill CS, Severgnini F, McKintosh E. How I do it: Awake craniotomy. Acta Neurochir (Wien) 2017;159:173-6. https://doi.org/10.1007/s00701-016-3021-z.

[41] Duffau H. The error of Broca: From the traditional localizationist concept to a connectomal anatomy of human brain. J Chem Neuroanat 2018;89:73-81. https://doi.org/10.1016/j.jchemneu.2017.04.003.

Chapter 6

Topographic Distribution of Intracranial Meningioma's Recurrences: Localized Versus Diffuse-Multicentric

Francesco Maiuri, Sergio Corvino, Elia Guadagno and Marialaura Del Basso De Caro

Abstract

Meningiomas recur with a rate of 10–32% at ten years. Several features influence the risk of recurrence. Our aim is to define the pathological and surgical features at risk of diffuse-multicentric versus local-peripheral recurrence. Thirty-three cases of multicentric-diffuse recurrence of intracranial meningiomas were retrospectively analyzed and compared with 50 cases who experienced local-peripheral recurrence. The analyzed factors included age and sex, tumor location and shape, brain-tumor interface, entity of resection, WHO grade, Ki67 MIB1, progesterone receptor (PR) expression, number of reoperations, progression of WHO grade, and outcome. The multicentric-diffuse recurrences were mainly related to flat-shaped and Ki67 Li greater than 4% features at first surgery. Among patients with multicentric-diffuse recurrences, 25 underwent one to three reoperations; among them, 17 are alive with local tumor control or slow progression 2 to 25 years after the initial surgery versus only 2 out of 8 who did not undergo surgery. We conclude that flat-shaped meningiomas and those with Ki67 Li greater than 4% are at higher risk to recur in multicentric-diffuse pattern. Even multiple reoperations over a period of several years may obtain rather long survivals in selected patients with prevalent intradural not anaplastic tumors and not too extensive dural infiltration.

Keywords: meningioma recurrence, diffuse recurrence, proliferation index, meningioma shape

1. Introduction

The recurrence's rate of intracranial meningiomas ranges from 10–32% at 10 years [1–3] .The main risk factors include the WHO grade [4–7], the extent of resection according to Simpson [8–10], the proliferation index Ki67-MIB1 [11–14] and mitotic index [15] and the postoperative adjuvant treatments [1, 16, 17]. Other factors have also been suggested, such as patient age and sex [4, 18], tumor size [19–21], location [22, 23] and morphology [19, 22, 24], brain invasion [10, 14], progesterone receptor (PR) expression [25–27].

Meningiomas may recur with different patterns of growth, from more localized to more extensive and sometimes diffuse forms. This carries several diagnostic and therapeutic implications. However, all published studies consider the overall recurrences, with no focusing on their topography and extension, which were first discussed only in our recent report [28].

2. Classification of the recurrences

According to their topography on the post-contrast magnetic resonance imaging (MRI) and surgical findings, the recurrences of meningiomas may be classified in 4 types [28]:

- type 1, local, at the previous dural site;
- type 2, peripheral, at the surrounding dura, contiguous to the previous site;
- type 3, multicentric, with multiple nodules both at the dural site and distant, with seemly normal interposed dura mater;
- type 4, diffuse, with multiple nodules with interposed dural infiltration, or diffuse dural and extradural infiltration.

Local type 1 is the most frequent regrowth pattern. It may occur after resection of Simpson grades 2 to 4; the tumor may growth both intradurally and at the bone. The recurrence may involve from a variable portion to the whole initial dural attachment and may extend to the contiguous previously normal dura.

Peripheral type 2 recurrences may be observed after initial resection of grade 1, but also of grade II when the dural attachment was carefully and extensively coagulated. The recurrence may involve a variable dural portion contiguous to the initial attachment and may often extend to it. In cases with larger recurrences the site of regrowth (local versus peripheral) is difficult to be defined.

Multicentric type 3 recurrences are characterized by tumor nodules or mass both at initial dural attachment or contiguous dura and in distal dural regions where no tumor nodules nor dural enhancement were visible on the magnetic resonance imaging at initial surgery. In this type the dura mater between local-peripheral and distal recurrent nodules seems to be normal.

Diffuse type 4 recurrences show multiple nodules of tumor regrowth even in very distal regions, with variable infiltration of the interposed dura and bone.

The above discussed patterns of recurrence suggest that multicentric and diffuse recurrences are two phases of the same pathological conditions.

3. Pathological origin of the multicentric-diffuse recurrences

The pathological mechanisms responsible for meningioma recurrence in distal dural regions are not well defined and deserve to be discussed.

The concept of regional multicentricity of meningiomas is known since about 35 years. Borovich and Doron [29] demonstrated in convexity meningiomas small tumor nodules as well as intradural clusters of tumor cells in the dural specimens taken up to 3 cm from the tumor. Qi et al. [30] found tumor invasion in 88% of dura adjacent to convexity meningioma up to 2,5 cm from the tumor origin. These observations may explain some "unexpected relapses" after an apparent complete resection (Simpson grade 1) of convexity meningiomas [29] and the frequent peripheral recurrences at the dura surrounding the initial attachment after resection od Simpson grades 1 and 2 in all locations.

These pathological findings support the concept of a wide dural excision 2-3 cm beyond the tumor base (grade zero resection), which was suggested for convexity [31] and falx meningiomas [32].

Mooney et al. [32] suggest that in the falcine meningiomas the tumor cells may spread from the site of origin to other falx regions between the two dural leaflets of the falx. However, this pattern of diffusion of the tumor cells cannot explain the very distant recurrences from other locations. For multiple meningiomas some studies [33, 34] have suggested that they may arise from a single progenitor cell and could then spread through the subarachnoid space. A similar mechanism may also be advocated for distant recurrences.

However, it is more like that multicentric-diffuse recurrences represent the progressive growth of multiple distant dural nodules with different growth potential. In this way the meningioma may be considered, at least in several cases, a diffuse disease of the meninges than a localized tumor.

4. Data of the personal series

Thirty-three patients with multicentric-diffuse recurrences of meningiomas are included in our series [28] (**Tables 1-3** and **Figures 1-3**). They are 22 females (67%) and 11 males (33%), with a median age of 52 years. The findings at initial surgery were as follows (**Table 1**). The most frequent location was non skull-base (55%), followed by lateral (36%) and medial skull-base (9%). The tumor was mostly flat-shaped (76%) and less frequently round (24%). Complete resection (Simpson grades 1 and 2) at initial surgery was obtained in 23 among 33 patients (70%).

The pathological findings at initial diagnosis (**Table 1**) showed 52% of WHO [35] grade I and 48% of grade II tumors; the Ki67-Li was <4% in 20% and ≥ 4%in 80%. The PR expression was ≤50% in 82% of specimens and > 50% in 9%.

When compared to the findings of meningiomas which showed localized-peripheral recurrences, only the higher rates of flat-shaped tumors ($p = 0.0008$) and tumors with Ki67-Li ≥4% ($p = 0.037$) were significant [28].

The management and outcome of the recurrences were as follows (**Table 2**). Twenty-five out of 33 patients (76%) were reoperated on and underwent one (48%) or two or three reoperations (52%) (**Figures 1** and **2**). The complete resection (Simpson grades I and II) was possible only in 5 among the 25 patients (20%). The histological WHO grade at first reoperation was similar to that of the initial surgery in 15 out of 25 patients (60%); progression to a higher grade was observed in 10 cases (40%).

Adjuvant treatments included external radiotherapy in 20 patients, stereotactic radiosurgery in 9 and chemotherapy in 5.

When compared to patients with localized-peripheral recurrences, those with multicentric-diffuse recurrences showed significantly higher number of reoperations ($p = 0.0034$), lower rate of gross total resection ($p = 0.00001$) and higher but not significant rate of cases with progression of the WHO grade ($p = 0.09$) [28].

The actual follow-up ranges from 2 to 25 years. One patient died postoperatively for respiratory failure. Among the other 24 patients operated on, eleven (34%) are alive with local tumor control versus none out of eight patients who did not undergo surgery ($p = 0.029$). Six (25%) show slow tumor progression with no symptoms in spite the surgery. Seven patients of the surgical group (29%) died during the follow-up (5 for tumor progression) versus 6 (for tumor progression) out of 8 (75%) of the non-surgical group ($p = 0.038$). Thus, among 25 patients reoperated on 17 (68%) are alive after one or more reoperations versus only 2 out of 8 (25%) who did not undergo surgery.

Covariates	Number of cases (rate)
Age (mean)	52 y
Sex	F 22 (67%) M 11 (33%)
Tumor location	
medial skull base	3 (9%)
lateral skull base	12 (36%)
non skull base	18 (55%)
Tumor shape	
flat	25 (76%)
round	8 (24%)
Brain-tumor interface	
preserved	15 (45%)
unclear- lost	18 (55%)
Extent of resection (Simpson grade)	
I	9 (28%)
II	14 (42%)
III	10 (30%)
Interval between initial surgery and recurrence (median)	4.7 y
WHO grade	
I	17 (52%)
II	16 (48%)
Ki67 Li	
< 4%	7 (20%)
≥ 4%	26 (80%)
P.R. expression	
≤ 15%	11 (33%)
16–50% 51–79%	16 (49%) 3 (9%)
≥ 80%	3 (9%)

Table 1.
Clinico-radiological, surgical and pathological findings at initial diagnosis (33 patients).

Covariates	Number of cases (rate)
• Surgery	25(76%)
• Number of surgeries	
One reoperation	12 (48%)
Two or three reoperations	13 (52%)
• Extent of resection	
Gross total	5 (20%)
Subtotal	20 (80%)
• WHO grade at the first reoperation	
Similar to the first surgery	15 (60%)
Progression from I to II	7 (28%)

Covariates	Number of cases (rate)
• Progression from II to III	3 (12%)
• Postoperative death	1 (4%)
• External radiotherapy	20 (60%)
• Stereotactic radiosurgery	9 (27%)
• Chemotherapy	5 (15%)

Table 2.
Management of 33 patients with multicentric-diffuse recurrences.

Covariates	Group 1-Surgery (24 pts)	Group 2-No-surgery (8 pts)	Statistical significance (Group 1 Vs Group 2)
Local control	11 (46%)	—	p = 0.029
Tumor progression	6 (25%)	2 (25%)	n.s.
Death during the follow-up	7 (29%)	6 (75%)	p = 0.038

Table 3.
Outcome of 33 patients with multicentric-diffuse meningioma recurrence.

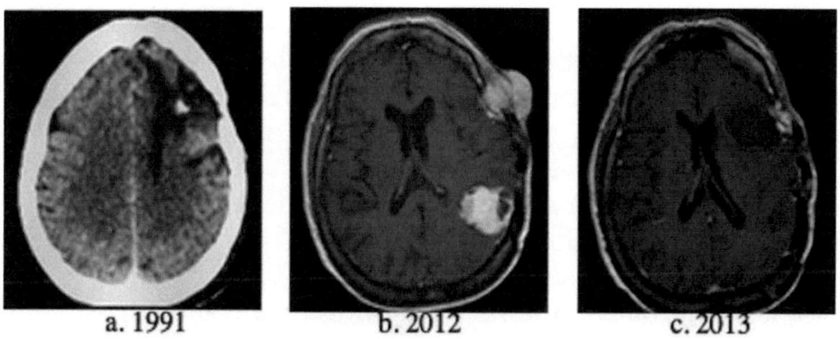

Figure 1.
58 years old woman with history of previous resection of a WHO I grade meningioma of the left frontal convexity in 1991. (a) Postoperative CT after the initial surgery: no residual tumor; (b) Post-contrast MRI 21 years later: local multicentric recurrence at the previous dural site and distal recurrence at the left parietal region; (c) Postoperative MRI showing resection of both nodules (WHO grade I) and interposed dura.

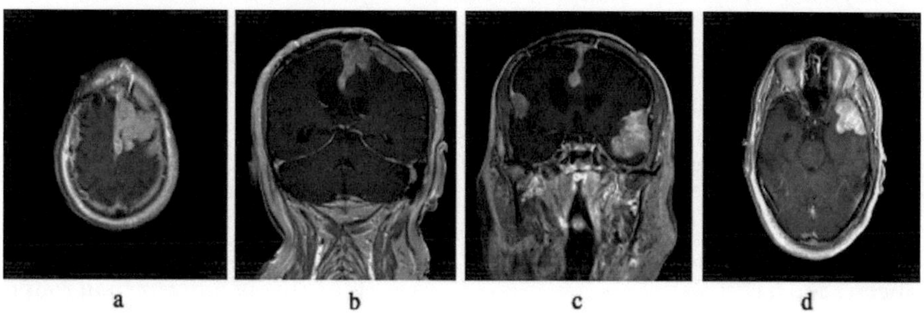

Figure 2.
68 years old man who underwent resection of an anterior parasagittal WHO grade II meningioma in 2010. (a-d) Post-contrast MRI, T1 axial (a, d) and coronal (b, c) sequences: diffuse recurrences of the parasagittal and both convexity regions with significant tumor masses, at the left parasagittal and convexity and at the anterior temporal convexity. Two-stage resection of the masses and irradiation.

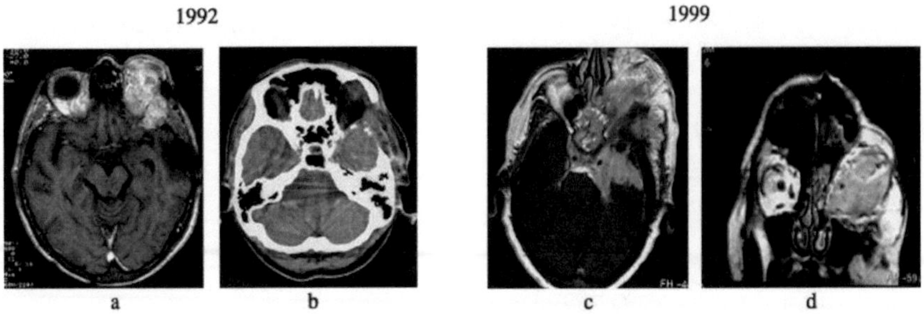

Figure 3.
(a-b) 72 years old man with history of a left spheno-orbital WHO grade II meningioma: a) preoperative T1 axial post-contrast MRI and (b) postoperative CT scan: complete resection. (c-d) Post-contrast T1 axial (c) and coronal (d) MRI sequences seven years after the initial surgery: large tumor recurrence involving the left orbital cavity and extending diffusely in the intracranial compartment at the suprasellar, left parasellar region and temporal fossa. Management by external radiotherapy.

5. Risk factors at initial diagnosis

Several pathological, neuroradiological and surgical findings at initial diagnosis are correlated to the meningioma recurrence. However, which factors may be considered at risk of multicentric-diffuse recurrence are not defined.

5.1 Location

The meningioma location is a significant risk factor of recurrence. Medial skull-base meningiomas include locations, such as olfactory groove, tuberculum sellae, anterior clinoid, foramen magnum, with low recurrence rates (0–15%) [36–38]. Besides, the low recurrence rate of spinal meningiomas is well known (0–10% in 15 among 19 reviewed series in our recent study [39]). On the other hand, the reported recurrence rates are higher for lateral skull-base (35–40% for lateral sphenoid wing and mainly spheno-orbital [38–40]) and for non-skull base meningiomas (16 to 24% for parasagittal and falcine) [23, 41].

However, when the rates of multicentric-diffuse recurrences are considered, the differences for intracranial tumor locations are not relevant. Although in our study [28] spheno-orbital and parasagittal meningiomas show higher rates of multicentric and diffuse recurrences, this finding does not reach significance. Our series does not include diffuse recurrences of spinal meningiomas; this agrees with the well known better biological behavior of this location.

Thus, the meningioma location is correlated with the rate but not with the growth pattern of the recurrences.

5.2 Shape

The shape of meningiomas may be variable. According to the rate height/base on magnetic resonance imaging, the meningiomas may be classified as round (rate > 1) and flat-shaped (rate ≤ 1). Flat-shaped meningiomas are characterized by prevalent and often extensive dural involvement as compared to round-shaped ones. Thus, it has been shown that flat-shaped meningiomas are more likely to recur than round ones [22, 24].

The flat-shaped morphology at initial diagnosis was the only radiological finding at significantly higher risk of multicentric diffuse recurrence as compared to local-peripheral recurrence in our study ($p = 0.0008$) [28]. Thus, it is like that flat-shaped meningiomas are associated to various degree of even distant microscopic dural infiltration.

5.3 Dural tail

The change of the peritumoral dura mater depicted on the postcontrast magnetic resonance studies and defined as "dural tail" is known since its description in 1989 [42]. It may correspond to various histopathological patterns, including increased loose connective tissue, angiogenesis, dilated vessels, reactive hyperplasia, tumor invasion [42, 43]. Qi et al. [30], in a large series of convexity meningiomas, described several types of dural tail with different histological aspects: smooth (uniformly extended) with tumor extension up to 1,5 cm; nodular, with nodular hyperplasia corresponding to tumor nodules and tumor extension to the distal dura up to 2,5 cm; mixed, with nodular enhancement proximal to the dural attachment and distal smooth enhancement. In spite of the presence of tumor cells nodules, the finding of dural tail was found to be not correlated to the meningioma recurrence in most studies [9, 19, 22]. We did not investigate this finding in our series of multicentric-diffuse recurrences; however, we suggest that further studies will define this aspect.

5.4 Brain-tumor interface

The brain-tumor interface, more often well preserved during meningioma surgery, may be unclear or lost, often with variable pial invasion, as in WHO grade II tumors. In such cases the tumor resection may be incomplete, with residual nodules mainly in critical regions. This may increase the risk of recurrence at the initial site or at the surrounding region [10, 14, 22]. On the other hand, the presence of the residual cell nests at the brain-tumor interface does not explain the recurrences in distal dural regions and the diffuse regrowths.

5.5 Extent of surgical resection

The entity of the resection at initial surgery is mostly considered a major risk factor for recurrence [23, 44, 45]. However, the clinical usefulness of the Simpson grading in general has been questioned, at least for benign meningiomas. Some studies found no statistically significant differences in progression-free survival between Simpson grades 1 to 4 [46] and 1 to 3 [13, 47] resections for WHO I grade meningiomas. This discrepancy may reflect the technical surgical improvement and the smaller tumor remnants in incomplete resections. In a recent report Haddad et al. [48]. found that patients with WHO grade I meningiomas and Ki67-MIB1 > 4,5% treated by gross total resection had similar risk of recurrence as those patients with subtotal resection. In this study, early recurrences were more significantly impacted by extent of resection, whereas the Ki67-MIB1 was more significant for later recurrences.

In our study on multicentric-diffuse recurrences [28], their rate is not impacted by the extent of resection at initial surgery.

5.6 Multiple meningiomas

Multiple meningiomas account for 2 to 8% of all meningiomas [49]. They may be diagnosed either initially or during the neuroradiological follow-up.

In a large metanalysis of the literature on multiple meningiomas, Pereira et al. [49] found recurrence rate of 8.07% and no higher with respect to single ones. On the other hand, in the study by Gousias et al. [45] multiple meningiomas showed higher recurrence rate and significantly lower progression-free survival than single ones.

Multiple meningiomas likely develop from multicentric dural tumor foci according to the Borovich [29] theory. A similar mechanism is suggested for multicentric recurrences. In our study on multicentric-diffuse recurrences two patients had multiple meningiomas (two lesions) at initial diagnosis, with no significant differences with local-peripheral ones. We think that further studies on the long-term follow-up of patients operated on for multiple meningiomas will defined the recurrence rates and patterns of these cases.

5.7 Pathological findings

In our study [28] meningiomas with values of Ki67 Li ≥ 4% are related to major risk of multicentric-diffuse recurrence, while the WHO grade (I versus II) is not significant. Several reports [7, 25–27] confirmed the relationship between higher Ki67-Li values and lower PR expression, and higher recurrence risk for intracranial meningiomas. However, in this study the PR expression is not correlated with the pattern of diffuse regrowth. Both these findings have not previously been reported.

The higher initial values of Ki67 Li of meningiomas recurring as diffuse forms suggest that even small dural tumor foci, even distant from the primary tumor site, may diffusely regrow.

Several studies have found that different genetic profiles and chromosomal abnormalities correspond to different meningioma subtypes with different aggressiveness and recurrence's rate [50–54], making speculate the existence of characteristic biomolecular profiles for meningiomas which recur in multicentric-diffuse pattern.

6. Management

The management of multicentric-diffuse recurrences of intracranial meningiomas is often difficult to be defined; there are not studies defining the guidelines. The management options include a second surgery, external radiotherapy, stereotactic radiosurgery, medical therapy.

The decision is based on several factors, including tumor location (non-skull base versus skull base; critical versus not critical), significant intradural mass versus prevalent dural infiltration (**Figures 4** and **5**), entity of bone extension, time to recurrence, WHO grade of the initial tumor, patient age and KPS, neurological symptoms and signs.

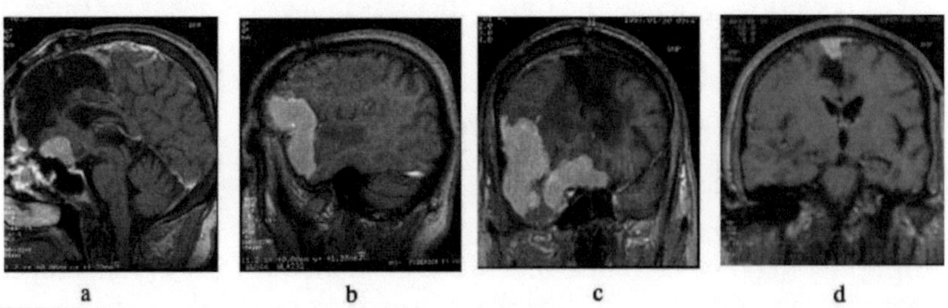

Figure 4.
Post-contrast MRI of a 58 years old man with history of previous surgery (5 years before) of gross-total resection of a bilateral meningioma of the anterior third of the falx (WHO grade II). Sagittal (a-b) and coronal (c-d) T1 sequences: distant and diffuse recurrence at the right fronto-temporal bone and suprasellar regions, with no recurrence at the initial tumor site. Reoperation and resection of the recurrent tumor (WHO grade II). Postoperative death for respiratory failure.

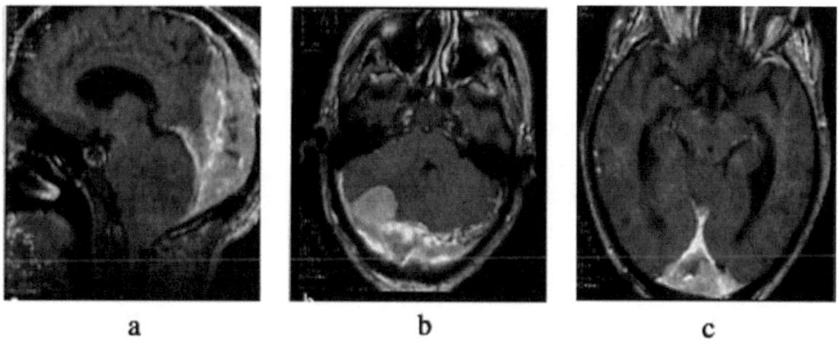

Figure 5.
Post-contrast MRI of a 70 years old woman with history of previous (7 year before) surgical resection (Simpson 3) of a WHO grade II meningioma of the posterior parasagittal region: sagittal (a) and coronal (b-c) sequences: diffuse recurrence with extensive dural and superior sagittal sinus involvement and tumor nodules at the posterior fossa. No reoperation was decided.

6.1 Surgery

The indication to reoperation is mainly posed for younger and middle-aged patients with symptomatic recurrences. According to the location and pattern of regrowth, surgery should be reserved to cases with prevalent intradural tumor growth, tumor nodules ≥3 cm and not extensive dural infiltration (**Figures 1**). Non skull-base meningiomas, mainly if limited to the brain convexity, are usually more favorable to surgery, because of the chance of more wide resection of the involved dura mater. For skull-base meningiomas a more wide resection is possible at the anterior cranial fossa and external sphenoid wing; on the other hand, diffuse recurrences at the suprasellar, parasellar and spheno-orbital regions (**Figure 3**), as well as clival and petroclival regions, are difficult to treat, because of the involvement of the cranial nerves and vessels; for such locations a second surgery is only justified for the resection of a large symptomatic intradural mass.

Elderly patients with comorbidities, particularly if with no or trivial neurological symptoms, must be treated conservatively with periodical radiological follow-up.

The WHO grade at initial diagnosis is obviously important. Only WHO grades I and II meningiomas are suitable for reoperation. On the other hand, anaplastic WHO grade III tumors at initial diagnosis must not be reoperated on.

In selected patients according to the above discussed criteria the reoperation results is satisfactory resection of the intradural tumor and involved dura. However, a really complete resection with no residual contrast enhancement on MRI (Simpson grades 1 and 2) is obtained only in some cases (20% in our series versus 76% of local-peripheral recurrences) [28].

Further recurrences may be reoperated on following the same criteria, if they occur after several years and if the tumor does not progress to anaplastic WHO III form.

6.2 Radiotherapy

All studies focusing on the irradiation of recurrent meningiomas include all recurrences; thus guidelines of radiotherapy management of diffuse recurrences are not available.

The external radiotherapy of multicentric-diffuse recurrences of meningiomas is in our opinion mandatory, independently from the entity of resection and the WHO grade, but mainly in subtotally or partially resected WHO grade II recurrences [55, 56].

The stereotactic radiosurgery is scarcely indicated, because of the extensive and diffuse tumor growth. It may sometimes be performed in association to the external radiotherapy to increase the control of smaller nodules and to treat the not infrequent second recurrences outside the radiotherapic field [57]. Besides, re-radiosurgery for recurrent meningiomas is advisable if the previous radiosurgical treatment was unsatisfactory [58].

6.3 Medical therapy

The medical therapy is reserved to recurrent meningiomas which show growth progression after surgery and irradiation and to malignant WHO III forms. Many clinical trials have studied the effects of cytotoxic chemotherapy [59, 60], hormone-directed therapy [61, 62], other targeted therapies [63–65] and molecular therapies [66]. Targeted and molecular therapies defined on the basis of the biomolecular profile of the meningioma may be useful in diffuse-multicentric recurrences showing progression after surgery and radiotherapy.

7. Conclusions

Meningiomas may sometimes recur as multicentric-diffuse forms, with dural infiltration and recurrent tumor mass distal to the initial site. These may result from the progressive growth of multiple tumor nodules with different growth potential.

Flat-shaped radiological aspect and Ki67 Li ≥4% at initial diagnosis are related to higher risk of recurrence in multicentric-diffuse pattern.

Patients with not anaplastic intracranial meningioma with prevalent intradural component and not extensive dural infiltration may undergone multiple surgical operations during years experimenting good postoperative quality of life.

Further studies will investigate whether the different patterns of regrowth and recurrence correspond to different biomolecular and genetic expression of the meningioma. This will aid to predict the tumor behavior and to detect the most appropriate molecular therapies.

Conflict of interest

The authors declare no conflict of interest.

Acronyms and abbreviations

WHO	World Health Organization
MRI	Magnetic Resonance Imaging

Author details

Francesco Maiuri[1]*, Sergio Corvino[1], Elia Guadagno[2] and Marialaura Del Basso De Caro[2]

1 Department of Neurosciences and Reproductive and Odontostomatological Sciences, Neurosurgical Clinic, "Federico" II University School of Medicine, Naples, Italy

2 Department of Advanced Biomorphological Sciences, "Federico II" University School of Medicine, Naples, Italy

*Address all correspondence to: frmaiuri@unina.it

References

[1] Aghi MK, Carter BS, Cosgrove GR, et al. Long-term recurrence rates of atypical meningiomas after gross total resection with or without postoperative adjuvant radiation. *Neurosurgery.* 2009;64(1): 56-60; discussion 60. https://doi.org/10.1227/01.NEU.0000330399.55586.63.

[2] Nakasu S, Fukami T, Jito J, Nozaki K. Recurrence and regrowth of benign meningiomas. *Brain Tumor Pathol.* 2009;26(2): 69-72. https://doi.org/10.1007/s10014-009-0251-2.

[3] van Alkemade H, de Leau M, Dieleman EM, et al. Impaired survival and long-term neurological problems in benign meningioma. *Neuro Oncol.* 2012;14(5): 658-666. https://doi.org/10.1093/neuonc/nos013.

[4] Mahmood A, Qureshi NH, Malik GM. Intracranial meningiomas: analysis of recurrence after surgical treatment. *Acta Neurochir (Wien).* 1994;126(2-4): 53-58.

[5] Matsuno A, Fujimaki T, Sasaki T, et al. Clinical and histopathological analysis of proliferative potentials of recurrent and non-recurrent meningiomas. *Acta Neuropathol.* 1996;91(5): 504-510.

[6] Yamasaki F, Yoshioka H, Hama S, Sugiyama K, Arita K, Kurisu K. Recurrence of meningiomas. *Cancer.* 2000;89(5): 1102-1110.

[7] Maiuri F, De Caro MB, Esposito F, et al. Recurrences of meningiomas: predictive value of pathological features and hormonal and growth factors. *J Neurooncol.* 2007;82(1): 63-68. https://doi.org/10.1007/s11060-005-9078-9.

[8] SIMPSON D. The recurrence of intracranial meningiomas after surgical treatment. *J Neurol Neurosurg Psychiatry.* 1957;20(1): 22-39.

[9] Hwang WL, Marciscano AE, Niemierko A, et al. Imaging and extent of surgical resection predict risk of meningioma recurrence better than WHO histopathological grade. *Neuro Oncol.* 2016;18(6): 863-872. https://doi.org/10.1093/neuonc/nov285.

[10] Champeaux C, Dunn L. World Health Organization Grade II Meningioma: A 10-Year Retrospective Study for Recurrence and Prognostic Factor Assessment. *World Neurosurg.* 2016;89: 180-186. https://doi.org/10.1016/j.wneu.2016.01.055.

[11] Abramovich CM, Prayson RA. MIB-1 labeling indices in benign, aggressive, and malignant meningiomas: a study of 90 tumors. *Hum Pathol.* 1998;29(12): 1420-1427.

[12] Abdelzaher E, El-Gendi SM, Yehya A, Gowil AG. Recurrence of benign meningiomas: predictive value of proliferative index, BCL2, p53, hormonal receptors and HER2 expression. *Br J Neurosurg.* 2011;25(6): 707-713. https://doi.org/10.3109/02688697.2010.522743.

[13] Oya S, Kawai K, Nakatomi H, Saito N. Significance of Simpson grading system in modern meningioma surgery: integration of the grade with MIB-1 labeling index as a key to predict the recurrence of WHO Grade I meningiomas. *J Neurosurg.* 2012;117(1): 121-128. https://doi.org/10.3171/2012.3.JNS111945.

[14] Sun SQ, Kim AH, Cai C, et al. Management of atypical cranial meningiomas, part 1: predictors of recurrence and the role of adjuvant radiation after gross total resection. *Neurosurgery.* 2014;75(4): 347-354; discussion 354-345; quiz 355. https://doi.org/10.1227/NEU.0000000000000461.

[15] Olar A, Wani KM, Sulman EP, et al. Mitotic Index is an Independent Predictor of Recurrence-Free Survival in Meningioma. *Brain Pathol.* 2015;25(3): 266-275. https://doi.org/10.1111/bpa.12174.

[16] Rogers L, Barani I, Chamberlain M, et al. Meningiomas: knowledge base, treatment outcomes, and uncertainties. A RANO review. *J Neurosurg.* 2015;122(1): 4-23. https://doi.org/10.3171/2014.7.JNS131644.

[17] Sun SQ, Hawasli AH, Huang J, Chicoine MR, Kim AH. An evidence-based treatment algorithm for the management of WHO Grade II and III meningiomas. *Neurosurg Focus.* 2015;38(3): E3. https://doi.org/10.3171/2015.1.FOCUS14757.

[18] Perry A, Stafford SL, Scheithauer BW, Suman VJ, Lohse CM. Meningioma grading: an analysis of histologic parameters. *Am J Surg Pathol.* 1997;21(12): 1455-1465.

[19] Ildan F, Erman T, Göçer AI, et al. Predicting the probability of meningioma recurrence in the preoperative and early postoperative period: a multivariate analysis in the midterm follow-up. *Skull Base.* 2007;17(3): 157-171. https://doi.org/10.1055/s-2007-970554.

[20] Domingues PH, Sousa P, Otero Á, et al. Proposal for a new risk stratification classification for meningioma based on patient age, WHO tumor grade, size, localization, and karyotype. *Neuro Oncol.* 2014;16(5): 735-747. https://doi.org/10.1093/neuonc/not325.

[21] Magill ST, Dalle Ore CL, Diaz MA, et al. Surgical outcomes after reoperation for recurrent non-skull base meningiomas. *J Neurosurg.* 2018: 1-9. https://doi.org/10.3171/2018.6.JNS18118.

[22] Nakasu S, Nakasu Y, Nakajima M, Matsuda M, Handa J. Preoperative identification of meningiomas that are highly likely to recur. *J Neurosurg.* 1999;90(3): 455-462. https://doi.org/10.3171/jns.1999.90.3.0455.

[23] McGovern SL, Aldape KD, Munsell MF, Mahajan A, DeMonte F, Woo SY. A comparison of World Health Organization tumor grades at recurrence in patients with non-skull base and skull base meningiomas. *J Neurosurg.* 2010;112(5): 925-933. https://doi.org/10.3171/2009.9.JNS09617.

[24] Nawashiro H. Tumor shape and recurrence. *J Neurosurg.* 2000;93(3): 528.

[25] Roser F, Nakamura M, Bellinzona M, Rosahl SK, Ostertag H, Samii M. The prognostic value of progesterone receptor status in meningiomas. *J Clin Pathol.* 2004;57(10): 1033-1037. https://doi.org/10.1136/jcp.2004.018333.

[26] Wolfsberger S, Doostkam S, Boecher-Schwarz HG, et al. Progesterone-receptor index in meningiomas: correlation with clinico-pathological parameters and review of the literature. *Neurosurg Rev.* 2004;27(4): 238-245. https://doi.org/10.1007/s10143-004-0340-y.

[27] Pravdenkova S, Al-Mefty O, Sawyer J, Husain M. Progesterone and estrogen receptors: opposing prognostic indicators in meningiomas. *J Neurosurg.* 2006;105(2): 163-173. https://doi.org/10.3171/jns.2006.105.2.163.

[28] Maiuri F, Mariniello G, Peca C, et al. Multicentric and diffuse recurrences of meningiomas. *Br J Neurosurg.* 2020: 1-8. https://doi.org/10.1080/02688697.2020.1754335.

[29] Borovich B, Doron Y. Recurrence of intracranial meningiomas: the role played by regional multicentricity. *J Neurosurg.* 1986;64(1): 58-63. https://doi.org/10.3171/jns.1986.64.1.0058.

[30] Qi ST, Liu Y, Pan J, Chotai S, Fang LX. A radiopathological classification of dural tail sign of meningiomas. *J Neurosurg.* 2012;117(4): 645-653. https://doi.org/10.3171/2012.6.JNS111987.

[31] Kinjo T, al-Mefty O, Kanaan I. Grade zero removal of supratentorial convexity meningiomas. *Neurosurgery.* 1993;33(3): 394-399; discussion 399. https://doi.org/10.1227/00006123-199309000-00007.

[32] Mooney MA, Abolfotoh M, Bi WL, et al. Is Falcine Meningioma a Diffuse Disease of the Falx? Case Series and Analysis of a "Grade Zero" Resection. *Neurosurgery.* 2020;87(5): 900-909. https://doi.org/10.1093/neuros/nyaa038.

[33] Larson JJ, Tew JM, Simon M, Menon AG. Evidence for clonal spread in the development of multiple meningiomas. *J Neurosurg.* 1995;83(4): 705-709. https://doi.org/10.3171/jns.1995.83.4.0705.

[34] von Deimling A, Kraus JA, Stangl AP, et al. Evidence for subarachnoid spread in the development of multiple meningiomas. *Brain Pathol.* 1995;5(1): 11-14. https://doi.org/10.1111/j.1750-3639.1995.tb00571.x.

[35] Louis DN, Ohgaki H, Wiestler OD, et al. The 2007 WHO classification of tumours of the central nervous system. *Acta Neuropathol.* 2007;114(2): 97-109. https://doi.org/10.1007/s00401-007-0243-4.

[36] Nanda A, Vannemreddy P. Recurrence and outcome in skull base meningiomas: do they differ from other intracranial meningiomas? *Skull Base.* 2008;18(4): 243-252. https://doi.org/10.1055/s-2007-1016956.

[37] Mansouri A, Klironomos G, Taslimi S, et al. Surgically resected skull base meningiomas demonstrate a divergent postoperative recurrence pattern compared with non-skull base meningiomas. *J Neurosurg.* 2016;125(2): 431-440. https://doi.org/10.3171/2015.7.JNS15546.

[38] Maiuri F, Mariniello G, Guadagno E, Barbato M, Corvino S, Del Basso De Caro M. WHO grade, proliferation index, and progesterone receptor expression are different according to the location of meningioma. *Acta Neurochir (Wien).* 2019;161(12): 2553-2561. https://doi.org/10.1007/s00701-019-04084-z.

[39] Maiuri F, Del Basso De Caro M, de Divitiis O, Guadagno E, Mariniello G. Recurrence of spinal meningiomas: analysis of the risk factors. *Br J Neurosurg.* 2019: 1-6. https://doi.org/10.1080/02688697.2019.1638886.

[40] Mariniello G, Maiuri F, Strianese D, et al. Spheno-orbital meningiomas: surgical approaches and outcome according to the intraorbital tumor extent. *Zentralbl Neurochir.* 2008;69(4): 175-181. https://doi.org/10.1055/s-2008-1077077.

[41] Giombini S, Solero CL, Morello G. Late outcome of operations for supratentorial convexity meningiomas. Report on 207 cases. *Surg Neurol.* 1984;22(6): 588-594. https://doi.org/10.1016/0090-3019(84)90436-1.

[42] Wilms G, Lammens M, Marchal G, et al. Thickening of dura surrounding meningiomas: MR features. *J Comput Assist Tomogr.* 1989;13(5): 763-768. https://doi.org/10.1097/00004728-198909000-00003.

[43] Tokumaru A, O'uchi T, Eguchi T, et al. Prominent meningeal enhancement adjacent to meningioma on Gd-DTPA-enhanced MR images: histopathologic correlation. *Radiology.* 1990;175(2): 431-433. https://doi.org/10.1148/radiology.175.2.2326470.

[44] Jääskeläinen J. Seemingly complete removal of histologically benign intracranial meningioma: late recurrence rate and factors predicting recurrence in 657 patients. A multivariate analysis. *Surg Neurol.* 1986;26(5): 461-469. https://doi.org/10.1016/0090-3019(86)90259-4.

[45] Gousias K, Schramm J, Simon M. The Simpson grading revisited: aggressive surgery and its place in modern meningioma management. *J Neurosurg.* 2016;125(3): 551-560. https://doi.org/10.3171/2015.9.JNS15754.

[46] Sughrue ME, Kane AJ, Shangari G, et al. The relevance of Simpson Grade I and II resection in modern neurosurgical treatment of World Health Organization Grade I meningiomas. *J Neurosurg.* 2010;113(5): 1029-1035. https://doi.org/10.3171/2010.3.JNS091971.

[47] Condra KS, Buatti JM, Mendenhall WM, Friedman WA, Marcus RB, Rhoton AL. Benign meningiomas: primary treatment selection affects survival. *Int J Radiat Oncol Biol Phys.* 1997;39(2): 427-436.

[48] Haddad AF, Young JS, Kanungo I, et al. WHO Grade I Meningioma Recurrence: Identifying High Risk Patients Using Histopathological Features and the MIB-1 Index. *Front Oncol.* 2020;10: 1522. https://doi.org/10.3389/fonc.2020.01522.

[49] Araújo Pereira BJ, Nogueira de Almeida A, Pires de Aguiar PH, Paiva WS, Teixeira MJ, Nagahashi Marie SK. Multiple Intracranial Meningiomas: A Case Series and Review of the Literature. *World Neurosurg.* 2019;122: e1536-e1541. https://doi.org/10.1016/j.wneu.2018.11.097.

[50] Pfisterer WK, Coons SW, Aboul-Enein F, Hendricks WP, Scheck AC, Preul MC. Implicating chromosomal aberrations with meningioma growth and recurrence: results from FISH and MIB-I analysis of grades I and II meningioma tissue. *J Neurooncol.* 2008;87(1): 43-50. https://doi.org/10.1007/s11060-007-9498-9.

[51] Monleón D, Morales JM, Gonzalez-Segura A, et al. Metabolic aggressiveness in benign meningiomas with chromosomal instabilities. *Cancer Res.* 2010;70(21): 8426-8434. https://doi.org/10.1158/0008-5472.CAN-10-1498.

[52] Pérez-Magán E, Campos-Martín Y, Mur P, et al. Genetic alterations associated with progression and recurrence in meningiomas. *J Neuropathol Exp Neurol.* 2012;71(10): 882-893. https://doi.org/10.1097/NEN.0b013e31826bf704.

[53] Serna E, Morales JM, Mata M, et al. Gene expression profiles of metabolic aggressiveness and tumor recurrence in benign meningioma. *PLoS One.* 2013;8(6): e67291. https://doi.org/10.1371/journal.pone.0067291.

[54] Olar A, Wani KM, Wilson CD, et al. Global epigenetic profiling identifies methylation subgroups associated with recurrence-free survival in meningioma. *Acta Neuropathol.* 2017;133(3): 431-444. https://doi.org/10.1007/s00401-017-1678-x.

[55] Klinger DR, Flores BC, Lewis JJ, et al. Atypical Meningiomas: Recurrence, Reoperation, and Radiotherapy. *World Neurosurg.* 2015;84(3): 839-845. https://doi.org/10.1016/j.wneu.2015.04.033.

[56] Bagshaw HP, Burt LM, Jensen RL, et al. Adjuvant radiotherapy for atypical meningiomas. *J Neurosurg.* 2017;126(6): 1822-1828. https://doi.org/10.3171/2016.5.JNS152809.

[57] Hardesty DA, Wolf AB, Brachman DG, et al. The impact of adjuvant stereotactic radiosurgery on atypical meningioma recurrence following aggressive microsurgical

resection. *J Neurosurg.* 2013;119(2): 475-481. https://doi.org/10.3171/2012.12.JNS12414.

[58] Kim M, Lee DH, Kim Rn HJ, Cho YH, Kim JH, Kwon DH. Analysis of the results of recurrent intracranial meningiomas treated with re-radiosurgery. *Clin Neurol Neurosurg.* 2017;153: 93-101. https://doi.org/10.1016/j.clineuro.2016.12.014.

[59] Mason WP, Gentili F, Macdonald DR, Hariharan S, Cruz CR, Abrey LE. Stabilization of disease progression by hydroxyurea in patients with recurrent or unresectable meningioma. *J Neurosurg.* 2002;97(2): 341-346. https://doi.org/10.3171/jns.2002.97.2.0341.

[60] Chamberlain MC, Johnston SK. Hydroxyurea for recurrent surgery and radiation refractory meningioma: a retrospective case series. *J Neurooncol.* 2011;104(3): 765-771. https://doi.org/10.1007/s11060-011-0541-5.

[61] Grunberg SM, Weiss MH, Spitz IM, et al. Treatment of unresectable meningiomas with the antiprogesterone agent mifepristone. *J Neurosurg.* 1991;74(6): 861-866. https://doi.org/10.3171/jns.1991.74.6.0861.

[62] Johnson DR, Kimmel DW, Burch PA, et al. Phase II study of subcutaneous octreotide in adults with recurrent or progressive meningioma and meningeal hemangiopericytoma. *Neuro Oncol.* 2011;13(5): 530-535. https://doi.org/10.1093/neuonc/nor044.

[63] Nayak L, Iwamoto FM, Rudnick JD, et al. Atypical and anaplastic meningiomas treated with bevacizumab. *J Neurooncol.* 2012;109(1): 187-193. https://doi.org/10.1007/s11060-012-0886-4.

[64] Raizer JJ, Grimm SA, Rademaker A, et al. A phase II trial of PTK787/ZK 222584 in recurrent or progressive radiation and surgery refractory meningiomas. *J Neurooncol.* 2014;117(1): 93-101. https://doi.org/10.1007/s11060-014-1358-9.

[65] Kaley TJ, Wen P, Schiff D, et al. Phase II trial of sunitinib for recurrent and progressive atypical and anaplastic meningioma. *Neuro Oncol.* 2015;17(1): 116-121. https://doi.org/10.1093/neuonc/nou148.

[66] Gupta S, Bi WL, Dunn IF. Medical management of meningioma in the era of precision medicine. *Neurosurg Focus.* 2018;44(4): E3. https://doi.org/10.3171/2018.1.FOCUS17754.

Chapter 7

Endoscopy in Neurosurgery

Khandkar Ali Kawsar

Abstract

Introduction of endoscope was undoubtedly a great advancement in neurosurgery. It minimises trauma to the brain tissue and maximises the vision around the remote areas. The access to the ventricle and cisterns has become much easier. Development in optics, lenses, long and angled instruments made the endoscopy in neurosurgery very versatile. In this chapter, the introduction of the endoscopy in neurosurgery has been described along with its use in different branches of neurosurgery like neuro-oncology, hydrocephalus, skullbase, aneurysms, craniosynostosis etc. The details of some common and important operation have been described. Some relevant anatomy, which can be encountered in endoscopic approach, has been described which will be helpful to the readers. This chapter will also act as an eye-opener to the vast use of neuroendoscopy and will help broaden the horizon of trainee neurosurgeons, following which the further details can be sought in relevant books and literature. In brief, this chapter will tell us about the evolution to revolution of the neuroendoscopy.

Keywords: Endoscopy, Neuroendoscopy, ETV, Arachnoid cyst, Hydrocephalus, Neuro-oncology, Skullbase, Pituitary, Transphenoidal, Aneurysm, Craniosynostosis

1. Introduction

Neuroendoscopy treats the pathologies of the central nervous system applying an endoscope. With the ever improving methods to treat cranial pathologies neuroendoscopy is being applied more and more to treat different pathologies. In this chapter, we will discuss the brief history, clinical application and important neuroendoscopic approaches along with the advantages, disadvantages, complications or important considerations in the procedures.

In **Table 1**, the events those revolutionized the endoscopic neurosurgery, are summarized.

In the early 1970s, both flexible fibreoptic and high-resolution rigid endoscopes could be developed based on the technological advances in optics and electronics. Those were used successfully for operating within the ventricles. From that point of treating hydrocephalus, the neuroendoscopy has progressed to endoscope-assisted surgical procedures which began in the 1980s and 1990s. This minimally invasive procedure retained its popularity and continued till now [6].

At the initial days of neuroendoscopy, as ventricles contain the ideal medium of crystal-clear CSF, the endoscopic procedures were confined to those. Currently, the field of neuroendoscopy has extended beyond ventricular procedures and is currently applied for all types of neurosurgically treatable diseases such as intracranial cysts, intraventricular tumors, hypothalamic hamartoma (HH), skull base tumors, craniosynostosis, degenerative spine disease, and rare subtypes of hydrocephalus [7].

IntechOpen

Year	Events	Performed by
1910	The first neurosurgical endoscopic procedure for choroid plexus fulguration using a cystoscope in two infants with hydrocephalus, one of them was successfully treated [1–3].	L'Espinasse
1922	Choroid plexectomy to treat hydrocephalus, which was unsuccessful [4].	Walter Dandy
1923	Successful endoscopic third ventriculostomy (ETV) in a 9-month-old girl with obstructive hydrocephalus, using a urethroscope [5].	Mixter
1935	Reported his initial results after using a novel endoscope equipped with a cauterizing electrode, an irrigation system to prevent ventricle collapse, and a movable operating tip to perforate the third ventricle floor [1, 3].	Scarff

Table 1.
Revolutionary events in endoscopic neurosurgery.

The benefit in minimally invasive endoscopic procedures is analogous to that of any endoscopic procedure and can be listed as follows:

1. Minimal tissue disruption

2. Enhanced visualization

3. Improved cosmetic results

4. Shorter hospital stay

5. Less surgical morbidity.

In neurosurgery, to minimize operative trauma, the surgeon tries hard to limit the size of the exposure and to avoid unnecessary brain retraction, which can cause damage by increasing pressure to the surrounding normal brain tissue and minimizing the regional cerebral blood flow [8] which has short-term and long-term knock on effect and these eventually may compromise the neurologic outcome following microneurosurgical procedures. The outcome can potentially be improved by the use of neuroendoscopy techniques. The endoscope enhances the surgeon's view by increasing illumination and magnification [9, 10], which makes it an excellent teaching tool. A comparison of endoscope and microscope from a survey of the neurosurgeons shows that microscope is superior only for less fatigue of the hand and 3D vision which are now removed with endoscope holder and 3D view of endoscopes. This 3D view is clearly more advantageous in looking at the areas, that were difficult to visualize with microscope. With the advent of different angled endoscopes, e.g. 30°, 45°, 70°, 110°, it is possible to have a panoramic view of the field [6].

2. Equipment

The endoscopy set should include: video camera, camera control units, light source, video recorder, video monitor and a computerized system for storage of video segments or single-picture capture as shown in **Figure 1**. Endoscope positioning and fixation arms help the surgeon to avoid arm fatigue, which can disturb eye–hand coordination and flexibility may be compromised [11]. With the fixation arms, sudden movement of the hand or hand tremor can be minimized.

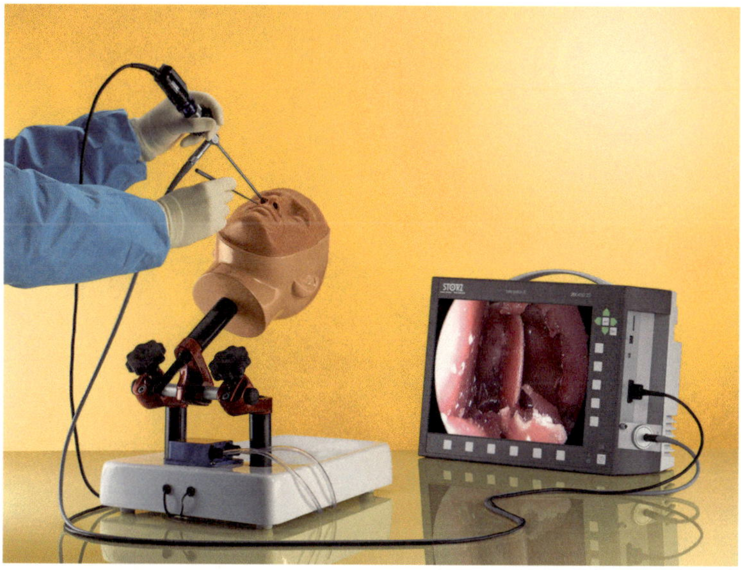

Figure 1.
Camera control units with light source and video monitor with video recorder.

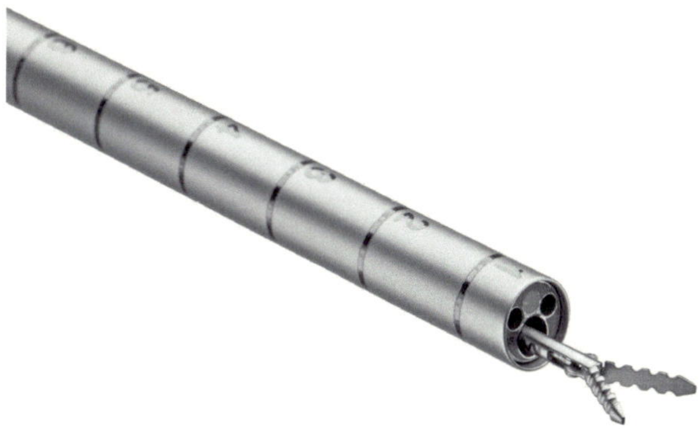

Figure 2.
Endoscopic grasping forceps.

Endoscopic instruments include a pair of grabbing forceps (**Figure 2**) and scissors, a monopolar or bipolar coagulation device, an irrigation system, and a straight and one or more scopes with various angles (**Figure 3**). When the endoscope holder is not used, a knowledgeable assistant is very helpful to show the difficult areas and the surgeon can work with both hands. Video recording equipment is very helpful for capturing images on video or digital format for training and later study [12]. The scope of neuroendoscopy has gone further with the help of flexible neuroendoscope (**Figure 4**).

Frameless computerized neuronavigation has been used more in intracranial endoscopic neurosurgery to increase the accuracy and precision. This has proven to be reliable and useful in selected intracranial neuroendoscopic procedures to improve the accuracy of the endoscopic approach [12].

Modern three-chip technology provides impressive color depth and brilliant red differentiation. The latest Full HD technology delivers lag-free images even with rapid camera movements. When we learn and understand more varieties of CNS pathologies, the targets and demands for endoscopic procedures will change

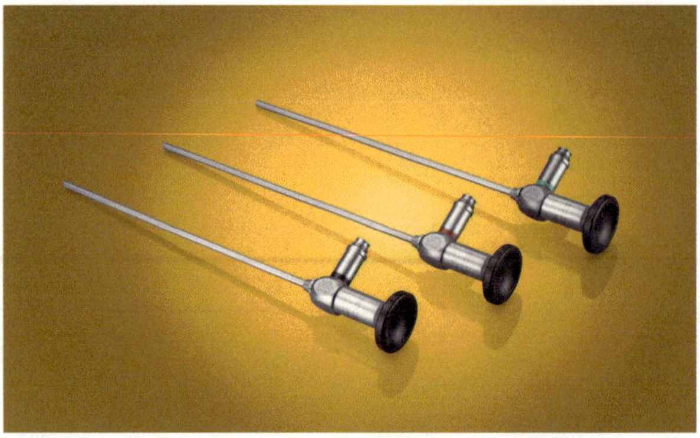

Figure 3.
Straight and angled scopes.

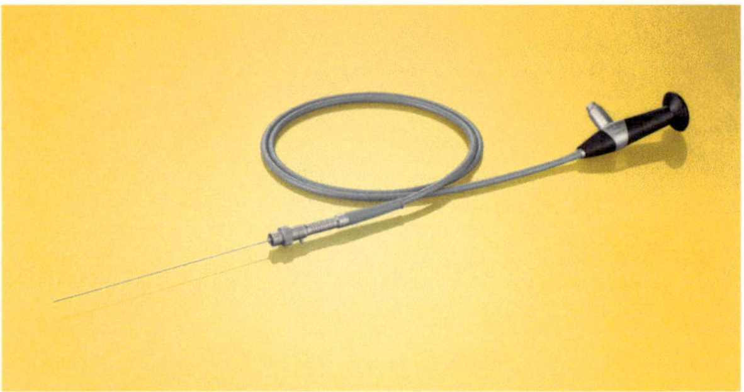

Figure 4.
Flexible endoscope.

accordingly. Telemanipulated neurosurgery, with supervisory-controlled robotic systems, or shared control systems, or even fully robotic telesurgery along with the recent advancement in nanotechnology will be needed to address future indications for minimally or even ultramicro-access neurosurgery [13]. The relentless work is going on to improve the endoscopic system which includes improved maneuverability of the scope by reduction of the bulk and integration of the camera and fiberoptic light components with an extensive viewing angle from 0 to 70 degrees, along with the provision of maintaining surgical orientation.

3. Endoscopic third ventriculostomy

3.1 History and background

In 1952, Nulsen and Spitz began the era of ventricular cerebrospinal fluid (CSF) shunting [14]. Due to the lack of initial encouraging results, not until 1970s, an interest in ETV for treating obstructive hydrocephalus was renewed when the imaging capability of endoscopes had a remarkable improvement. In 1978, Vries described his experience treating five patients with hydrocephalus, in whom he demonstrated that ETVs were technically feasible using a fiberoptic endoscope [15]. In the small series of 24 patients with various forms of hydrocephalus, Jones and colleagues described a 50% shunt-free success rate for ETV, initially in 1990 [16]. They reported a better success rate of 61% in a series of 103 patients 4 years later [17]. Obstructive hydrocephalus which has resulted from either benign aqueductal stenosis or compressive periaqueductal benign or malignant mass lesions are being treated primarily with ETV in the modern era. In the current time, the shunt-free success rate ranges from 80 to 95% [2].

The indications for ETV are expanding to meningomyelocele, Chiari malformation or Dandy-Walker-related hydrocephalus cases. Few studies reported fairly good success rates after ETV for cases of communicating hydrocephalus in idiopathic normal pressure hydrocephalus [18]. In selected cases, ETV is becoming more and more preferable to ventriculoperitoneal (VP) shunt placement due to avoidance of shunt dependency and complications that come with the shunting [19]. With introduction of improved endoscopic techniques, ETV is now used to treat hydrocephalus following shunt malfunction or infection and refractory slit-ventricle syndrome [18].

3.2 Important landmarks

Recognition of critical landmarks and structures in the ventricles is very important to achieve a successful ETV. **Figure 5** is showing the instruments required for ETV and an endoscopic view showing some important landmarks. In **Table 2**, we discuss few important landmarks with which the surgeons need to be familiar to accomplish the procedure safely.

The supraoptic and paraventricular arcuate nuclei are the structures most prone to injury, which may give rise to endocrine disturbances [20].

To increase the success of the ETV endoscope needs to be progressed and Lilliequest membrane needs fenestration. Basilar artery will be seen during this stage (**Figure 7**).

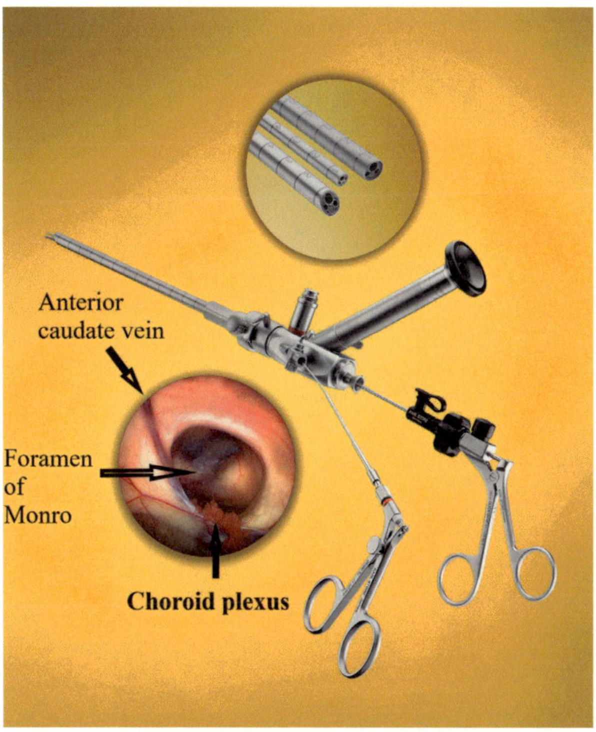

Figure 5.
In the middle, ETV endoscope with side channel with working instrument (forceps for fenestration). In the upper circle, end of the ETV endoscopes. In lower circle, the endoscopic view before entering into the foramen of Monro.

Anatomical landmark	Reason of importance	Comments
Choroid plexus	This remains at choroidal fissure and gives the surgeon an important navigational tool, even with gross distortions in the ventricular anatomy.	Anterior part of choroid plexus extends to the foramen of Monro and then to the third ventricle.
Fornix	This forms the superior and anterior margin of the foramen of Monro.	Endoscope needs to be carefully advanced from lateral to third ventricle to avoid the injury to fornix and resultant memory impairment the chance of which increases with multiple passages because of the location of the fornix.
Thalamostriate vein	Being usually the largest tributary of the Internal Cerebral Veins, it is a prominent structure. It goes down to the foramen of Monro with the choroid plexus.	During advancement in third ventricle, too much deviation of endoscope laterally towards this vein, may damage the hypothalamus as it forms the lateral walls of the third ventricle.
Mamillary Bodies	Paired structure visible underneath the floor of the third ventricle.	Floor of the third ventricle is usually thinned out which needs to be fenestrated behind this paired mamillary bodies (**Figure 6**).

Table 2.
Landmarks for ETV [20].

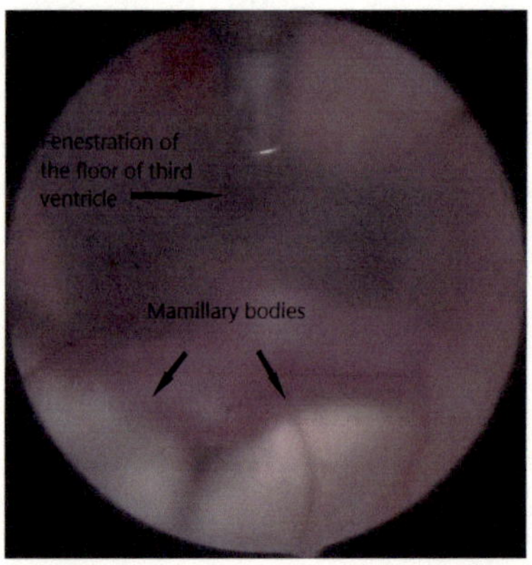

Figure 6.
Endoscopic view of the floor of the third ventricle before fenestration of the floor of the ventricle.

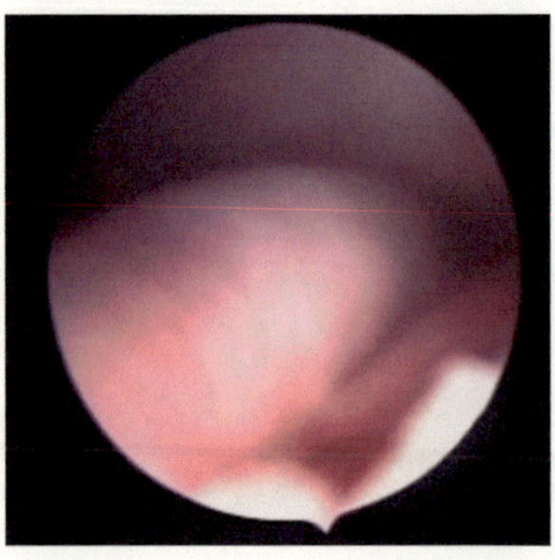

Figure 7.
Endoscopic view of basilar artery following fenestration of the floor of the third ventricle and Liliequist membrane.

3.3 Precautions

There are several precautions to take when performing ETV when there is history of previous tumors, shunting procedure or thickened floor of third ventricle. The anatomy may be difficult to interpret as it can be altered by tumors e.g. a brainstem glioma. Floor of the third ventricle may be distorted and basilar artery may be displaced forward, minimizing the safe zone of the floor for penetration. The onset of hydrocephalus resulting from tumor obstruction may be relatively acute and the floor of the third ventricle may appear opaque and non-attenuated. The procedure will pose more challenges as the penetration of the floor will be difficult and invariably requires a sharper technique without visualization of the neurovascular structures underneath the membrane for penetration, which obviously increases the risk.

3.4 Consideration for success of ETV

Patients, who have been previously shunted, are technically more difficult to perform ETV upon, because -

i. Less marked ventricular dilatation because of shunt assisted drainage

ii. A thicker ventricular floor

iii. Abnormal anatomy which is not an infrequent finding.

An ETV procedure may have to be abandoned in some cases for the following reasons –

i. Thick floor of the third ventricle

ii. Endoscopic view is obstructed by blood and cannot be cleared

iii. The basilar artery is very close or just under the planned site of fenestration.

iv. The anatomy is really unclear.

Despite all these, ETV has an overall success rate of approximately 75% after 3 years. Though the success depends not only on patient selection, but also on the experience of the surgeons. The results of ETV is better than shunting specially in patients with posterior fossa tumors [21]. In addition if the expenses are taken into account; ETV is superior to shunting [22].

Early failure of ETV can occur for mostly peroperative events such as

i. Bleeding around the fenestration site

ii. Unnoticed additional arachnoid membranes occluding the flow of CSF

iii. Inadequate size of the fenestration.

Late failure is the result of subsequent closure of the fenestration by gliotic tissue or arachnoid membrane. This problem is potentially serious because the failure can occur in a short period of time, may be unpredictable and presentation may be late due to a false sense of security. There are now several reports in the literature of death following late failure of ETV [23] and this remains a management problem. Tumor progression and inadequate CSF absorption at the level of the arachnoid villi may result in early or late failure. A cohort of patients with open fenestrations who remained well for months, exhibits deterioration, the reasons of which are still not understood [24].

Procedure-related complications reported in the literature include bradycardia, hypothalamic dysfunction and hemorrhage from damage to arteries, ependymal veins, or the choroid plexus. The complications are divided into two main categories; short-term complications, which mostly resolve from intraoperative and technique-related, and long-term complications which occur at a much lower rate [25].

4. Simplifications of complex hydrocephalus and intracranial cysts

4.1 Multiloculated hydrocephalus

Multiloculated hydrocephalus is a condition in which there is isolated CSF compartments within the ventricular system that tend to enlarge even if the patient has a functioning V-P shunt. Multiloculation usually develops as a complication of meningitis, intraventricular hemorrhage, post shunt infection, head injury, ependymal trauma during shunt insertion and other inflammatory processes [26].

Following neonatal meningitis in infants, more than 30% of the survivors will develop hydrocephalus, most of these neonates have a risk of having multiloculated hydrocephalus [27]. The compartments are separated by septa that prevent accumulated CSF from being absorbed by either the ventricular catheter or normal sites of CSF absorption [28]. Even with multiple shunts, all compartments may not be drained properly. As a consequence, shunts are associated with high failure rates. There is also the risk of subsequent infections.

Endoscopy offers a simple means of communicating isolated CSF spaces and ventricles by membrane fenestration. A good analysis of the preoperative MRI scans will help to achieve a good outcome in these cases. Entry points are to be determined in a way, so that through the least number of burr holes, maximum number of cysts can be fenestrated and communication among them can be established [29]. Same burr hole as that for the placement of a ventricular catheter can also be taken into account for the fenestration procedure. Fenestration of the septum pellucidum to connect the two lateral ventricles in patients with loculated ventricles will preclude the need for two shunts in the majority of patients [20].

Spennato et al., explained high incidence of shunt obstruction in multiloculation by the chronic inflammation of the ependyma and appearance of new septa. They considered multiloculated hydrocephalus as progressive disease [30]. Akbari et al., found that 38.5% of patients with multiloculated hydrocephalus required additional endoscopic fenestrations after the initial surgery, while El-Ghandour found that in 33% of patients endoscopic fenestration was repeated during the follow-up period [31, 32].

Aqueductoplasty can be used for the treatment of trapped fourth ventricle syndrome. There is a high closure rate, which can be prevented by stenting. In these cases, endoscopic third ventriculostomy should also be done. Applied neuroendoscopic techniques have been extended to foraminoplasty of the foramens of Monro and Magendie, as well as endoscopic fourth ventriculostomy [1, 2, 11].

4.2 Intracranial cysts

The ventricular system may lodge many types of cysts like arachnoid cysts (AC), choroid plexus cysts, neoplastic cysts and infected cysts (e.g. hydatid and cysticercotic cysts). ACs, although typically extra-axial, may occur within the ventricles.

ACs can be treated with either endoscopic resection or fenestration to achieve a successful outcome in many patients [33].

Intracranial ACs comprise about 1% of all intracranial space-occupying lesions [34]. In the recent years with increased availability of computed tomography (CT) and magnetic resonance imaging (MRI), the incidence has seem to be increased as more are detected [35, 36]. Different surgical techniques are recommended. Because of the development of neuroendoscopy, pure endoscopic AC fenestration has become increasingly popular, where a communication can also be established with either ventricles or cisterns, and is actually preferred by many neurosurgeons [36, 37], especially in cases of cysts located in the suprasellar or quadrigeminal as well as in the posterior fossa [38–40].

Walker et al. reported in their preliminary series that 9 of 14 children (64%) with arachnoid cysts were successfully treated by endoscopic fenestration through a burr hole, thereby avoiding the need for craniotomy and brain manipulation [41]. Even cysts confined to the pituitary fossa are ideally suited to endoscopic transsphenoidal surgery. Ventriculo-cysto-cisternostomy offers long-term decompression of suprasellar arachnoid cysts without the need for shunting. Most patients with intraventricular cyst or tumors have concomitant hydrocephalus. These cases are better managed by endoscopic surgery rather than open, as procedures can be performed for both CSF diversion and tumor management simultaneously [42, 43]. Teo et al. had successful outcome in fenestrating ACs, cysts of the cavum velum interpositum, neuroepithelial cysts of the ventricle, colloid cysts and large pineal region cysts. While operating in smaller ventricles, frameless stereotactic guidance has been useful in planning the site(s) of the burr hole(s) and to plan the trajectory to these cysts. The current advancement of neuronavigation with electromagnetic guidance helps the endoscopic surgery more precise and well directed. The goal of surgery for arachnoid cysts is symptomatic improvement. This is particularly pertinent with endoscopic fenestration, as the appearance of the cyst on postoperative imaging may be only slightly diminished, despite marked clinical improvement [6].

5. Application of endoscopy to neuro-oncology

Endoscopy can be applied to neuro-oncology as it provides an ideal venue for this. The advancement of visualization of intraventricular pathology, management of tumor-related hydrocephalus, safer techniques of biopsies, and minimally invasive surgery for removal of intraventricular tumors are very useful adjuncts to traditional tumor management [6].

Once a tumor is removed, the surgeon can use the endoscope to assess the degree of resection. With the advantage of looking at the remote corners, the same surgery can be accomplished through a smaller craniotomy with the help of the endoscopes, may be with different angles, in keeping with the concept of minimally invasive surgery with maximally effective results [44]. By removing more tumor intraoperatively, endoscopy may improve the rate of survival for patients with benign tumors by reducing the less chance of recurrence and less requirement of adjuvant treatment [45, 46]. Adjunctive procedures, like third ventriculostomy and septostomy, can easily be performed through the same access points to manage concomitant problems like secondary hydrocephalus, where shunt placement can be avoided [6].

Endoscopic visualization and removal of intraaxial brain tumors using stereotactic guidance was first described in 1980 [47, 48]. In addition, stereotactic endoscopy for tumor removal through a conduit created by a bullet shaped dilator was reported in 1990 [49]. Kassam et al. described the development of a completely endoscopic system for resection of intraaxial tumors through a dilatable conduit.

The channel is created by dilatation of white matter, minimizing the neural structures by attempting to create a parafascicular approach to the tumor. The port creates an air medium that allows bimanual dissection. The instruments work parallel to the endoscope and the technique is safe as this does not deviate from the proven microsurgical principles [50].

Dr. Kelly pioneered a 20 mm diameter stereotactic tubular retraction system for the microscopic resection of deep brain tumors. Based on his work, the concept of endoscopic resection was initially developed [51–53]. As the microscope delivers a cone of light, tapering from the source until it reaches the target, the conduit that is required to deliver microscopic visualization is larger than an endoscopic conduit. In contrast, the endoscope delivers light and magnification via an inverted cone of light. Therefore, a much smaller port (11.5 mm) or conduit can be used to deliver the endoscope only very few millimeters from the target to visualize the tumor, creating a "flashlight" effect to illuminate the tumor. This advantage of the endoscope can be exploited to perform intraaxial tumor resections [50].

Although the conventional endoscope does not provide binocular vision, it has not been a major issue. Bimanual dissection allows proprioceptive feedback by which the loss of binocular vision can easily be compensated. This is similar to working from the observer's perspective during microscopic neurosurgery. Once adequate experience is gained, the surgeon develops a good perception relying on tactile feedback from touch and movement. The development of 3D technology overcomes this limitation. Kassam et al. reported that endoscopic approach may prove to be superior to microscopic one for subcortical tumors, because the endoscope allows unrestricted and better illumination in deep regions with a closer view of the pathology. For cortical lesions, due to its location, microscope has got obvious advantages and it is preferred. But for deep-seated brain tumors, direct endoscopic view can add lot more details and significant advantages for removal. Many surgeons now prefer to have a final endoscopic visualization to confirm adequate resection for intraparenchymal tumors once the microscope has been taken out of the field [54].

Selected primary and metastatic brain tumors may be safely removed with this approach. Using dynamic retraction of the port and the method of piecemeal extirpation, a small conduit can be used for an effective removal of tumors that are much larger than the conduit itself can be effectively removed. Obviously, the long-term prognosis will ultimately be determined by the biology of the tumor. However, in the group of appropriately selected patients the port may offer a viable option to achieve the goals of surgery—that is, partial removal with a view of cytoreduction or complete removal of tumor with an acceptable level of morbidity, minimizing both corticectomy volume and white-matter dissection required for the resection of the tumor [8].

The burr hole is placed in an area of skull so that the scope should enter the ventricle from a furthest possible point towards the tumor so that the scope is directly viewing the tumor, not looking from one corner. The distal approach helps the surgeon to perceive the abnormal anatomy following an orientation of normal anatomical structures while passing the scope through non-pathological part of the brain. As most of the distal part of the scope is within the ventricle, the surgeon can move the scope in multiple directions with more flexibility without damaging the normal surrounding neural structures [6].

Endoscopic approach is not ideal for all intraventricular tumors. The suitability criteria for endoscopic removal include –

i. Moderate to low vascularity

ii. Soft consistency

iii. Associated secondary hydrocephalus

iv. Histologically low grade [6].

Even with the advancement of the MRI, all these criteria may always not be possible to confirm preoperatively.

Few principles should be followed during removal of the intraventricular tumor safely. The surgeon needs to choose a trajectory that avoids eloquent structures but allows a good view of the tumor. The outside of the tumor is coagulated with either monopolar electrocautery or a laser to ease the removal of the tumor. Profuse irrigation is needed for clearing the blood and debris and to prevent building up of too much heat inside the ventricle. Cysts need to be opened and the contents are either drained or sucked or removed as piecemeal. Remaining wall is removed piecemeal which allows removal of the whole pathology with a smaller access. With completion of the procedure, the scope is withdrawn while inspecting the tract for intraparenchymal bleeding [6]. Hemostasis is obtained with copious irrigation. If there is a clot noted, a cut-end foley catheter can be used with gentle aspiration to remove blood clot during intraventricular hemostasis [55].

Endoscopic tumor biopsy is a well-known procedure for the management of intraventricular tumors. It has a high diagnostic yield of more than 90% and low risk of less than 3.5%. Germ cell tumor, infiltrative hypothalamic/optic pathway glioma, and Langerhans cell histiocytosis can be addressed with endoscopic biopsy [2]. Endoscopic removal is well-established procedure for colloid cysts or tumors that are also pedunculated at the ependymal surface. Endoscopic excision of a colloid cyst is accessible and technically possible through the lateral ventricle in most cases unless the cyst is very large, which poses more risk of venous injury at the foramen of Monro [2, 56]. Transventricular endoscopic decompression of tumor cyst can temporarily or permanently treat the obstructive hydrocephalus or prevent the visual loss [7].

Hypothalamic hamartoms are rare non-neoplastic congenital malformations that arises from inferior hypothalamus and give rise to the symptoms of gelastic seizures, precocious puberty and cognitive problems. Surgical treatment is required for all patients except those with precocious puberty. Single or combination treatment are supposed to be used according to HH type as per the classification of Delalande and Fohlen [57] or Choi et al. [58] Endoscopic resection guided by stereotactic navigation has been attempted for surgical removal of small HHs, but parts of the tumors remained. Surgical resection of HHs is typically carried out in multiple steps. Despite that, recent reports indicate that endoscopic disconnection of HHs seems to be more effective and safer than other modalities [58, 59]. In spite of good visualization of the endoscopes, navigation assistance is recommended, in most cases, for obvious reason of precision in normal sized lateral and third ventricles [7].

6. Endoscope-assisted microsurgery

Endoscope-assisted microsurgery is the most rapidly growing area in endoscopic neurosurgery. Use of endoscope is the next step for surpassing the limitations of traditional microsurgery and allows the neurosurgeon to view tumor remnants such as those hidden behind eloquent brain tissue, a cranial nerve, or the tentorial edge.

Microsurgery evolved to maximize visualization and minimize retraction. Endoscopy allows the neurosurgeon to move another step further towards achieving these goals. Rigid endoscopes with various angles and flexible endoscopes help the surgeon to look around the remote corners which can be very useful in the removal of tumors and the clipping of cerebral aneurysms. Several approaches to the extra-axial structures of the skull base have been described to improve visualization with strict adherence to the principles of standard microsurgical techniques. The most commonly adopted method is to insert the scope down the same operative field. This, obviously, creates no further morbidity but tends to clutter the already limited surgical field, which can be avoided by inserting instruments through a contralateral burr hole. The subarachnoid space can be accessed through a small supra-orbital incision and then standard microsurgical dissection is carried out to identify the pathology. Once the pathology is identified under direct vision, the endoscope should be fixed in place and the attention is focused on the ipsilateral side. This technique offers excellent visualization of the tips of an aneurysm clip or the contralateral extent of a tumor. Endoscopes are increasingly used to inspect tumors, tumor beds following resection, aneurysms and other pathologies. Various authors have described the advantages of endoscopes for these purposes [25, 60, 61].

The endoscope offers a superior and often novel view of the anatomy, which can be extremely useful for the understanding of the operative approach for the trainee neurosurgeons. Furthermore, the trainer and the learner share the same view of the surgical field, which may not always be possible even with an operating microscope.

There are risks, the most problematic of which of using the scope is the risk of friction upon structures while introducing the scope. It is of crucial importance to guide the endoscope by visualizing it along the length of its shaft, rather than watching the images on the monitor. Following placement of the scope into the surgical field, if the scope is not fixed, then small, barely noticeable movements at the tip can be the result of larger excursions at the back of the scope. Obviously, this can have potentially disastrous consequences. Hence, the endoscopic field of work should be observed and the movement of the shaft of the endoscope has to be delicate at the same time. A fixed endoscope holder can stop the unnecessary movement of the endoscope and aid the surgeon to work with both hands and to use more complex instruments, and will also prevent the endoscope from drifting against vital structures located superficially along the operative corridor [6].

7. Endoscopy for skull base lesions

The pioneering work of neuroendoscopy for skull base tumors was done by Carrau and colleagues [62], who reported their original experience of endonasal transsphenoidal hypophysectomy at the University of Pittsburgh. The endoscopic approach was expanded by de Divitiis and colleagues [4] to include other lesions of the sellar and parasellar regions. The bilateral endonasal endoscopic approach now allows for visualization of tumors at the anterior skull base up to the crista galli and down to the level of C2 [7]. **Figure 8** shows how endoscope can access and treat the pathologies in

a. the crista galli to tuberculum sella,

b. sella and suprasellar region,

c. upper clival region and

d. lower clival region upto the level of axis vertebra (C2).

The application of endoscopic endonasal surgery (EES) for excision of pituitary adenoma and craniopharyngioma has been reported with encouraging results and low morbidity [7]. The surgical corridor for the endoscopic approach for sellar or suprasellar tumors should be tailored on the basis of the extent of lesion.

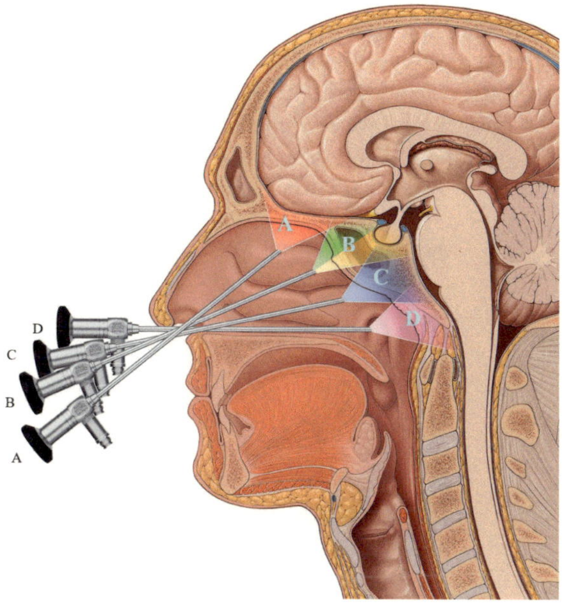

Figure 8.
Angles of endoscope by which the broad area of skull base (A. Frontal base, B. Sella, C. upper clivus, D. lower clivus) can be approached.

Supradiaphragmatic lesions can be removed via the endonasal route. On the other hand the suprasellar prechiasmatic preinfundibular lesions can be removed with the transtuberculum-transplanum sphenoidale approach [2].

Tumors of the tuberculum sellae region present different type of difficulties for endoscopic endonasal surgery. It is a compact anatomic region where fine and critical microvasculature can be seen with the potential involvement of the Circle of Willis. The endoscopic procedure may leave high flow CSF leaks which may require the use of a vascularized flap, the most common example of which is the nasal septal flap [63, 64]. A natural extension for the endoscopic endonasal approach is anteriorly along the skull base to the planum and cribriform for resection of planum/cribriform [65].

EES has become a powerful tool for treating pathology of the clivus, the petro-clival region, along with the intradural posterior fossa lesions immediately adjacent to the clivus. Traditionally, the pathologies in the clival and paraclival regions have been difficult to approach, especially for those, which have significant extension in the sagittal plain and/or had significant bilateral extension. For these tumors, often a combination of open approaches was required, as evidenced by dividing the clivus into thirds, each requiring a separate approach [66].

Expanded Endonasal Approaches (EEA) is versatile in the sagittal plain so much so that the ventral surgical corridor provides access to lesions that extend bilaterally across the midline. A single endonasal corridor can be sufficient to access large tumors that span the entire clival region. An endoscopic approach to the upper clivus provides midline access to the interpeduncular cistern, basilar artery, mammillary bodies and the floor of the third ventricle. The upper clivus or "sellar clivus" is formed by the posterior clinoid processes and the dorsum sella, which needs to be accessed and resected during this approach. A middle transclival approach provides access to the ventral pons and prepontine cistern, the basilar trunk and anterior inferior cerebellar artery, as well as the cisternal segment of the abducens nerve. The paraclival ICAs and the petroclival fissure set the lateral limit of the sphenoidal clivus. Laterally, the middle transclival exposure is limited by the interdural segment of cranial nerve VI [67].

Meckel's cave lesions can be approached by expanding the exposures laterally and inferiorly to the cavernous sinus [68–70]. The lower transclival approach through the lower segment of the clivus, which lies below the roof of the choana, allows access to the premedullary cistern and ventral medullary surface, the vertebral arteries, vertebrobasilar junction and posterior inferior cerebellar arteries and the cranial nerves IX–XII [9]. **Figures 9–11** are showing an endoscopic view of the cerebellopontine angle [71].

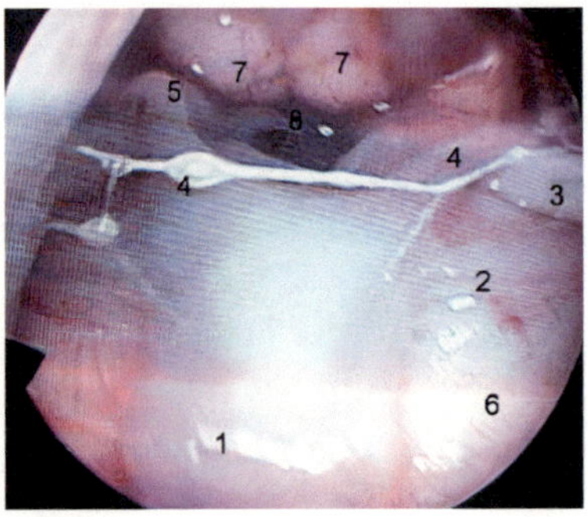

Figure 9.
Endoscopic view of interpeduncular fossa and posterior part of CW. 1-basilar trunk, 2- superior cerebellar artery (SCA), 3- oculomotor nerve, 4-P1 artery, 5-posterior communicating artery, 6-basilar pons, 7-mamillary bodies & 8-Thalamoperforators.

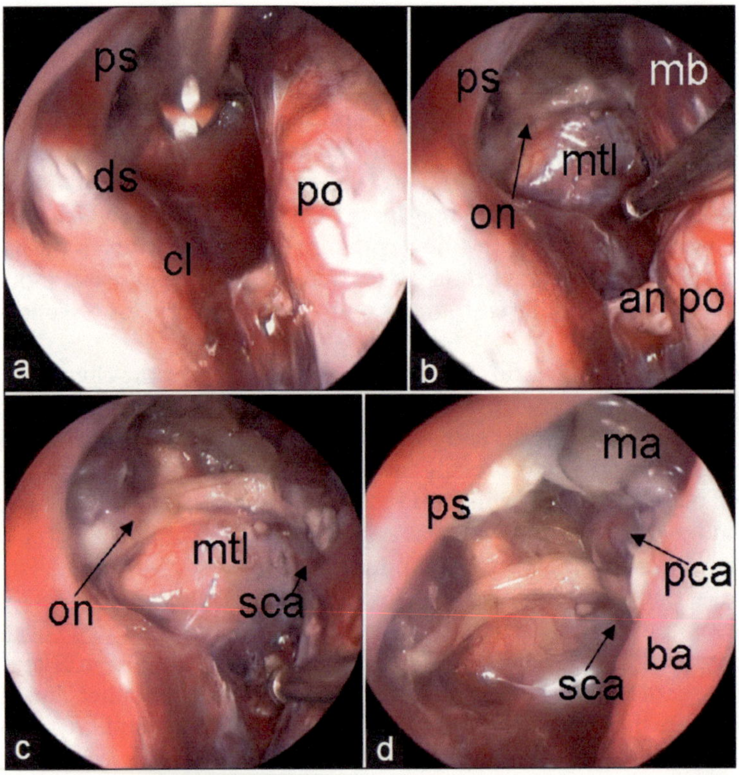

Figure 10.
Endoscopic view through a cerebellopontine angle approach showing part of interpeduncular fossa and right sided medial temporal lobe. (a) Ps-pituitary stalk; po-pons; ds - dorsum sellae; and cl-clivus. (b) Ps-pituitary stalk; mtl - medial temporal lobe; on - oculomotor nerve; mb-midbrain; an-abducent nerve; po-pons. (c) On-oculomotor nerve; mtl-medial temporal lobe; and sca-superior cerebellar artery. (d) Ps-pituitary stalk; ma-right mamillary body; ba- basillar artery; pca-posterior cerebral artery; and sca-superior cerebellar artery.

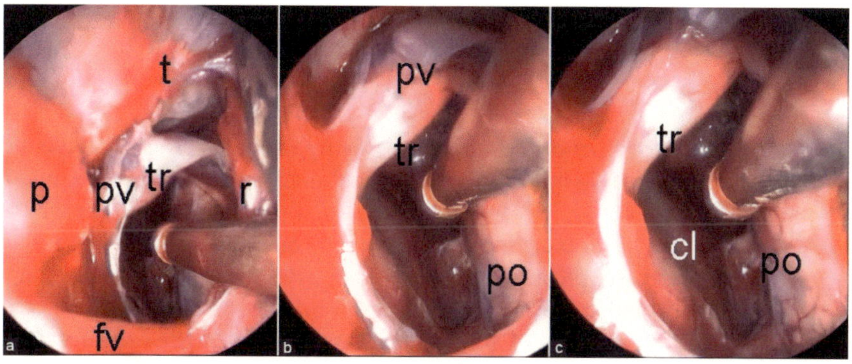

Figure 11.
Endoscopic view through a cerebellopontine angle approach showing upper pons. Fv-facial and vestibulo cochlear nerve complex; p - petrous; r-retractor; pv - petrosal vein, Tr -trigeminal nerve; Po - pons; Cl - clivus; and t – tentorium cerebelli.

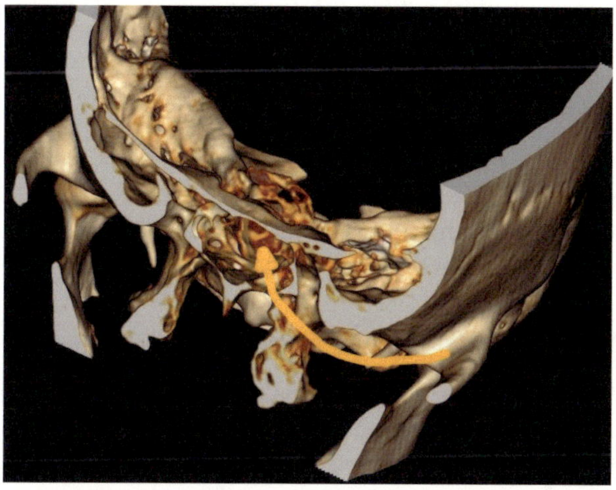

Figure 12.
Route of endoscopic transposition of vascularized TPTMF flap for CSF leak repair on a 3D reconstructed skull.

CSF rhinorrhoea, which commonly occurs as the result of trauma and iatrogenic disruption of the skull base as in EES & EEA and secondary to inflammation, neoplasm and pseudotumour syndromes, can be treated with endoscopic treatment. Skull base defects can be repaired with endoscopic remodeling of tissue planes and complete separation of the sinonasal cavities from the cranial space to carry out a multilayered reconstruction. Single layer of autologous fat or fascia, followed by tissue sealant may well be sufficient for small bony defects. Larger skull base defects with a high-volume intraoperative CSF leaks require robust closure with multiple layers. This multilayered closure can be achieved with an autologous fat graft in the bony defect followed by fascia lata, bony buttress and tissue sealant. These larger defects of skull base can be supplemented with a gasket seal closure [2, 63]. Currently, there are options of using multilayer closure with artificial dural substitutes and tissue sealants which work nicely in many cases. Sometimes, lack of vascularity may affect the integrity of the closure. Fortes et al. described endoscopic repair of CSF leak by transpterygoid transposition of a temporoparietal fascia flap [72] and Kawsar et al. showed good long-term outcome ranging from 6 months to 4 years in their small series. The pathway of the flap through the endoscopic route has been shown in **Figure 12** [73].

8. Endoscopic transsphenoidal surgery

8.1 Introduction

Gerard Guiot is recognized as the first neurosurgeon to use the endoscope in the transsphenoidal approach, although he abandoned the procedure because of inadequate visualization [74, 75]. In the late 1970s Apuzzo, et al. [76], as well as Bushe and Halves [77, 78], resurrected the application of endoscopes as a technical adjunct in the microscopic extirpation of pituitary lesions with extrasellar extension. Application of endoscopes was started initially to augment microsurgery, allowing the visualization of structures that were out of the line of vision; a view that were acquired with angled mirrors by other surgeons [75, 79]. Axel Perneczky, introduced the use of the endoscope in intracranial neurosurgery. He emphasized that endoscopic appreciation of micro-anatomy which may not be appreciated with microscope and pioneered the concept of minimally invasive neurosurgery [9, 80].

In the early 1990s, the pure endoscopic transsphenoidal technique was introduced as a result of the collaboration between neurological and otorhinolaryngological surgeons. In 1992 Jankowski and coworkers from the Central Hospital of the University of Nancy shared the experience of 3 cases of pituitary tumor in which they carried out a pure endoscopic transsphenoidal approach [81].

More recently, with other technical adjuncts such as neuronavigation and microvascular Doppler ultrasonography, endoscopic transsphenoidal surgery has been extended to the treatment of lesions outside the sella turcica, introducing the concept of extended approaches to the skull base [82, 83].

8.2 Operative procedure

The patient is intubated under general anesthesia, in supine position with the trunk elevated 10^0 and the head turned 10^0 towards the surgeon and fixed with three pin or tape in a horse-shoe headrest. Some surgeons prefer to fix with 3 pin rigid fixation and some do not; navigation is possible either way. Just before entering with the endoscope, the nasal cavities are packed with pledgets soaked in a diluted adrenaline. Some surgeons prefer cocaine or a mixture of cocaine and adrenaline. The operation can be divided in the following 3 phases.

8.2.1 Nasal phase

On entering with the endoscope, the main anatomical landmarks can be identified, such as the nasal septum medially and the inferior turbinate laterally (**Figure 13**). Following the tail of the inferior turbinate with the endoscope, choana can be reached, that is limited medially by the midline marker, vomer and, superiorly, by the floor of the sphenoid sinus.

The middle turbinate is gently pushed laterally to enlarge the virtual surgical corridor between the nasal septum and the middle turbinate. For a greater passage, some surgeons prefer to break and take the middle turbinate out, which can easily be avoided by lateralizing the turbinate. Looking upward with the endoscope, it is possible to identify the sphenoid ostium, usually located approximately 1.5 cm above the roof of the choana. If the sphenoid ostium is covered by either the superior or the supreme turbinate, these can be gently lateralized or removed, protecting the lateral lamella of the cribriform plate on which they are inserted. The removal or the lateral luxation of these turbinates should be done with extreme care in order to avoid ethmoidal plate injuries resulting in cerebrospinal fluid (CSF) leak.

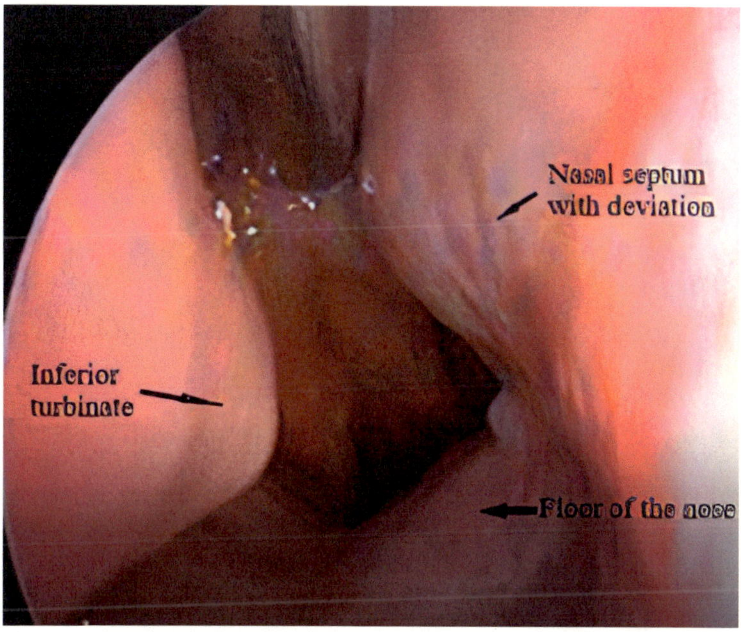

Figure 13.
Nasal stage of endoscopic pituitary surgery.

8.2.2 Sphenoid phase

To avoid arterial bleeding from septal branches of the sphenopalatine artery, the sphenoid phase of the procedure starts with the coagulation of the spheno-ethmoid recess and the area around the sphenoid ostium. The nasal septum is detached from the sphenoid rostrum by means of a microdrill. Subsequently, the anterior wall of the sphenoid sinus is widely opened with microdrill and Kerrison punches, proceeding circumferentially, with a caution not to overextend the opening in the inferolateral direction to avoid the damage to the sphenopalatine artery or its major branches.

It is important to widely expose and open the anterior face of the sphenoid to allow a proper working angle for the entire instrument when inside the sphenoid with their tips in the sella. After the removal of all the sphenoid septa, the posterior and lateral walls of the sphenoid sinus, with the sellar floor at the center, the spheno-ethmoid planum above it, and the clival indentation below, become visible. The bony prominences of the intracavernous carotid artery, the optic nerve and, between them, the optico-carotid recess can be visualized lateral to the sellar floor (**Figure 14**). The bony protuberances of the intracavernous carotid artery should be recognized to define the sellar floor boundaries, though the bony landmarks may not be properly identified in all cases. The superior and inferior intercavernous sinuses should be identified, bearing in mind that there are variations in anatomy and number of the intercavernous sinuses.

The sphenoid sinuses were classified into conchal, presellar and sellar types (there is also a description of mixed types) initially by Hammer and Radberg [84], a widely accepted classification as it can predict the surgical corridor used in transsphenoidal surgeries. Guldner *et al.* subdivided the sellar type into incomplete and complete types that were based on the extension of the pneumatization beyond the posterior wall of the sella [85, 86]. The modifications and the traditional system focus on the posterior extent of pneumatization and the ease of accessibility of the sellar floor during endoscopic endonasal resection.

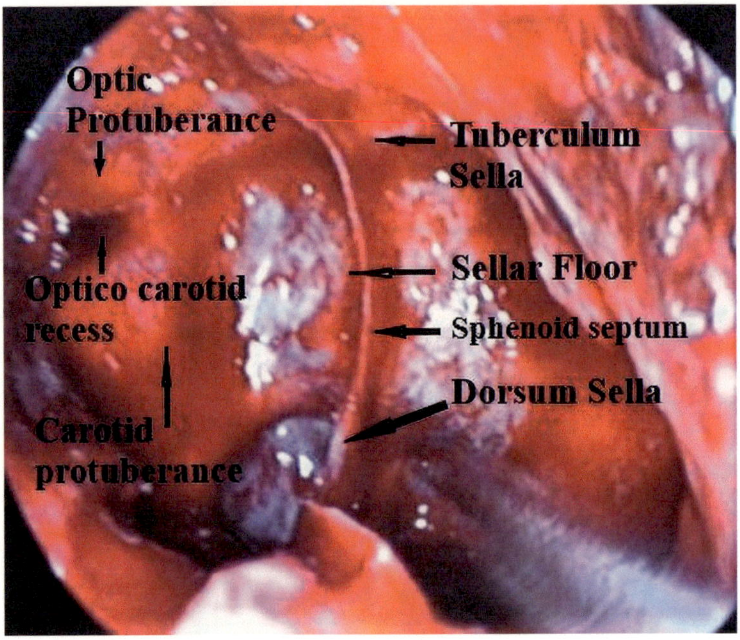

Figure 14.
End of sphenoidal phase of the pituitary surgery. The sellar floor is seen.

8.2.3 Sellar phase

From this phase of the procedure, the endoscope can be fixed to the holder, in order to free both of the surgeon's hands. Actually, it is our practice to continue using the endoscope free-hand, which is held dynamically by an assistant, while the surgeon can move the two instruments through one or both nostrils.

The sellar phase of the procedure (**Figure 15**) follows the same rules of the microsurgical transsphenoidal approach. Sellar floor opening is performed using a high-speed microdrill and a Kerrison rongeur usually extending the bone removal from one cavernous sinus to the other and from the tuberculum to the floor of the sella, although its shape and size could be tailored depending on lesion. Microdebrider can be another instrument which can be very helpful in removing the unwanted mucosal and bony debris. During such maneuvers a Doppler ultrasound probe will easily identify the carotid arteries, which will allow a safer opening of the dura that thereafter is incised in a midline position and in a rectangular, linear or cruciate fashion. In case of a macroadenoma, the inferior and lateral components of the lesion are removed before the superior aspect. This sequence will reduce the possibility of

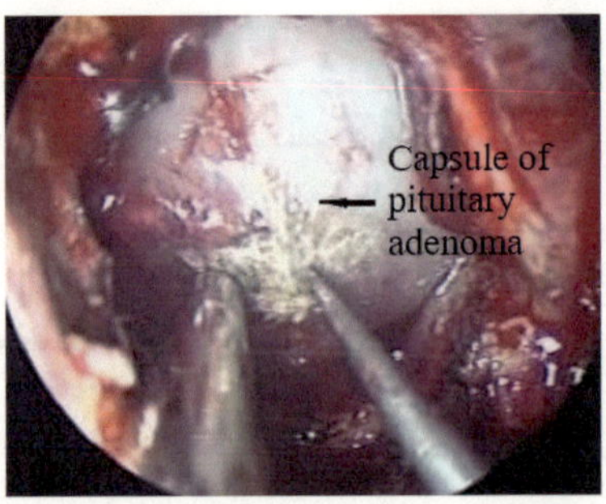

Figure 15.
Sellar stage of pituitary surgery. The capsule of pituitary tumor is exposed.

suprasellar cistern and the redundant diaphragma falling into the operative field and the lateral portions of the lesion will be less difficult to remove. Nevertheless, if the descent of the suprasellar portion of the lesion is not noted, a Valsalva maneuver is helpful to check the protrusion of the suprasellar cistern into the sellar cavity.

Besides, in case of microadenoma, dissecting tumor pseudocapsule from pituitary gland tissue is preferable for a complete 'en bloc' removal of the tumor, when possible, rather than performing an internal debulking [87]. This increases the chances of cure.

Finally, after removal of the lesion, an endoscopic exploration of the tumor cavity, by the means of a 0^0 and/or angled scope, is performed to assess for the presence of any tumor remnants. In case of hormone secreting tumors, the whole tumor needs to be removed to get a better outcome and angled scopes can contribute a great deal.

8.2.4 Sellar reconstruction

At the end of the procedure, especially in case of an intraoperative CSF leak, sellar repair is mandatory. Different methods of repair techniques are used (intra and/or extradural closure of the sella and packing of the sellar cavity with or without packing of the sphenoid sinus), based on the size of osteo-dural defect and of the space created following removal of the tumor inside the sella [88]. A number of dural substitute, tissue sealant and nasal packing are now available to secure the sellar reconstructions in place.

The aim of such a repair is to guarantee a watertight closure reducing the chance of CSF leak, reduce the dead space and prevent the descent of the chiasm into the sellar cavity. Nevertheless, overpacking has to be avoided to prevent compression of the optic system. Lumbar drainage is currently avoided, except in case of a minimal, unexpected post-operative CSF leak occurs. The endoscope is removed gradually, and the middle turbinate is gently put back in a medial direction. Packing of the nasal cavity is not used by most of the surgeons, though there are absorbable and non-absorbable packing are available.

8.3 Advantages

Transsphenoidal endoscopic resection of pituitary tumor brings a number of advantages to the patient like less nasal trauma, no nasal packing, less post-operative pain and usually quick recovery. The surgeon enjoys some advantages too, like wider and closer view of the surgical target area, recording of the operation for training and studying purposes for future improvement and more interdisciplinary cooperation etc. [89–91].

8.4 Complications

The study by Ciric et al. [92] which is regarded as the benchmark transsphenoidal surgery complication questionnaire pertaining to perioperative complications reported major morbidity in 1–2% of cases and postoperative CSF leaks in 3.9% of cases. The most experienced surgeons had better results with lower complication rates [93].

Lobatto et al. reported the postoperative incidence rates of CSF leaks between 1.4 and 16.9% in their systematic review where the higher body mass index (BMI) and younger age were risk factors for postoperative CSF leaks [94]. The reported incidence of DI ranges from 0.3–45% and is variable in part because of inconsistent definitions [95]. Two experienced pituitary groups who used accepted definitions for DI and whose surgical experience predominantly focused on endoscopic resection of pituitary adenomas have recently published their postoperative DI rates with fairly comparable results [96, 97]. In 178 and 271 patients respectively, both studies reported a DI incidence rate of 26% and 16.6% with only 10% and 4% progressing to permanent DI [96, 97].

While hypernatremia can lead to severe morbidity in the perioperative phase, delayed hyponatremia is the most common cause of unplanned readmission following pituitary tumor surgery [98]. Most delayed hyponatremia is a secondary consequence of inappropriate release of antidiuretic hormone (SIADH) and usually occurs between post-operative day 4 and 7 with a reported incidence of 3.6% to 19.8% [99–101].

Dysfunction of the hypothalamic–pituitary axis (HPA) remains a recognized clinical problem. The most life threatening of these problems is adrenal insufficiency with contemporary cases series reporting rates between 3% and 21% [102].

Excessive removal of nasal septum can result in loss of nasal structural support, resulting in external nasal deformity. This risk can be increased when extended approaches requiring nasal septal flap reconstruction are employed [103, 104]. Removal of significant posterior-superior portions of the nasal septum, its mucosa, and the adjacent superior and middle turbinate mucosa (structures which make up the olfactory cleft) can result in hyposmia, or worse, anosmia. Therefore, an adequate surgical corridor needs to be carefully created towards the sellar region while trying to preserve the above structures specially when nasoseptal flap is harvested [105, 106].

Injury to the ICA during sellar exposure or removal of the tumor is rare with reported incidence between 0.2 to 0.4% and is associated with significant morbidity [107]. The iatrogenic injury can result in severe stroke, disability or death [108]. Significant epistaxis requiring additional intervention can occur in the range of 3% of cases [109, 110].

Ciric et al. reported from the self –reported questionnaire survey that the mean operative mortality for all three groups was 0.9% [92]. Agam et al. recently (2019)

Surgery related complications	Sellar: • CSF rhinorrhoea • Internal carotid artery injury
	Orbital • Optic nerve injury • Diplopia • Blindness
	Nasal • Epistaxis
	Endocrinologic • Diabetes insipidus • Hypernatremia • Delayed Hyponatremia (SIADH) • Hypopituitarism
Medical complications (related to surgery)	• Bacterial Meningitis
Medical complications (indirectly related to surgery)	• Deep vein thrombosis • Pulmonary embolism

Table 3.
Complications of pituitary surgery.

reported only one case of mortality among 1153 cases, which is 0.1% perioperative death in their series [111].

Agam et al. reported patients with visual deficits and tumors which invades any surrounding structures are at higher risk of complication, is likely a caveat of more severe underlying disease [111]. Revision surgeries for prior transsphenoidal surgery, craniotomy and radiosurgery were also at higher risk for complications, likely because of fibrosis, adhesions and scarring that make the surgical environment more difficult (**Table 3**) [112].

9. Endoscopic application in aneurysm surgery

9.1 General roles of endoscope

The advantages of better illumination, clear views of regional anatomic features at close range and the extended viewing angles make the use of the endoscope a good adjunct or an independent alternative of microscope. Endoscope can be used in and around the operative field of aneurysms easier and safer. Furthermore, the endoscope facilitates confirmation of optimal clip positions [113].

In a cadaveric study by Chowdhury et al. the variations were identified and the authors concluded endonasal extended transsphenoidal approach can fully expose CW with brain in situ to observe the circle for variations and asymmetry (**Figures 16** and **17**) [114]. Taniguchi et al. reported in their series of 54 cases, the endoscope was used for further clarification of the detailed additional anatomy in 9 cases (16.7%). The surgeons reapplied the clip on the basis of endoscopic information which was gained after the initial clipping in 5 cases (9.3%) [115]. In a series of studies by Kalavakonda et al., the endoscope was used to observe anatomical features in 26 (33%) and clip position in 75 of 79 cases (95%). In 15 (19%) aneurysms, the important information like the neck and back wall of the aneurysm, parent artery, branches, perforators and the completeness of clipping of the neck and inclusion of the parent artery in the clip could be visualized via the endoscope. To complete the clipping of the residual neck or to avoid the inclusion of parent artery within the clip, the clip was repositioned in six cases, and to avoid compression of the optic nerve the clip position was reapplied in 1 case [116]. Fischer et al. reported, the endoscope was used to obtain additional topographic information before clipping in 150 of 180 cases (83%) [5, 117]. In 4 cases, clipping was achieved under endoscopic view. Following the clip application, endoscopic inspection was performed in 130 out of 180 procedures [113].

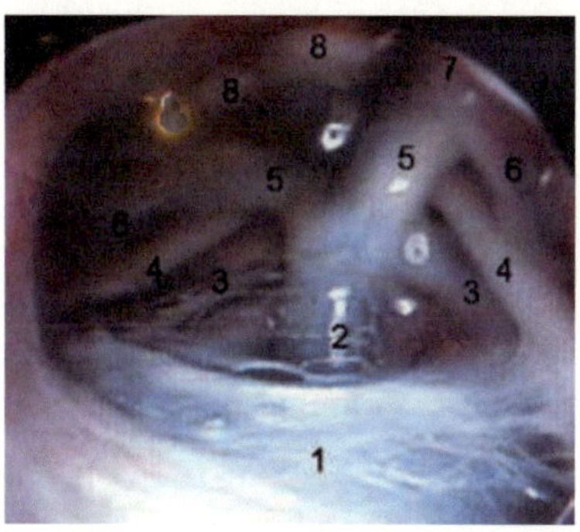

Figure 16.
Endoscopic view of posterior part of circle of Willils showing a number of anatomical variations. 1-Liliequist membrane, 2-basilar trunk, 3-SCA (left>right), 4-oculomotor nerve, 5-P1 (left>right), 6-P2 (left>right), 7-fetal type of Pcom & 8-mamillary bodies.

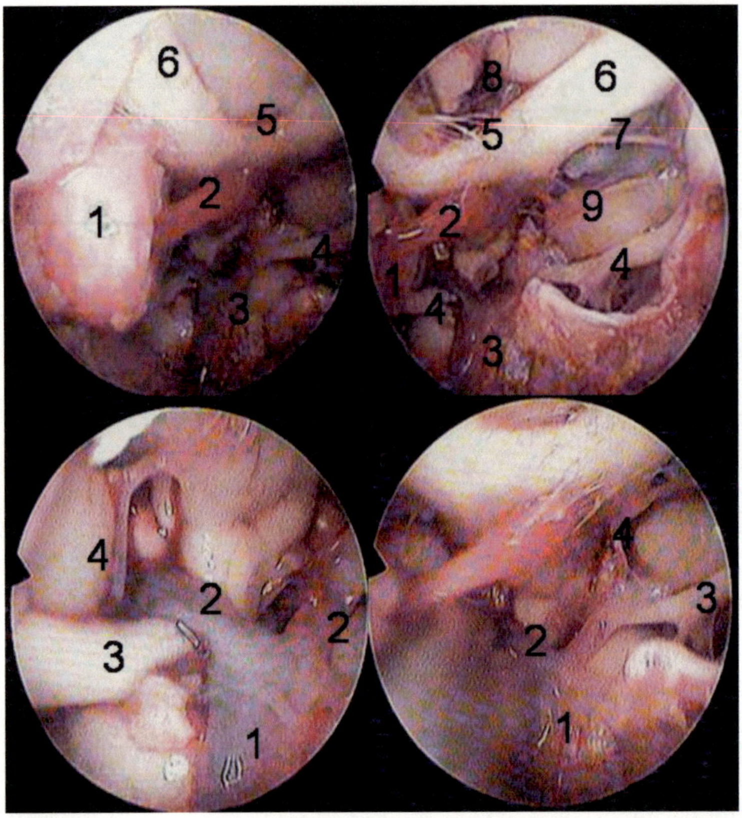

Figure 17.
Endoscopic view of interpeducular fossa and posterior part of CW after mobilization of pituitary gland to right cavernous sinus area. A) 1-pituitary gland (mobilized), 2-pituitary stalk. 3-basilar artery, 4 - oculomotor nerve, 5- optic chiasma & 6-optic nerve. B) 1- pituitary gland (mobilized), 2- pituitary stalk. 3- basilar artery, 4 - oculomotor nerve, 5- optic chiasma, 6-optic nerve, 7-proximal A1 and internal carotid artery, 8-Acom complex, & 9-medial temporal lobe. C) 1-basilar artery, 2-P1, 3-oculomotor nerve, & 4- medial temporal lobe. D) 1-basilar artery, 2-P1, 3-oculomotor nerve & 4-posterior communicating artery (Pcom)).

In general, very large and giant aneurysms gain fewer benefits from the endoscope than smaller ones in the same location, because the mass of the lesion compromises insertion and fixation of the endoscope in the operative field [118]. The endoscope is especially useful in the treatment of deeply located cerebral aneurysm. Hence the location is another important factor. The effectiveness of the endoscope for these aneurysms is limited in case of superficially located aneurysms like middle cerebral artery aneurysms and distal aneurysms such as pericallosal aneurysms [113]. The detailed approach to the aneurysms are beyond the scope of this chapter.

Endoscopic application may be associated with some disadvantages. The endoscope can cause rupture of the aneurysm during initial inspection. Blood in the operative field may make the endoscope useless and clot must be removed before proceeding. There is still a lack of instrumentation specifically designed for endoscopic surgery [116]. Three dimensional views were not available before, which has now been circumvented by newer version of 3D endoscopes.

10. Microvascular decompression

The presence of offending vessels, which often compress the relevant nerve at the root entry/exit zone (REZ) generally cause the primary trigeminal neuralgia

(TN), hemifacial spasm (HFS), and glossopharyngeal neuralgia [119–121]. Microvascular decompression (MVD) is a well-established and effective treatment supported by many studies [122, 123].

Endoscopic techniques such as endoscopic or endoscope-assisted MVD (EMVD) have been used for MVD operations. Meanwhile, as the technique matures and the surgeons attain experience with endoscopic operation, some disadvantages of Microscopic MVD (MMVD) can be overcome. Though many neurosurgeons have not find EMVD is superior to MMVD as the access for MMVD can be small and the offending vessels can be separated easily through that, several authors indicated the superior efficacy of endoscopic or endoscope assisted surgery in locating the offending site of neurovascular conflict when compared with the microscopic surgery [124–126].

Regarding TN, the lateral pontomesencephalic segment of the SCA usually runs medial to the trigeminal nerve and the nerve can be compressed in a rostromedial direction [127, 128]. Through an endoscopic approach, the lateral pontomesencephalic segment of the SCA can be transposed rostromedially and fixed at the cerebellar tentorium. An approach with the thirty degree endoscope through the lateral tentorial surface of the cerebellum via a keyhole provides excellent exposure of the trigeminal nerve from the REZ to the Meckel's cave. This can also show the course of the lateral pontomesencephalic segment of the SCA as the offending artery along the midbrain while requiring neither brain retraction nor ligation of the petrosal vein [129]. A clear endoscopic view also allows visualization of the perforators from the lateral pontomesencephalic segment of the SCA. Perforators from the lateral pontomesencephalic segment of the SCA are relatively long which helps transposition to fixation at the tentorium.

For HFS, the REZ of the facial nerve is located immediately medial to cranial nerve VIII in the supraolivary fossette, and the flocculus exits just lateral to cranial nerve VIII [127, 128]. The REZ of the facial nerve is often compressed by the lateral pontomedullary segment of the AICA from a caudal direction [127, 128]. The AICA can be transposed caudally and fixed at the petrosal dura mater by endoscopic approach. A 30^0 or 45^0 view of endoscopes through the petrosal surface of the cerebellum via a retrosigmoid keyhole clearly demonstrates the neurovascular structures and relationship around the supraolivary fossette behind the flocculus. The REZ of the facial nerve is readily identified after mobilization of the AICA as the offending artery. The endoscope also clearly demonstrates small perforators even behind obstacles [130], and secure recognition of perforators contributes to avoidance of injury during decompression procedures, especially for the transposition technique.

In the meta-analysis by Li et al., it is shown that, EMVD was superior considering the perioperative safety as with less perioperative complications [131]. Facial paralysis was significantly low in EMVD, and CSF leak and dysaudia (defective articulation stemming from auditory disability) also showed a similar trend with the previous discussions [132, 133]. Postoperative efficacy like recent remission rate, long-term remission rate, and offending vessel discovery rate was also superior to MMVD. The data from the series of Li et al. favored EMVD as the preferred method of surgery for MVD for the management of trigeminal or glossopharyngeal neuralgia and facial spasm [131].

11. Endoscopic operation for craniosynostosis

Jimenez and colleagues [134, 135] pioneered MIS treatment of craniosynostosis. Endoscopy-assisted craniosynostosis surgery (EACS) before the age of 6 months can correct this condition while combined with postoperative helmet molding therapy. The optimal age for EACS is 3 months. The procedure is essentially strip craniectomy and can be carried out with a standard surgical instrument and a 0° endoscope with a working shaft used for endoscopic facial lift surgery without irrigation.

In scaphocephaly, the craniectomy is performed from the anterior fontanelle to the posterior one. The softer skull bone at this young age can be cut with strong scissors. The removed strip should be 4–5 cm wide and 11 cm long. Lateral barrel stave osteotomies or wedge-shaped osteotomies can be added behind the coronal suture and in front of the lambdoid sutures. Moreover the complication rate is reportedly low. Blood transfusion was required only in 9% of 139 patients. The children required to wear a helmet within 3 weeks postoperatively for 10 months. Special attention is given for possible pressure ulcerations or eczema, but skin complications are rare [2, 7, 135]. The reported studies showed that endoscopic approach has a good outcome with low reported complication rate and good success rate.

12. Evacuation of ICH: endoscopic and endoscope-assisted

Endoscope-Assisted Evacuation describes the creation of a small craniotomy or craniectomy with stereotactic introduction of a port or sheath to the hematoma followed by evacuation with the endoscope and a suction device or a combination device where the suction device is there side by side in the lumen of the sheath which is even less traumatic. Kim et al. performed a prospective study in 2009 evaluating endoscope-assisted evacuation in the treatment of patients with small ICH of less than 30 cm^3 of volume and limited to the basal ganglia and thalamus [136]. Between the two groups, 204 patients in one group underwent stereotactic guided active evacuation and 103 patients in the other group were managed with conservative management. Patients that underwent endoscope assisted evacuation had mRS scores of 1.2 and medically managed group has an mRS scores of 3.0 at 180 days after initial presentation which obviously representing superiority of endoscopic assisted surgery [137].

Endoscopic evacuation is one of the earliest studies to investigate active MIS ICH evacuation using only endoscopes. Auer et al. published in 1989 demonstrating a significant benefit in favor of endoscopic evacuation, though in a single-center trial [138]. Investigators randomized 100 patients (within 48 hours from onset) with CT-proven supratentorial ICH greater than 10 cm^3 and altered level of consciousness. Most patients had a 50 to 70% reduction of the volume of hematoma after endoscope-assisted surgery and experienced significantly lower mortality and morbidity rates when compared to the medically managed cohort (30 and 60% versus 70 and 75%). The cohort of patients, who were benefitted most from the procedure, had hemorrhages with a volume under 50 cm^3 and age under 60 years [137].

13. Future perspectives

In this era of minimally invasive surgery, the future of neuroendoscopic surgery is likely to be bright as in other surgical superspecialities. The field will benefit from further miniaturization of cameras and optical technology with improvement of lenses with 3D technological improvement, innovations in surgical instrumentation design, the introduction of new navigation or robotics systems, new technological advances such as multiport endoscopic surgery, and an enhanced ability to perform endoscope-assisted microsurgery with bimanual microdissection. With ongoing development of endoscopic instruments and advanced surgical techniques including multiport approaches, endoscopic surgery will be expanded beyond intraventricular and skull base lesions to intraparenchymal brain lesions. Other goals are telemanipulated neurosurgery with supervisory-controlled robotic systems, shared control systems, and even fully robotic telesurgery which can be operated by a panel of surgeons from different parts of the country or the world. Nanotechnology developments are needed to address future indications for minimally or even ultramicro-access neurosurgery.

In the future, neuroendoscopy is expected to become routine with further expansion in various aspects of modern neurosurgical practice. Institutions should develop training programs for young neurosurgeons [7].

14. Conclusion

From this chapter we learn how versatile the endoscopic approach can be in neurosurgery. As the scope of the chapter is limited, elaborate details could not be described. But the common approaches are mentioned and recent advancements are described. Some future directions are also described. This is how this chapter should benefit the trainees and the neurosurgeons.

Author details

Khandkar Ali Kawsar
Consultant Neurosurgeon, The Royal Infirmary of Edinburgh, UK

*Address all correspondence to: drkawsar@yahoo.com

References

[1] Li KW, Nelson C, Suk I, Jallo GI. Neuroendoscopy: past, present, and future. Neurosurg Focus. 2005;19:E1.

[2] Sgouros S. Neuroendoscopy: current status and future trends. ed 1. Heidelberg: Springer Science & Business Media; 2013.

[3] Walker ML. History of ventriculostomy. Neurosurg Clin N Am. 2001;12:101-110. viii.

[4] de Divitiis E, Cappabianca P, Cavallo LM. Endoscopic transsphenoidal approach: adaptability of the procedure to different sellar lesions. Neurosurgery. 2002;51:699-705. discussion 705-707.

[5] Mixter WJ. Ventriculoscopy and puncture of the floor of the third ventricle: preliminary report of a case. Boston Med Surg J. 1923;188:277-278.

[6] Teo C & Mobbs R: Neuroendoscopy / Chapter 10 / Principals of Neurosurgery. Available from: https://www.researchgate.net/publication/306379195_ Neuroendoscopy_ Chapter_10_Principals_of_ Neurosurgery

[7] Shim KW, Park EK, Kim DS, Cho JU. Neuroendoscopy : Current and Future Perspectives. J Korean Neurosurg Soc 60 (3) : 322-326, 2017

[8] Yokoh A, Sugita K, Kobayashi S. Intermittent versus continuous brain retraction: an experimental study. *J Neurosurg* 1983; 58: 918-23.

[9] Perneczky A, Fries G. Endoscope-assisted brain surgery: Part I Evolution, basic concept, and current technique. *Neurosurgery* 1998; 42: 219-25.

[10] Teo C. Endoscopic-assisted tumour and neurovascular procedures. *Clin Neurosurg* 2000; 46: 515-25.

[11] Siomin V & Constantini S, Basic principles and equipment in neuroendoscopy. Neurosurg Clin N Am 15 (2004) 19-31.

[12] Alberti O, Riegel T, Hellwig D, Bertalanffy H. Frameless navigation and endoscopy. *J Neurosurg* 2001; 95: 541-3.

[13] André Grotenhuis Neuroendoscopic Instruments and Surgical Technique. S. Sgouros (ed.), Neuroendoscopy, 81 DOI 10.1007/978-3-642-39085-2_7, © Springer-Verlag Berlin Heidelberg 2014.

[14] Nulsen FE, Spitz EB : Treatment of hydrocephalus by direct shunt from ventricle to jugular vain. Surg Forum 1951 : 399-403.

[15] Vries JK : An endoscopic technique for third ventriculostomy. Surg Neurol 9 : 165-168, 1978.

[16] Jones RF, Stening WA, Brydon M : Endoscopic third ventriculostomy. Neurosurgery 26 : 86-91; discussion 91-92, 1990.

[17] Jones RF, Kwok BC, Stening WA, Vonau M : Neuroendoscopic third ventriculostomy. A practical alternative to extracranial shunts in non-communicating hydrocephalus. Acta Neurochir Suppl 61 : 79-83, 1994.

[18] Mugamba J, Stagno V, Indication for Endoscopic Third Ventriculostomy, World Neurosurgery, Volume 79, Issue 2, Supplement, 2013, Pages S20.e19-S20.e23, ISSN 1878-8750, https://doi.org/10.1016/j.wneu.2012.02.016.

[19] Sufianov A, Sufianova G, Iakimov I. Neuroendoscopic procedures in achievement of shunt independence: Outcome analysis of 28 patients with shunt malfunction. Minimally Invasive Neurosurgery. 2008;51:158-164.

[20] Unal TC, Aydoseli A; Endoscopic Third Ventriculostomy. 2018, Intechopen.75394.

[21] Saint-Rose C, Cinalli G, Roux FE, et al. Management of hydrocephalus in paediatric patients with posterior fossa tumours; the role of endoscopic third ventriculostomy. J Neurosurg 2001; 95: 791-7.

[22] Barlow P, Ching HS. An economic argument in favour of endoscopic third ventriculostomy as a treatment for obstructive hydrocephalus. Minim Invas Neurosurg 1997; 40: 37-9.

[23] Hader WJ, Drake J, Cochrane D, Sparrow O, Johnson ES, Kestle J. Death after late failure of third ventriculostomy in children. Report of three cases. J Neurosurg 2002; 97: 211-15.

[24] Tisell M, Almstrom O, Stephenson H, Tullberg M, Wikkelson C. How effective is endoscopsic third ventriculostomy in treating adult hydrocephalus caused by primary aqueductal stenosis? Neurosurgery 2000; 46: 104-9.

[25] Brockmeyer D, Abtin K, Carey L, Walker ML. Endoscopic third ventriculostomy: an outcome analysis. Paediatr Neurosurg 1998; 28: 236-40.

[26] Andresen M. and Juhler M.: Multiloculated hydrocephalus: A review of current problems in classification and treatment. Childs. Nerv. Syst., Mar., 28 (3): 357-62, 2012.

[27] Reinprecht A., Dietrich W. and Berger A.: Posthemorrhagic hydrocephalus in preterm infants: Long term follow-up and shunt related complications. Child's Nerv. Syst., 17: 663-9, 2001.

[28] Spennato P, Cinalli G, Carannante G., Ruggiero C. and Del ML: Multiloculated hydrocephalus. In: Cinalli G., Maixner W.J., Sainte-Rose C., editors. Pediatric Hydrocephalus. Milan: Springer, p. 219-44, 2004.

[29] El-Tantawy MH, Endoscopic Fenestration of Multiloculated Post-Infectious Hydrocephalus, Med. J. Cairo Univ., Vol. 86, No. 6, September: 2995-3002, 2018 www. medicaljournalofcairouniversity.net

[30] Spennato P, Cinalli G, Ruggiero C, Aliberti F, Trischitta V., Cianciulli E. and Maggi G.: Neuroendoscopic treatment of multiloculated hydrocephalus in children. J. Neurosurg., 106: 29-35, 2007.

[31] El-Ghandour NM: Endoscopic cyst fenestration in the treatment of multiloculated hydrocephalus in children. J. Neurosurg. Pediatr., Mar., 1 (3): 217-22, 2008.

[32] Akbari SH, Holekamp TF, Murphy TM, Mercer D, Leonard JR, Smyth MD, Park TS and Limbrick DD. Jr.: Surgical management of complex multiloculated hydrocephalus in infants and children. Childs. Nerv. Syst., Feb., 31 (2): 243-9, 2015.

[33] Oi S, Abbott R : Loculated ventricles and isolated compartments in hydrocephalus: their pathophysiology and the efficacy of neuroendoscopic surgery. Neurosurg Clin N Am 15 : 77-87, 2004.

[34] Robinson RG. Congenital cysts of the brain: arachnoid malformations. Prog Neurol Surg. 1971;4: 133-174 (doi:10.1159/000391818).

[35] Hanieh A, Simpson DA, North JB. Arachnoid cysts: a critical review of 41 cases. Childs Nerv Syst. 1988;4(2):92-96.

[36] Fernández Molina G. Neuroendoscopic management of middle fossa arachnoid cysts. World Neurosurg. 2013;79(2):S19.e19-23.

[37] Oertel J, Linsler S, Wagner W, Gaab M, Schroeder H, Rediker J. Endoscopic Treatment of Intracranial Arachnoid Cysts: A Retrospective Analysis of a 25-Year Experience (Case Series), Operative Neurosurgery. October, 2020. Downloaded from https://academic.oup.com/ons/advance-article/doi/10.1093/ons/opaa292/5918037

[38] Gangemi M, Seneca V, Colella G, Cioffi V, Imperato A, Maiuri F. Endoscopy versus microsurgical cyst excision and shunting for treating intracranial arachnoid cysts. J Neurosurg Pediatr. 2011;8(2):158-164.

[39] Karabagli H, Etus V. Success of pure neuroendoscopic technique in the treatment of Sylvian arachnoid cysts in children. Childs Nerv Syst. 2012;28(3):445-452.

[40] Wang C, Liu C, Xiong Y, Han G, et al. Surgical treatment of intracranial arachnoid cyst in adult patients. Neurol India. 2013;61(1):60-64.

[41] Guiot G. Ventriculo-cisternostomy for stenosis of the aqueduct of Sylvis. *Acta Neurochir (Wien)* 1973; 28: 275-89.

[42] Di Rocco F, Yoshino M, Oi S : Neuroendoscopic transventricular ventriculocystostomy in treatment for intracranial cysts. J Neurosurg 103(1 Suppl) : 54-60, 2005

[43] Fukushima T, Ishijima B, Hirakawa K, Nakamura N, Sano K : Ventriculofiberscope: a new technique for endoscopic diagnosis and operation. Technical note. J Neurosurg 38 : 251-256, 1973.

[44] Perneczky A, Muller-Forell W, van Lindert E, Fries G. Keyhole Concept in Neurosurgery. Stuttgart: Thieme; 1999: 120-48.

[45] Wallner KR, Gonzales M, Sheline GE. Treatment of oligodendrogliomas with or without post-operative irradiation. J Neurosurg 1988; 68: 684-8.

[46] Garcia DM, Fulling KH. Juvenile pilocytic astrocytomas of the cerebrum in adults. A distinctive neoplasm with favorable prognosis. J Neurosurg 1985; 63: 382-6.

[47] Jacques S, Shelden CH, McCann GD, Freshwater DB, Rand R: Computerized three-dimensional stereotaxic removal of small central nervous system lesions in patients. J Neurosurg 53:816-820, 1980.

[48] Shelden CH, McCann G, Jacques S, Lutes HR, Frazier RE, Katz R, et al: Development of a computerized microstereotaxic method for localization and removal of minute CNS lesions under direct 3-D vision: technical report. J Neurosurg 52:21-27, 1980.

[49] Otsuki T, Jokura H, Yoshimoto T: Stereotactic guiding tube for open-system endoscopy: a new approach for the stereotactic endoscopic resection of intra-axial brain tumours. Neurosurgery 27:326-330, 1990

[50] Kassam AB, Engh JA, Mintz AH, Prevede llo DM. Completely endoscopic resection of intraparenchymal brain tumours J. Neurosurg. / Vol 110 / January, 2009

[51] Kelly PJ, Goerss SJ, Kall BA: The stereotaxic retractor in computer-assisted stereotaxic microsurgery. J Neurosurg 69:301– 306, 1988

[52] Kelly PJ, Kall BA, Goerss S, Earnest F: Computer-assisted stereotaxic laser resection of intra-axial brain neoplasms. J Neurosurg 64:427-439, 1986

[53] Russell SM, Kelly PJ: Volumetric stereotaxy and the supratentorial occipitosubtemporal approach in the resection of posterior hippocampus and

parahippocampal gyrus lesions. Neurosurgery 50:978-988, 2002

[54] Teo C, Nakaji P: Application of endoscopy to the resection of intra-axial tumours. Op Tech Neursurg 8: 179-185, 2005

[55] Kawsar KA, Haque MR, Chowdhury FH. Avoidance and management of perioperative complications of endoscopic third ventriculostomy: the Dhaka experience. J Neurosurg. 2015 Dec;123(6):1414-9.

[56] Yamini B, Refai D, Rubin CM, Frim DM : Initial endoscopic management of pineal region tumours and associated hydrocephalus: clinical series and literature review. J Neurosurg 100(5 Suppl Pediatrics) : 437-441, 2004.

[57] Delalande O, Fohlen M : Disconnecting surgical treatment of hypothalamic hamartoma in children and adults with refractory epilepsy and proposal of a new classification. Neurol Med Chir (Tokyo) 43: 61-68, 2003.

[58] Choi JU, Yang KH, Kim TG, Chang JH, Chang JW, Lee BI, et al. : Endoscopic disconnection for hypothalamic hamartoma with intractable seizure. Report of four cases. J Neurosurg 100(5 Suppl Pediatrics) : 506-511, 2004.

[59] Rekate HL, Feiz-Erfan I, Ng YT, Gonzalez LF, Kerrigan JF : Endoscopic surgery for hypothalamic hamartomas causing medically refractory gelastic epilepsy. Childs Nerv Syst 22 : 874-880, 2006.

[60] Lewis AI, Crone KR, Taha J, *et al*. Surgical resection of third ventricle colloid cyst. Preliminary results comparing transcallosal microsurgery with endoscopy. *J Neurosurg* 1994; 81: 174-8.

[61] Gamea A, Fathi M, el-Guindy A. The use of the rigid endoscope in trans-sphenoidal pituitary surgery. *J Laryngol Otol* 1994; 108: 19-22.

[62] Carrau RL, Jho HD, Ko Y : Transnasal-transsphenoidal endoscopic surgery of the pituitary gland. Laryngoscope 106 : 914-918, 1996.

[63] Hadad G, Bassagasteguy L, Carrau RL et al (2006) A novel reconstructive technique after endoscopic expanded endonasal approaches: vascular pedicle nasoseptal flap. Laryngoscope 116(10):1882-1886.

[64] El-Sayed IH, Roediger FC, Goldberg AN, Parsa AT, McDermott MW (2008) Endoscopic reconstruction of skull base defects with the nasal septal flap. Skull Base 18(6):385-394.

[65] Roxbury CR, Ishii M, Gallia GL, Reh DD (2016) Endoscopic management of esthesioneuroblastoma. Otolaryngol Clin N Am 49(1):153-165.

[66] Sekhar LN, Sen C, Snyderman CH (1993) Anterior, anterolateral, and lateral approaches to extradural petroclival tumours. In: Sekhar LN, Janecka IP (eds) Surgery of cranial base tumours. Raven Press, New York.

[67] Zwagerman NT, Zenonos G, Lieber S, Wang WH, Wang EW, Fernandez-Miranda JC, Snyderman CH, Gardner PA. Endoscopic transnasal skull base surgery: pushing the boundaries, J Neurooncol, 2016.

[68] Wang X, Zhang X, Hu F et al (2016) Image-guided endoscopic endonasal transmaxillary transpterygoid approach to meckel's cave. Turkish Neurosurg 26(2):309-314.

[69] Raza SM, Donaldson AM, Mehta A, Tsiouris AJ, Anand VK, Schwartz TH (2014) Surgical management of trigeminal schwannomas: defining the role for endoscopic endonasal approaches. Neurosurg Focus 37(4):E17.

[70] Jouanneau E, Simon E, Jacquesson T et al (2014) The endoscopic endonasal approach to the Meckel's cave tumours: surgical technique and indications. World Neurosurg 82(6 Suppl):S155–S161.

[71] Chowdhury FH, Haque MR. Endoscopic assisted microsurgical removal of cerebello-pontine angle and prepontine epidermoid. J Neurosci Rural Pract. 2012 Sep;3(3):414-9. doi: 10.4103/0976-3147.102647. PMID: 23189019; PMCID: PMC3505358.

[72] Fortes FS, Carrau RL, Snyderman CH, Kassam A, Prevedello D, Vescan A, Mintz A, Gardner P. Transpterygoid transposition of a temporoparietal fascia flap: a new method for skull base reconstruction after endoscopic expanded endonasal approaches. Laryngoscope. 2007 Jun;117(6):970-6. doi: 10.1097/MLG.0b013e3180471482. PMID: 17417106.

[73] Kawsar KA, Land T, Tsermoulas G, Paluzzi A, Ahmed S. Novel Surgical Treatment of Recurrent CSF Leak by Temporoparietal Temporalis Myofascial Flap: A Series of 6 Cases. World Neurosurg. 2021 Mar;147:1-6. doi: 10.1016/j.wneu.2020.11.156. Epub 2020 Dec 5. PMID: 33290899.

[74] Guiot G, Rougerie J, Fourestier M, et al: Explorations endoscopiques intracraniennes. Presse Med 71: 1225-1228, 1963.

[75] Liu JK, Das K, Weiss MH, et al: The history and evolution of transsphenoidal surgery. J Neurosurg 95:1083-1096, 2001.

[76] Apuzzo MLJ, Heifetz M, Weiss MH, Kurze T: Neurosurgical endoscopy using the side-viewing telescope. Technical note. J Neurosurg 16:398-400, 1977.

[77] Bushe KA, Halves E: Modifizierte Technik bei transnasaler Operation der Hypophysengeschwulste. Acta Neurochir (Wien) 41:163-175, 1978.

[78] Halves E, Bushe KA: Transsphenoidal operation on craniopharyngiomas with extrasellar extensions. The advantage of the operating endoscope [proceedings]. Acta Neurochir Suppl 28: 362, 1979.

[79] Hardy J: La chirurgie de l'hypophyse par voie transspénoïdale. Union Med Can 96:702-712, 1967.

[80] Fries G, Perneczky A: Endoscope-assisted brain surgery: part 2— analysis of 380 procedures. Neurosurgery 42:226-232, 1998.

[81] Jankowski R, Auque J, Simon C, et al: Endoscopic pituitary tumour surgery. Laryngoscope 102:198-202, 1992

[82] Kaptain GJ, Vincent DA, Sheehan JP, et al: Transsphenoidal approaches for the extracapsular resection of midline suprasellar and anterior cranial base lesions. Neurosurgery 49:94-100, 2001.

[83] Locatelli D, Castelnuovo P, Santi L, et al: Endoscopic approaches to the cranial base: perspectives and realities. Childs Nerv Syst 16:686-691, 2000.

[84] Hammer G, Radberg C. The sphenoidal sinus. An anatomical and roentgenologic study with reference to transsphenoid hypophysectomy. Acta Radiol. 1962;56:401-22.

[85] Güldner C, Pistorius SM, Diogo I, Bien S, Sesterhenn A, Werner JA. Analysis of pneumatization and neurovascular structures of the sphenoid sinus using cone-beam tomography (CBT) Acta Radiol. 2012;53:214-9.

[86] Hiremath SB, Gautam AA, Sheeja K, Benjamin G. Assessment of variations in sphenoid sinus pneumatization in Indian population: A multidetector computed tomography study. Indian J

Radiol Imaging. 2018 Jul-Sep; 28(3): 273-279.

[87] Oldfield EH, Vortmeyer AO (2006) Development of a histological pseudocapsule and its use as a surgical capsule in the excision of pituitary tumours. J Neurosurg 104:7-19 (Medline)

[88] Cappabianca P, Cavallo LM, Esposito F, Valente V, de Divitiis E (2002) Sellar repair in endoscopic endonasal transsphenoidal surgery: results of 170 cases. Neurosurgery 51:1365-1371 (discussion 1371-1362, Medline).

[89] Spencer WR, Das K, Nwagu C et al (1999) Approaches to the sellar and parasellar region: anatomic comparison of the microscope versus endoscope. Laryngoscope 109:791-794 (Medline).

[90] Snyderman C, Kassam A, Carrau R, Mintz A, Gardner P, Prevedello DM (2007) Acquisition of surgical skills for endonasal skull base surgery: a training program. Laryngoscope 117:699-705.

[91] Cappabianca P, Cavallo LM, Divitiis OD, Solari D, Esposito F, Colao A. Endoscopic pituitary surgery. Pituitary (2008) 11:385-390.

[92] Ciric I, Ragin A, Baumgartner C, Pierce D: Complications of transsphenoidal surgery: results of a national survey, review of the literature, and personal experience. Neurosurgery 40:225-237, 1997.

[93] Barker FG II, Klibanski A, Swearingen B: Transsphenoidal surgery for pituitary tumours in the United States, 1996-2000: mortality, morbidity, and the effects of hospital and surgeon volume. J Clin Endocrinol Metab 88:4709-4719, 2003.

[94] Lobatto, D.J., de Vries, F., Zamanipoor Najafabadi, A.H. *et al.* Preoperative risk factors for postoperative complications in endoscopic pituitary surgery: a systematic review. *Pituitary* **21,** 84-97 (2018).

[95] Abhinav K, Tyler M, Dale OT, Mohyeldin A, Fernandez-Miranda JC & Katznelson L. (2020) Managing complications of endoscopic transsphenoidal surgery in pituitary adenomas, Expert Review of Endocrinology & Metabolism, 15:5, 311-319.

[96] Ajlan AM, Abdulqader SB, Achrol AS, et al. Diabetes Insipidus following Endoscopic Transsphenoidal Surgery for Pituitary Adenoma. J Neurol Surg B Skull Base. 2018 Apr;79(2):117-122. doi: 10.1055/s-0037-1604363.

[97] Nayak P, Montaser AS, Hu J, et al. Predictors of Postoperative Diabetes Insipidus Following Endoscopic Resection of Pituitary Adenomas. J Endocr Soc. 2018 Sep 1; 2(9):1010-1019.

[98] Bohl MA, Ahmad S, Jahnke H, et al. Delayed Hyponatremia Is the Most Common Cause of 30-Day Unplanned Readmission After Transsphenoidal Surgery for Pituitary Tumours. Neurosurgery. 2016 Jan;78(1):84-90.

[99] Barber SM, Liebelt BD, Baskin DS. Incidence, Etiology and Outcomes of Hyponatremia after Transsphenoidal Surgery: Experience with 344 Consecutive Patients at a Single Tertiary Center. J Clin Med. 2014 Oct 28;3(4):1199-219. doi: 10.3390/jcm3041199.

[100] Hussain NS, Piper M, Ludlam WG, et al. Delayed postoperative hyponatremia after transsphenoidal surgery: prevalence and associated factors. JNeurosurg. 2013 Dec;119(6):1453-60. doi: 10.3171/2013.8.JNS13411. PubMed PMID: 24053496.

[101] Jahangiri A, Wagner J, Han SW, et al. Morbidity of repeat transsphenoidal surgery assessed in more than 1000 operations. J Neurosurg. 2014 Jul;121(1):67-74. doi: 10.3171/2014.3.JNS131532. PubMed PMID: 24834943.

[102] Little AS, Kelly DF, White WL, et al. Results of a prospective multicenter controlled study comparing surgical outcomes of microscopic versus fully endoscopic transsphenoidal surgery for nonfunctioning pituitary adenomas: the Transsphenoidal Extent of Resection (TRANSSPHER) Study. J Neurosurg. 2019 Mar 22:1-11.

[103] Rowan NR, Valappil B, Chen J, et al. Prospective characterization of postoperative nasal deformities in patients undergoing endoscopic endonasal skull-base surgery. Int Forum Allergy Rhinol. 2019 Oct 30. doi: 10.1002/alr.22466. PubMed PMID: 31665569.

[104] Rowan NR, Wang EW, Gardner PA, et al. Nasal Deformities Following Nasoseptal Flap Reconstruction of Skull Base Defects. J Neurol Surg B Skull Base. 2016 Feb;77(1):14-8. doi: 10.1055/s-0035-1555136. PubMed PMID: 26949583; PubMed Central PMCID: PMCPMC4777617.

[105] Harvey RJ, Malek J, Winder M, et al. Sinonasal morbidity following tumour resection with and without nasoseptal flap reconstruction. Rhinology. 2015 Jun;53(2):122-8. doi: 10.4193/Rhin14.247. PubMed PMID: 26030034.

[106] Harvey RJ, Winder M, Davidson A, et al. The Olfactory Strip and Its Preservation in Endoscopic Pituitary Surgery Maintains Smell and Sinonasal Function. J Neurol Surg B Skull Base. 2015 Dec;76(6):464-70.

[107] Perry A, Graffeo CS, Meyer J, et al. Beyond the Learning Curve: Comparison of Microscopic and Endoscopic Incidences of Internal Carotid Injury in a Series of Highly Experienced Operators. World Neurosurg. 2019 Nov;131:e128-e135. doi: 10.1016/j.wneu.2019.07.074. PubMed PMID: 31319187.

[108] Chin OY, Ghosh R, Fang CH, et al. Internal carotid artery injury in endoscopic endonasal surgery: A systematic review. Laryngoscope. 2016 Mar;126(3):582-90. doi: 10.1002/lary.25748. PubMed PMID: 26525334.

[109] De Los Reyes KM, Gross BA, Frerichs KU, et al. Incidence, risk factors and management of severe post-transsphenoidal epistaxis. J Clin Neurosci. 2015 Jan;22(1):116-22. doi: 10.1016/j.jocn.2014.07.004. PubMed PMID: 25150759.

[110] Alzhrani G, Sivakumar W, Park MS, et al. Delayed Complications After Transsphenoidal Surgery for Pituitary Adenomas. World Neurosurg. 2018Jan;109:233-241.

[111] Agam MS, Wedemeyer MA, Wrobel B, Weiss MH, Carmichael JD, Zada G. Complications associated with microscopic and endoscopic transsphenoidal pituitary surgery: experience of 1153 consecutive cases treated at a single tertiary care pituitary center. J Neurosurg 130:1576-1583, 2019

[112] Esquenazi Y, Essayed WI, Singh H, Mauer E, Ahmed M, Christos PJ, et al: Endoscopic endonasal versus microscopic transsphenoidal surgery for recurrent and/or residual pituitary adenomas. World Neurosurg 101:186-195, 2017.

[113] Yoshioka H, Kinouchi H. The Roles of Endoscope in Aneurysmal Surgery. Neurol Med Chir (Tokyo). 2015;55(6):469-478. doi:10.2176/nmc.ra.2014-0428.

[114] Chowdhury FH, Haque MR, Kawsar KA, Ara S, Mohammod QD,

Sarker MH, Goel AH. Endoscopic endonasal transsphenoidal exposure of circle of Willis (CW); can it be applied in vascular neurosurgery in the near future? A cadaveric study of 26 cases. Turk Neurosurg. 2012;22(1):68-76. doi: 10.5137/1019-5149.JTN.4887-11.2. PMID: 22274974.

[115] Taniguchi M, Takimoto H, Yoshimine T, Shimada N, Miyao Y, Hirata M, Maruno M, Kato A, Kohmura E, Hayakawa T: Application of a rigid endoscope to the microsurgical management of 54 cerebral aneurysms: results in 48 patients. J Neurosurg 91: 231– 237, 1999.

[116] Kalavakonda C, Sekhar LN, Ramachandran P, Hechl P: Endoscope-assisted microsurgery for intracranial aneurysms. Neurosurgery 51: 1119– 1126; discussion 1126-1127, 2002.

[117] Fisher G, Oertel J, Perneczky A. Endoscopy in aneurysm surgery. Neurosurgery 70(ONS Supple 2): ons184– ons191, 2012.

[118] Galzio RJ, Di Cola F, Raysi Dehcordi S, Ricci A, De Paulis D: Endoscope-assisted microneurosurgery for intracranial aneurysms. Front Neurol 4: 201, 2013.

[119] Haines SJ, Jannetta PJ, Zorub DS. Microvascular relations of the trigeminal nerve. An anatomical study with clinical correlation. J Neurosurg. 1980;52: 381-386.

[120] Antonini G, Di Pasquale A, Cruccu G, et al. Magnetic resonance imaging contribution for diagnosing symptomatic neurovascular contact in classical trigeminal neuralgia: a blinded casecontrol study and meta-analysis. Pain. 2014;155: 1464-1471.

[121] Campos-Benitez M, Kaufmann AM. Neurovascular compression findings in hemifacial spasm. J Neurosurg. 2008;109:416-420.

[122] Pollock BE, Schoeberl KA. Prospective comparison of posterior fossa exploration and stereotactic radiosurgery dorsal root entry zone target as primary surgery for patients with idiopathic trigeminal neuralgia. Neurosurgery. 2010;67:633-638 [discussion: 8-9].

[123] Apra C, Lefaucheur JP, Le Guerinel C. Microvascular decompression is an effective therapy for trigeminal neuralgia due to dolichoectatic basilar artery compression: case reports and literature review. Neurosurg Rev. 2017;40:577-582.

[124] Duntze J, Litre CF, Eap C, et al. Adjunctive use of endoscopy during microvascular decompression in the cerebellopontine angle: 27 case reports. Neurochirurgie. 2011;57:68-72 [in French].

[125] Chen MJ, Zhang WJ, Yang C, Wu YQ, Zhang ZY, Wang Y. Endoscopic neurovascular perspective in microvascular decompression of trigeminal neuralgia. J Craniomaxillofac Surg. 2008;36:456-461.

[126] Burchiel KJ, Clarke H, Haglund M, Loeser JD. Long-term efficacy of microvascular decompression in trigeminal neuralgia. J Neurosurg. 1988;69: 35-38.

[127] Hitotsumatsu T, Matsushima T, Inoue T. Microvascular decompression for treatment of trigeminal neuralgia, hemifacial spasm, and glossopharyngeal neuralgia: three surgical approach variations: technical note. Neurosurgery 2003;53(6):1436-1441; discussion 1442-1443.

[128] Martin RG, Grant JL, Peace D, Theiss C, Rhoton AL Jr. Microsurgical relationships of the anterior inferior cerebellar artery and the facialvestibulocochlear nerve complex. Neurosurgery 1980;6(5):483-507.

[129] Komatsu F, Komatsu M, Di Ieva A, Tschabitscher M. Endoscopic approaches to the trigeminal nerve and clinical consideration for trigeminal schwannomas: a cadaveric study. J Neurosurg 2012;117(4):690-696.

[130] Ishikawa M, Tanaka Y, Watanabe E. Microvascular decompression under neuroendoscopic view in hemifacial spasm: rostral-type compression and perforator-type compression. Acta Neurochir (Wien) 2015;157(2):329-332; discussion 332.

[131] Li Y, Mao F, Cheng F, Peng C, Guo D, Wang B. A meta-analysis of endoscopic microvascular decompression versus microscopic microvascular decompression for the treatment for cranial nerve syndrome caused by vascular compression. World neurosurgery. 2019 Jun 1;126:647-55.

[132] Kabil MS, Eby JB, Shahinian HK. Endoscopic vascular decompression versus microvascular decompression of the trigeminal nerve. Minim Invasive Neurosurg. 2005;48:207-212.

[133] Badr-El-Dine M, El-Garem HF, Talaat AM, Magnan J. Endoscopically assisted minimally invasive microvascular decompression of hemifacial spasm. Otol Neurotol. 2002;23:122-128.

[134] Jimenez DF, Barone CM : Endoscopic craniectomy for early surgical correction of sagittal craniosynostosis. J Neurosurg 88 : 77-81, 1998.

[135] Jimenez DF, Barone CM, McGee ME, Cartwright CC, Baker CL : Endoscopy-assisted wide-vertex craniectomy, barrel stave osteotomies, and postoperative helmet molding therapy in the management of sagittal suture craniosynostosis. J Neurosurg 100(5 Suppl Pediatrics) : 407- 417, 2004.

[136] Kim YZ, Kim KH. Even in patients with a small hemorrhagic volume, stereotactic-guided evacuation of spontaneous intracerebral hemorrhage improves functional outcome. J Korean Neurosurg Soc. 2009;46:109-15.

[137] Hersh EH, Gologorsky Y, Chartrain AG, Mocco J, Kellner CP. Minimally invasive surgery for intracerebral hemorrhage. Current neurology and neuroscience reports. 2018 Jun 1;18(6):34.

[138] Auer LM, Deinsberger W, Niederkorn K, Gell G, Kleinert R, Schneider G, et al. Endoscopic surgery versus medical treatment for spontaneous intracerebral hematoma: a randomized study. J Neurosurg. 1989;70:530-5

Section 3

Cerebrovascular Diseases

Chapter 8

The History of Neurosurgical Management of Ischemic Stroke

Lydia Kaoutzani and Scott Y. Rahimi

Abstract

Stroke remains a major public health issue and the second leading cause of death worldwide. The Hippocratic Corpus used the word apoplexy to describe a person collapsing while retaining pulse and respiration. This is believed to be the first written description of stroke. The theories of what caused stroke evolved over the years. When autopsies were performed stroke was attributed to emboli and thrombi formation. Carotid endarterectomies (CEA) were then performed for the treatment of stroke. Originally CEA were seen with skepticism but the North American Symptomatic Carotid Endarterectomy trial (NASCET) and the European Carotid Surgery trial (ECS) helped restore their efficacy in the management of ischemic stroke. A milestone in the management of ischemic stroke was the use of intravenous tissue plasminogen activator (tPA). Secondary to the limitations of the use of tPA other avenues were sought which included intraarterial recombinant prourokinase and mechanical thrombectomy. The field of mechanical thrombectomy continues to be rapidly changing and evolving. Various randomized controlled trials and meta-analysis have been conducted in order to evaluate who will benefit from mechanical thrombectomies, the timing, the best device to use and the role of combining this intervention with the administration of intravenous tPA.

Keywords: Ischemic stroke, history of stroke, carotid endarterectomy, intravenous tissue plasminogen activator, endovascular mechanical thrombectomy

1. Introduction

The World Health Organization in 1980 defined stroke as "the rapidly developed clinical signs of focal (or global) disturbance of cerebral function, with symptoms lasting 24 hours or longer or leading to death, with no apparent cause other than of vascular origin" [1]. In 2013, the American Stroke Association for the 21st century came up with a new broader definition of stroke [2]. The new definition of stroke includes "brain, spinal cord, or retinal cell death attributable to ischemia, based on 1. pathological, imaging, or other objective evidence of cerebral, spinal cord, or retinal focal ischemic injury in a defined vascular distribution; or 2. clinical evidence of cerebral, spinal cord, or retinal focal ischemic injury based on symptoms persisting ≥24 hours or until death, and other etiologies excluded" [2]. Stroke is a major cause of morbidity and it remains the second leading cause of death worldwide after ischemic heart disease [3, 4]. Stroke is also the third most common cause of disability with significant increase in stroke burden in the world and especially in developing countries [5]. On average in the United States (U.S.) someone has a stroke every 40 seconds [6].

Stroke is divided into ischemic and hemorrhagic stroke. Hemorrhagic stroke is further divided into intracerebral and subarachnoid hemorrhage. Approximately 85% of all strokes are ischemic with the remaining 15% being hemorrhagic [7]. We have currently moved away from using terms such as "cerebrovascular accident" and "reversible ischemic neurologic deficit" [7].

Transient ischemic attacks (TIA) also known as "warning strokes" are defined by the American Heart Association and American Stroke association as "brief episodes of neurological dysfunction resulting from focal cerebral ischemia not associated with permanent cerebral infarction" [8]. Although it is difficult to count the exact numbers of patients suffering from TIAs, in the U.S. this number has been estimated to be 200,000–500,000 per year [8].

Ischemic stroke is the result of a blockade of the arteries that supply the brain. The most common criteria used for classifying the causes of ischemic stroke are the Trial of ORG 10172 in Acute Stroke Treatment (TOAST) criteria [9]. The TOAST criteria group the causes for ischemic stroke into five main groups which include: 1) large-artery atherosclerosis, 2) cardioembolic, 3) small-vessel occlusion, 4) stroke of other determined etiology and 5) stroke of undetermined etiology [9].

Hemorrhagic stroke results from the rupture of a blood vessel resulting in blood outside the vessel in the brain parenchyma. Intracerebral hemorrhage has an annual incidence of 10–30 per 100,000 population and there has been an 18% increase in intracerebral hemorrhage in the last ten years [10]. Subarachnoid hemorrhage is the presence of blood in the subarachnoid space, the space between the arachnoid mater and the pia mater. Common causes of subarachnoid hemorrhage include trauma, rupture of an intracranial aneurysm and perimesencephalic hemorrhage [11]. The overall global incidence of aneurysmal subarachnoid hemorrhage is 7.9 per 100,000 people per year [12]. Rupture of a cerebral aneurysm resulting in subarachnoid hemorrhage remains a neurosurgical emergency. The mortality rate for patients hospitalized with non-traumatic subarachnoid hemorrhage can be higher than 25% [13].

Risk factors of stroke have been well established some of which are hypertension, hyperlipidemia, diabetes and smoking [14]. Prevention of stroke can be achieved by managing the above risk factors. Prevention of stroke is key as survivors of stroke often face poor functional outcome as well as cognitive and physiological impairment [15].

The National Institutes of Health Stroke Scale (NIHSS) is a scale used by medical personnel to determine the severity of the neurological deficit following a stroke [16]. The scale ranges from 0 to 42 with higher scores reflecting a worse neurological impairment [16]. The NIHSS can also be used after treatment to assess any improvement in clinical symptoms. The NIHSS is probably the most widely used stroke scale. However due to some limitations efforts are made to improve and modify it [17]. Another widely used scale to predict functional outcome following a stroke is the modified Ranking Scale (mRS) [18]. The mRS is a categorical scale ranging from 0 to 6 with score 0 referring to a fully independent patient and score 6 referring to someone being dead [18].

The key in managing a patient who is experiencing a stroke is early recognition of symptoms. Any patient who is suspected of having a stroke should undergo emergent computed tomography of the brain in order to determine whether the stroke is ischemic or hemorrhagic in nature. If hemorrhagic stroke is excluded, ischemic stroke is suspected and if there are no contraindications intravenous tissue plasminogen (tPA) activator should be administered. Computed tomography perfusion (CTP) is necessary to identify the salvageable brain region. Computed cerebral angiography (CTA) should also be performed to look for any large vessel occlusion. If a proximal large vessel occlusion in the anterior circulation is identified patients who meet the criteria can undergo endovascular mechanical thrombectomy to relieve the obstruction.

Following mechanical thrombectomy the modified Thrombolysis in Cerebral Infarction (mTICI) grade is used to determine the percent of arterial revascularization. Over the years the scale has been modified. The original scale had scores ranging from 0 to 4 [19]. The scores on the most recent scale range from 0 to 3 with score 2 being divided into a, b and c [20]. mTICI 0 refers to no perfusion or anterograde flow beyond the site of occlusion [20]. mTICI 1 refers to penetration but no perfusion [20]. mTICI 2a refers to some perfusion with distal branch filling of less than 50% of territory visualized [20]. mTICI 2b refers to substantial perfusion with distal branch filling of more than equal to 50% of territory visualized [20]. mTICI 2c refers to near complete perfusion except for slow flow in a few distal cortical vessels, or presence of small distal cortical emboli [20]. mTICI 3 refers to complete perfusion with normal filling of distal branches [20].

Stroke is a health condition that neurosurgeons deal with on an everyday basis. Over the years the management of ischemic stroke is a field that has been rapidly evolving and advancing. The focus of this book chapter will be to discuss the history that has led to the current techniques used by neurosurgeons for treating ischemic stroke.

2. Early understanding of stroke

The word "apoplexy" was first documented in the Hippocratic Corpus and refers to a person collapsing while retaining pulse and respiration [21]. In Greek language the word αποπληξία (apoplixia) means to be struck with violence. The following extract from the Hippocratic writings gives a description of apoplexy: "The healthy subject is taken with a sudden pain; he immediately loses his speech and rattles in his throat. His mouth gapes and if one calls him or stirs him he only groans but understands nothing. He urinates copiously without being aware of it. If fever does not supervene, he succumbs in seven days, but if it does he usually recovers." [22]. In the Greco-Roman period apoplexy was a term used to describe strokes, epilepsy and migraines [21, 23]. The four humours (blood, phlegm, yellow bile and black bile) were first mentioned in the Hippocratic treatise called *The Nature of Man*, and it was actually the work of Polybus, Hippocrates' student [24]. According to Hippocrates, apoplexy was secondary to heating of the head blood vessels that brought phlegm or caused the flow of black bile to the head [22]. Aretaeus was the first to document the concept that apoplexy to one side of the brain results to the contralateral paralysis of the body [25]. Galen claimed that stroke was the result of humors imbalance resulting in blocking the transmission of the animal spirit [26]. Specifically, Galen believed that blood accumulated in the brain whereas phlegm and black bile accumulated in the cerebral ventricles [26].

During the Medieval era the concepts around apoplexy remained grossly unchanged [21]. The ideas of apoplexy in the Medieval era remained influenced by ideas from Greco-Roman works [21].

More information into the cause of apoplexy was obtained during the Renaissance era, between the 14th and 17th century [21]. During the Renaissance era autopsies were permitted and the ancient works were translated in this way expanding the knowledge of apoplexy [21]. In 1599, the Oxford English Dictionary gave a synonym for the "stroke of the palsy" as the "stroke of God's hands" [27].

From the 17th century and onwards the various conditions that made up the term apoplexy started to be individually explored [21]. In 1658, Johan Jakob Wepfer published "*Historiae apoplecticorum*" which was the first time that apoplexy was related to intracerebral hemorrhage [28]. Wepfer performed an autopsy on a patient who suffered from "apoplexy" and found that the brain and the ventricles were filled with blood and no signs of external trauma were evident [28]. In 1689, William Cole was the first to use the term stroke to refer to apoplexy [21]. Others such as Morgagni (1761), Biumi (1765), Blackall (1814), Rochoux (1814) and Rostan (1819) shed light into diseases ranging from unruptured to ruptured aneurysms, as well as the difference between ischemic and hemorrhagic stroke [21].

3. The development of carotid endarterectomy

In 1852, Rudloph Virchow played an important role in shaping our understanding of stroke as he was the first to identify that stroke was the result of an embolism and/or thrombus [21, 29]. In fact Virchow was the first to use the term "thrombosis" and "embolus" that can lead to decrease blood flow in distal vessels and can result in stroke [30].

Approximately 8% of all ischemic strokes are due to extracranial internal carotid artery stenosis [31]. Chiari in 1906 and Hunt in 1914 performed autopsies in patients who had suffered from cerebral infarction and noted that lesions in the cervical carotid artery could be the culprit for the stroke [32]. Fisher in 1951, published case reports that showed that the cause of cerebral infarction was secondary to occlusion of internal carotid artery [32]. The introduction of cerebral angiography in 1927 by Moniz played a crucial role in the understanding of carotid artery disease and the subsequent development of carotid endarterectomy (CEA) [33]. The first carotid artery reconstruction was completed in 1951 in Buenos Aires and it was the result of the combined work of Fisher, Murphy, Carrea and Mollins [34]. In 1953, Debakey successfully completed the first CEA surgery for a patient with cerebrovascular insufficiency [35]. However, Debakey did not publish this case report until 1975 [36]. In the meanwhile, in 1956 Cooley was the first to publish a case report on a patient undergoing a successful CEA [37]. This was also the first report of the application of a temporary shunt during a CEA [37].

In 1969, the Joint Study of Extracranial Arterial Occlusion was published that showed that in 2,400 operations performed between 1961 and 1968 there was a 4.5% surgical mortality [38]. The indications for CEA remained unclear and given the surgical risk associated with the surgery, it took years before it became the standard of care [39]. In 1991, The North American Symptomatic Carotid Endarterectomy trial (NASCET) and the European Carotid Surgery (ECS) trial proved that patients with symptomatic carotid stenosis of 70–99% who underwent CEA had better outcomes when compared to patients who were treated medically [40, 41]. Specifically, the NASCET study showed that there was an absolute risk reduction of 17 ± 3.5 percent ($P < 0.001$) of having any ipsilateral stroke at two years and an absolute risk reduction of 10.6 ± 2.6 percent ($P < 0.001$) for a major or fatal ipsilateral stoke when comparing patients who underwent CEA versus those who underwent medical management [42]. The ECS trial showed that patients with carotid artery stenosis of 70–99% ($P < 0.0001$) had a six fold reduction in their risk of experiencing stroke during the next three years if they underwent surgical treatment versus medical management [43].

In addition, in 1995 the Asymptomatic Carotid Artery Stenosis (ACAS) trial showed that patient with asymptomatic carotid artery stenosis of 60% or greater benefited from CEA [44]. In this study there was a 53% risk reduction of having a stroke in patients treated surgically versus those treated medically [44].

Subsequently there was also interest as to whether carotid artery stenting (CAS) could replace CEAs. In 2010, a randomized controlled trial showed that CAS was associated with a significant higher periprocedural risk of stroke, whereas CEA was associated with a higher risk of myocardial infarction [45]. This study also showed that in the four year follow up there was no significant difference of further strokes between the two groups [45].

4. Intravenous tissue plasminogen activator

A milestone in the management of ischemic stroke occurred in 1995 when the National Institute of Neurological Disorders and stroke rt-PA Stroke Study (NINDS) showed that administering intravenous recombinant tissue plasminogen activator (tPA) within 3 hours of symptoms onset had favorable outcomes in stroke management [46]. Intravenous tPA is a thrombolytic agent used to break down a clot [47]. In particular, it converts the inactive plasminogen into plasmin a proteolytic enzyme that breaks down fibrin [47]. The NINDS study was a randomized, double-blind trial with patients either randomized to receiving intravenous tPA or placebo, within 3 hours of the onset of symptoms [46]. The results of the study showed that neurological improvement was similar between the two groups 24 hours after treatment and better in the group that received intravenous tPA at three months [46]. The major adverse effect in the treatment group was symptomatic intracerebral hemorrhage within 36 hours after treatment that occurred in 6.4% of the treatment group versus 0.6% of the placebo group ($P < 0.001$) [46].

The European Cooperative Acute Stroke Study (ECASS) I published in 1995 was a randomized controlled study that divided subjects into two groups those receiving 1.1 mg per kg of body weight of intravenous tPA or placebo [48]. Patients were included in the study if they presented within 6 hours from onset of symptoms and had moderate to severe neurological deficit [48]. Patients receiving intravenous tPA had better mRS at 90 days and better neurological recovery in comparison to the placebo group [48]. The incidence of intracerebral hemorrhage and mortality rate was similar between the groups [48]. However, the group receiving intravenous tPA had a higher incidence of large intracerebral hemorrhage [48].

Other randomized controlled studies including the ECASS II in 1998 and the Alteplase Thrombolysis for Acute Noninterventional Therapy in Ischemic Stroke (ATLANTIS) B in 1999 urged against the use of intravenous tPA beyond 3 hours in management of ischemic stroke [49, 50]. This conclusion was based on the high incidence of intracerebral hemorrhage that was observed in those who received intravenous tPA [49, 50].

In 2008, ECASS III study, a randomized controlled study, showed that administration of intravenous tPA to patients with ischemic stroke up to 4.5 hours after the onset of stroke symptoms was beneficial [51]. Patients were randomly assigned to either receive intravenous tPA or placebo and the median time for administration of the medication was 3 hours and 59 minutes [51]. The study showed that the group that received tPA had better outcomes than the placebo group (52.4% vs. 45.2%, confidence interval (CI), 1.02 to 1.76; $P = 0.04$) [51]. Both incidences of any intracerebral hemorrhage and symptomatic intracerebral hemorrhage were higher in the treatment group versus the placebo group with results being 27% vs. 17.6%, $P = 0.001$ and 2.4% vs. 0.2%, $P = 0.008$ respectively [51]. Mortality and other serious adverse events were similar between the groups [51].

Intracerebral hemorrhage following intravenous tPA remains a concern that can lead to devastating results. To decrease the risk of intracerebral hemorrhage following intravenous tPA, the American Heart Association and American Stroke Association issued guidelines with strict criteria for which patients are eligible for receiving intravenous tPA [52]. Other limitations to consider is that larger and more proximally located thrombi might not respond to intravenous tPA [53]. It has been reported that restoration of blood flow in large vessel occlusion after intravenous tPA ranges between 10 and 30% depending on the large vessel that is occluded [53].

Given the limitations of intravenous tPA other avenues for management of ischemic stroke were needed. The Prourokinase (Prolyse) in Acute Cerebral Thromboembolism (PROACT II) study, a randomized controlled study aimed to determine the effects of administrating intraarterial recombinant prourokinase (r-proUK) compared to heparin within 6 hours of onset of symptoms [54]. The PROACT II study showed an increase in recanalization rate and improvement in modified Rankin score in patients treated with r-proUK versus those who were treated with heparin alone [54]. The major limitation of r-proUK was an increase in intracerebral hemorrhage 24 hours after administration that was associated with neurological deterioration (10% in treatment group versus 2% in control group, $P < 0.06$) [54].

Another medication that has been considered for the management of acute ischemic stroke is tirofiban [55]. Tirofiban is a glycoprotein IIb/IIIa platelet receptor antagonist [55]. The Safety of Tirofiban in acute Ischemic Stroke (SaTIS) trial aimed to determine whether tirofiban could be used for the treatment of acute ischemic stroke [55]. SaTIS was a prospective, open-labeled treatment, blinded outcome reading multicenter trial [55]. Patients that were included in the study had an NIHSS between 4 and 18 and received either intravenous tirofiban or placebo up to 48 hours from onset of symptoms [55]. There was no difference between the two groups in terms of intracerebral hemorrhage or neurological outcome up to five months of treatment [55]. Five months following intervention mortality was lower in the treatment group [55].

5. Endovascular Mechanical Thrombectomy

In 2005, the Mechanical Embolus Removal in Cerebral Ischemia (MERCI) trial revolutionized the way ischemic strokes are managed [56]. This was the first study that showed how endovascular embolectomy using a first generation device can improve outcomes of ischemic stroke [56]. The MERCI trial used the embolectomy device (Merci Retriever) for patients who presented within 8 hours of onset of stroke and were otherwise ineligible for intravenous tPA administration [56]. The study showed that recanalization was achieved in 48% of patients who underwent embolectomy and the risk of intracranial hemorrhage was significantly lower, only 7.8%, in comparison to 10% in the PROACT II study [56]. In 2008, after the development of the Merci Retriever the Penumbra System was developed. The Penumbra device is a second generation thrombectomy device that is inserted all the way through the clot followed by application of mechanical aspiration with the use of a suction pump [39]. By using the Penumbra System partial to normal reperfusion was achieved in 81.6% of patients, a percentage higher than that achieved by using the Merci Retriever [56, 57]. Intracranial hemorrhage was observed in 28% of patients on post procedural 24 hour CT scan however only 11.2% were symptomatic [57]. Despite the increase in intracranial hemorrhage observed with the Penumbra device in comparison to the Merci Retriever the 90-day mRS of less than or equal 2 was similar between the two groups, with 25% for the Penumbra system and 27.7% for the Merci Retriever [56, 57]. Shortly thereafter stent retrievers were developed for the use as thrombectomy devices.

In 2012, a third generation mechanical thrombectomy device was introduced. The Solitaire Flow Restoration device versus the Merci Retriever in patients with acute ischemic stroke was studied [58]. The SWIFT study was a randomized, parallel-group, non-inferiority trial that showed that Solitaire Flow Restoration device is significantly better than the Merci retriever device [58]. In particular, patients treated with the Solitaire Flow Restoration device had a rate of recanalization of 61% in comparison to 24% in those treated with the Merci Retriever device [58]. With the use of the Solitaire flow restoration device the rate of symptomatic intracranial hemorrhage was decreased and the overall neurological outcomes were better [58].

Another area of interest was whether devices that combined direct aspiration with thrombectomy would be beneficial in the management of ischemic stroke. The MAX reperfusion catheters as well as a direct aspiration first pass technique (ADAPT) enabled direct aspiration with thrombectomy [53]. In 2018, a randomized controlled study aimed to determine whether there was a difference in ischemic stroke outcomes when the novel 3-dimensional (3-D) stent retriever was used in conjugation with an aspiration-based mechanical thrombectomy device (Penumbra System; Penumbra) versus the aspiration-based thrombectomy alone [59]. The results of the study showed that 87.2% in the 3-D stent retriever with aspiration group versus 82.3% in the aspiration based thrombectomy alone group had a mTICI of 2–3 [59]. The 90-day mRS score of 0 to 2, device-related serious adverse events and procedure-related serious adverse events were similar between the two groups [59].

The next step in the management of acute ischemic stroke was to determine whether endovascular thrombectomy was superior to standard medical care alone [60]. There were five key randomized control studies that aimed to answer this question: MR CLEAN, ESCAPE, REVASCAT, SWIFT PRIME, and EXTEND IA [61–65].

The MR CLEAN trial aimed to determine whether patients who presented within 6 hours after onset of ischemic symptoms and proximal intracranial occlusion of the anterior circulation would benefit from mechanical thrombectomy [61]. In particular, all patients in the study received intravenous tPA and were subsequently randomized to receive either intraarterial treatment or not [61]. The study showed that there was improvement in functional independence in the treatment group but no changes in mortality or the occurrence of symptomatic intracerebral hemorrhage between the two groups [61].

The ESCAPE study assessed whether patients who presented within 12 hours of onset of symptoms would benefit from mechanical thrombectomy [62]. The patients included in the study had a proximal vessel occlusion in the anterior circulation and they all received intravenous tPA [62]. The experimental group also received mechanical thrombectomy [62]. The results of the study showed that patients who received mechanical thrombectomy had substantial increase of functional independence (53% in the treatment group versus 29.3% in the control group; $P < 0.001$), decreased mortality in the intervention group and similar intracerebral hemorrhage rates [62].

The REVASCAT study examined whether there is a difference in outcome in patients when treated with a combination therapy of both intravenous tPA (if eligible) and mechanical thrombectomy than those treated with medical therapy alone [63]. The patients who were included in the study had to present within 8 hours of onset of symptoms and had to have a proximal anterior circulation occlusion [63]. Solitaire stent retriever was the device used for the thrombectomy group [63]. The results of the study showed that functional independence was increased in the experimental group, with 43.7% having functional independence (mRS score of 0–2) in 90 days versus 28.2% in the control group [63]. The rates of intracerebral hemorrhage remained the same in both groups [63].

The SWIFT PRIME study aimed to determine whether patients treated with both intravenous tPA and Solitaire Revascularization Device within 6 hours of symptoms onset had better outcome than those who were treated with intravenous tPA alone [64]. The results of the study showed that there was a greater proportion of patients in the experimental group that were functional independent at 90 days in comparison to the control group [64]. Secondary outcomes such as functional independence at 90 days, improvement in NIHSS score and successful reperfusion at 27 hours were better in the treatment group versus the control group [64]. There was no significant difference in complications between the two groups [64].

The EXTEND IA study aimed to determine whether patients treated with both intravenous tPA and Solitaire Revascularization Device within 4.5 hours of symptom onset had better outcome than those who were treated with intravenous tPA alone [65]. The results of the study showed that reperfusion at 24 hours was better in the experimental group versus the control group (median, 100% vs. 37%, $P < 0.001$) [65]. The neurological improvement at 3 days and the functional outcome was better in the experimental group versus the control group [65]. With regards to adverse consequences such as death and intracerebral hemorrhage the results were similar between the two groups [65].

Subsequently, a meta-analysis published in 2016 looked at the results from the above five randomized controlled trials [60]. There were 1287 patients that were included in the study and who had an acute proximal anterior circulation stroke [60]. Prior to randomization to the two groups patients received intravenous tPA if they met the inclusion criteria [60]. The major results of this meta-analysis were: 1) endovascular thrombectomy led to reduced disability at 90 days, 2) the risk of intracerebral hemorrhage and symptomatic hemorrhage did not differ between the groups and 3) the mortality rate was similar between groups [60].

In 2018, two major randomized controlled studies the DAWN and the DEFUSE 3 were published [66, 67]. The data collected from these studies showed that mechanical thrombectomy can be extended to 24 hours from onset of stroke symptoms [66, 67]. The DAWN study randomized patients to receive either intravenous tPA alone (control group) or thrombectomy plus intravenous tPA (experimental group) [66]. The patients had an intracranial internal carotid artery or proximal middle cerebral artery occlusion and were last known well 6–24 hours prior [66]. The patients included in the study had disproportionately worse neurological exam in comparison to the infarct volume that was observed on imaging [66]. The study showed that at 90 days the thrombectomy group had a better mRS score and improved functional independence [66]. Adverse effects such as intracerebral hemorrhage and death were similar between the two groups [66].

The DEFUSE 3 study was a multicenter, randomized, open-label trial, in which the control group received intravenous tPA and the experimental group received endovascular therapy plus intravenous tPA [67]. Patients who were included in the study had onset of symptoms 6–16 hours prior to presentation, were found to have proximal middle cerebral artery or internal carotid artery occlusion with initial infarct size less than 70 ml and a ratio of the volume of ischemic tissue on perfusion imaging to infarct volume of 1.8 [67]. The study showed that patients who underwent mechanical thrombectomy had an increase chance of being functionally independent (45% vs. 17%, $P < 0.001$) and the 90-day mortality rate was 14% in the experimental group versus 26% in the control group [67]. Symptomatic intracerebral hemorrhage and adverse effects were similar between the groups [67].

It is worth mentioning that acute ischemic stroke can be managed by artery stenting. The Stent-Assisted Recanalization in Acute Ischemic Stroke (SARIS) trial was a prospective trial the goal of which was to determine whether cerebral arterial stenting would be beneficial in the management of acute ischemic stroke [68]. In a series of twenty patients the mRS score of 3 was achieved in 60% and that of 1 was achieved in 45% [68]. Symptomatic intracerebral hemorrhage was present in 5% of the patients and asymptomatic intracerebral hemorrhage was present in 10% [68]. There is, however, no consensus on whether the benefits of arterial stenting in acute stroke outweigh the risks primarily due to the lack of randomized controlled trials [69].

6. Decompressive hemicraniectomy for malignant middle cerebral artery territory infarct

Patients who suffer from middle cerebral artery infarction can have a mortality rate secondary to elevated intracranial pressure. Neurosurgeons often perform decompressive craniectomies when such situations arise. Multiple studies were conducted over the years to determine the efficacy of this practice. There were three randomized controlled landmark studies and a meta-analysis of these studies that aimed to address this issue.

The first trial was the "Decompressive Surgery for the Treatment of Malignant Infarction of the Middle Cerebral Artery (DESTINY)" that was published in 2007 [70]. The second trial was the "Sequential-Design, Multicenter, Randomized, Controlled Trial of Early Decompressive Craniectomy in Malignant Middle Cerebral Artery Infarction (DECIMAL Trial)" that was published in 2007 [71]. The third trial was the "Hemicraniectomy after middle cerebral artery infarction with life-threatening Edema trial (HAMLET)" published in 2009 [72].

In 2007 a meta-analysis of the above three randomized controlled studies was conducted while the above studies were ongoing [73]. The aim of the study was to determine whether performing decompressive hemicraniectomy in patients who had suffered malignant middle cerebral artery territory infarct had good long-term outcomes [73]. The study showed that more patients in the hemicraniectomy group had an mRS of less than equal to 4 in comparison to the control group [73]. The study also showed that survival rate in the hemicraniectomy group was higher than in the control group [73]. This meta-analysis favored decompressive hemicraniectomy in patients with malignant middle cerebral artery infarction who underwent surgery within 48 hours of stroke onset in order to reduce mortality and improve mRS score in survivors [73].

7. Conclusion

Stroke is a medical entity that was known in ancient Greece as apoplexy. Hippocrates was the first to describe a patient with stroke like symptoms followed by Areteus and Galen. Ischemic stroke was once a disease process of which we had a scarce understanding. Efficient treatments were, however, made possible with more insight into the anatomical and pathophysiological changes that are associated with ischemic stroke. These developments were attributed to Wepfer, Virchow, Murphy, Cooley and others. The advancement in technology, such as the development of cerebral angiography, CTA and CTP, were also crucial in the advancements made in treating ischemic stroke.

Neurosurgeons are able to perform a wide range of procedures to manage ischemic stroke and thus their role in this disease remains pivotal. For prevention of stroke, CEAs are performed; for reperfusion of salvageable brain tissue, mechanical thrombectomies improve outcomes; and for management of brain herniation hemicraniectomies are carried out. Additionally, endovascular mechanical thrombectomies have undoubtedly revolutionized the way ischemic stroke is managed. But, more progress remains to be made, with several previous and on-going randomized controlled studies attempting to find the gold standard for treating ischemic stroke.

Ischemic stroke remains a major public health concern that can undoubtedly cause severe disability. Even with increase efforts for public education and primary prevention, neurosurgeons still need to be able to manage ischemic strokes efficiently.

Conflict of interest

The authors declare no conflict of interest.

Author details

Lydia Kaoutzani* and Scott Y. Rahimi
Department of Neurosurgery, Augusta University Medical Center, Augusta, Georgia, USA

*Address all correspondence to: lkaoutzani@augusta.edu

References

[1] K. Aho, P. Harmsen, S. Hatano, J. Marquardsen, V. E. Smirnov, and T. Strasser, "Cerebrovascular disease in the community: results of a WHO collaborative study," Bull. World Health Organ., 1980.

[2] R. L. Sacco *et al.*, "An Updated Definition of Stroke for the 21st Century," Stroke, 2013, doi: 10.1161/str.0b013e318296aeca.

[3] P. B. Gorelick, "The global burden of stroke: persistent and disabling," The Lancet Neurology. 2019, doi: 10.1016/S1474-4422(19)30030-4.

[4] M. A. Khan *et al.*, "Global Epidemiology of Ischemic Heart Disease: Results from the Global Burden of Disease Study," Cureus, 2020, doi: 10.7759/cureus.9349.

[5] V. L. Feigin, B. Norrving, and G. A. Mensah, "Global Burden of Stroke," Circ. Res., 2017, doi: 10.1161/CIRCRESAHA.116.308413.

[6] S. S. Virani *et al.*, "Heart disease and stroke statistics—2020 update: A report from the American Heart Association," *Circulation*. 2020, doi: 10.1161/CIR.0000000000000757.

[7] T. D. Musuka, S. B. Wilton, M. Traboulsi, and M. D. Hill, "Diagnosis and management of acute ischemic stroke: Speed is critical," CMAJ. 2015, doi: 10.1503/cmaj.140355.

[8] J. D. Easton *et al.*, "Definition and Evaluation of Transient Ischemic Attack," Stroke, 2009, doi: 10.1161/strokeaha.108.192218.

[9] H. . Adams *et al.*, "Classification of Subtype of Acute Ischemic Stroke," *Stroke*, 1993.

[10] A. I. Qureshi, A. D. Mendelow, and D. F. Hanley, "Intracerebral haemorrhage," The Lancet. 2009, doi: 10.1016/S0140-6736(09)60371-8.

[11] C. P. Marder, V. Narla, J. R. Fink, and K. R. Tozer Fink, "Subarachnoid hemorrhage: Beyond aneurysms," American Journal of Roentgenology. 2014, doi: 10.2214/AJR.12.9749.

[12] N. Etminan *et al.*, "Worldwide Incidence of Aneurysmal Subarachnoid Hemorrhage According to Region, Time Period, Blood Pressure, and Smoking Prevalence in the Population: A Systematic Review and Meta-analysis," JAMA Neurol., 2019, doi: 10.1001/jamaneurol.2019.0006.

[13] A. M. Shea, S. D. Reed, L. H. Curtis, M. J. Alexander, J. J. Villani, and K. A. Schulman, "Characteristics of nontraumatic subarachnoid hemorrhage in the United States in 2003," Neurosurgery, 2007, doi: 10.1227/01.neu.0000306090.30517.ae.

[14] A. K. Boehme, C. Esenwa, and M. S. V. Elkind, "Stroke Risk Factors, Genetics, and Prevention," Circulation Research. 2017, doi: 10.1161/CIRCRESAHA.116.308398.

[15] S. L. Crichton, B. D. Bray, C. McKevitt, A. G. Rudd, and C. D. A. Wolfe, "Patient outcomes up to 15 years after stroke: Survival, disability, quality of life, cognition and mental health," J. Neurol. Neurosurg. Psychiatry, 2016, doi: 10.1136/jnnp-2016-313361.

[16] P. Lyden, "Using the National Institutes of Health Stroke Scale," Stroke. 2017, doi: 10.1161/STROKEAHA.116.015434.

[17] P. D. Lyden, M. Lu, S. R. Levine, T. G. Brott, and J. Broderick, "A modified national institutes of health stroke scale for use in stroke clinical trials preliminary reliability and validity," Stroke, 2001, doi: 10.1161/01.str.32.6.1310.

[18] J. L. Banks and C. A. Marotta, "Outcomes validity and reliability of the modified rankin scale: Implications for stroke clinical trials - A literature review and synthesis," Stroke. 2007, doi: 10.1161/01.STR.0000258355.23810.c6.

[19] R. T. Higashida *et al.*, "Trial design and reporting standards for intra-arterial cerebral thrombolysis for acute ischemic stroke.," Stroke, 2003, doi: 10.1161/01.str.0000082721.62796.09.

[20] M. Goyal *et al.*, "2C or not 2C: Defining an improved revascularization grading scale and the need for standardization of angiography outcomes in stroke trials," Journal of NeuroInterventional Surgery. 2014, doi: 10.1136/neurintsurg-2013-010665.

[21] E. Engelhardt, "Apoplexy, cerebrovascular disease, and stroke: Historical evolution of terms and definitions," Dement. Neuropsychol., 2017, doi: 10.1590/1980-57642016dn11-040016.

[22] E. CLARKE, "APOPLEXY IN THE HIPPOCRATIC WRITINGS.," Bull. Hist. Med., 1963.

[23] A. P. Coupland, A. Thapar, M. I. Qureshi, H. Jenkins, and A. H. Davies, "The definition of stroke," J. R. Soc. Med., 2017, doi: 10.1177/0141076816680121.

[24] J. Jouanna, "The Legacy of the Hippocratic Treatise The Nature of Man: The Theory of the Four Humours," in *Greek Medicine from Hippocrates to Galen*, 2012.

[25] J. M. S. Pearce, "The Neurology of Aretaeus: Radix Pedis Neurologia," Eur. Neurol., 2013, doi: 10.1159/000352031.

[26] A. Karenberg, "Blood, Phlegm and Spirits: Galen on Stroke," Istor. meditsiny, 2015, doi: 10.17720/2409-5583.t2.2.2015.15k.

[27] F. Schiller, "Concepts of stroke before and after Virchow," Med. Hist., 1970, doi: 10.1017/S0025727300015325.

[28] J. M. Pearce, "Johann Jakob Wepfer (1620-95) and cerebral haemorrhage.," J. Neurol. Neurosurg. Psychiatry, 1997, doi: 10.1136/jnnp.62.4.387.

[29] S. Safavi-Abbasi et al., "Rudolf Ludwig Karl Virchow: pathologist, physician, anthropologist, and politician. Implications of his work for the understanding of cerebrovascular pathology and stroke.," Neurosurg. Focus, 2006, doi: 10.3171/foc.2006.20.6.1.

[30] J. M. Pearce, "Rudolf Ludwig Karl Virchow (1821-1902).," J. Neurol., 2002, doi: 10.1007/s004150200049.

[31] M. L. Flaherty *et al.*, "Carotid artery stenosis as a cause of stroke," Neuroepidemiology, 2012, doi: 10.1159/000341410.

[32] S. P. Saha, S. Saha, and K. S. Vyas, "Carotid endarterectomy: Current concepts and practice patterns," Int. J. Angiol., 2014, doi: 10.1055/s-0035-1558645.

[33] M. Artico *et al.*, "Egas Moniz: 90 years (1927-2017) from cerebral angiography," Front. Neuroanat., 2017, doi: 10.3389/fnana.2017.00081.

[34] C. J. Estol, "Dr C. Miller Fisher and the history of carotid artery disease," Stroke, 1996, doi: 10.1161/01.STR.27.3.559.

[35] M. E. Debakey, "Successful Carotid Endarterectomy For Cerebrovascular Insufficiency: Nineteen-Year Follow-up," JAMA J. Am. Med. Assoc., 1975, doi: 10.1001/jama.1975.03260100053020.

[36] S. G. Friedman and N. M. Rich, "The first carotid endarterectomy," J. Vasc. Surg., 2014, doi: 10.1016/j.jvs.2014.08.059.

[37] F. Robicsek, T. S. Roush, J. W. Cook, and M. K. Reames, "From Hippocrates to Palmaz-Schatz, The History of Carotid Surgery," Eur. J. Vasc. Endovasc. Surg., 2004, doi: 10.1016/j.ejvs.2004.01.004.

[38] W. F. Blaisdell, R. H. Clauss, J. G. Galbraith, A. M. Imparato, and E. J. Wylie, "Joint Study of Extracranial Arterial Occlusion: IV. A Review of Surgical Considerations," JAMA J. Am. Med. Assoc., 1969, doi: 10.1001/jama.1969.03160250045010.

[39] J. Withrow, N. Todnem, and S. Rahimi, "The Evolution of the Neurosurgical Treatment of Ischemic Stroke," J. Cerebrovasc. Endovasc. Neurosurg., 2018, doi: 10.7461/jcen.2018.20.1.53.

[40] G. G. Ferguson *et al.*, "The North American Symptomatic Carotid Endarterectomy Trial: Surgical results in 1415 patients," Stroke, 1999, doi: 10.1161/01.STR.30.9.1751.

[41] C. Warlow, B. Farrell, A. Fraser, P. Sandercock, and J. Slattery, "Randomised trial of endarterectomy for recently symptomatic carotid stenosis: Final results of the MRC European Carotid Surgery Trial (ECST)," Lancet, 1998, doi: 10.1016/S0140-6736(97)09292-1.

[42] NASCET, "Beneficial effect of carotid endarterectomy in symptomatic patients with high-grade carotid stenosis. North American Symptomatic Carotid Endarterectomy Trial Collaborators," *N. Engl. J. Med.*, 1991.

[43] C. Warlow, "MRC European Carotid Surgery Trial: interim results for symptomatic patients with severe (70-99%) or with mild (0-29%) carotid stenosis," Lancet, 1991, doi: 10.1016/0140-6736(91)92916-P.

[44] "Endarterectomy for asymptomatic carotid artery stenosis. Executive Committee for the Asymptomatic Carotid Atherosclerosis Study," *JAMA J. Am. Med. Assoc.*, 1995, doi: 10.1001/jama.273.18.1421.

[45] T. G. Brott *et al.*, "Stenting versus endarterectomy for treatment of carotid-artery stenosis," N. Engl. J. Med., 2010, doi: 10.1056/NEJMoa0912321.

[46] "Tissue plasminogen activator for acute ischemic stroke," *N. Engl. J. Med.*, 1995, doi: 10.1056/NEJM199512143332401.

[47] S. Bhaskar, P. Stanwell, D. Cordato, J. Attia, and C. Levi, "Reperfusion therapy in acute ischemic stroke: Dawn of a new era?," BMC Neurology. 2018, doi: 10.1186/s12883-017-1007-y.

[48] W. Hacke et al., "Intravenous Thrombolysis With Recombinant Tissue Plasminogen Activator for Acute Hemispheric Stroke: The European Cooperative Acute Stroke Study (ECASS)," JAMA J. Am. Med. Assoc., 1995, doi: 10.1001/jama.1995.03530130023023.

[49] W. Hacke *et al.*, "Randomised double-blind placebo-controlled trial of thrombolytic therapy with intravenous alteplase in acute ischaemic stroke (ECASS II)," Lancet, 1998, doi: 10.1016/S0140-6736(98)08020-9.

[50] W. M. Clark, S. Wissman, G. W. Albers, J. H. Jhamandas, K. P. Madden, and S. Hamilton, "Recombinant tissue-type plasminogen activator (Alteplase) for ischemic stroke 3 to 5 hours after symptom onset the ATLANTIS study: A randomized controlled trial," J. Am. Med. Assoc., 1999, doi: 10.1001/jama.282.21.2019.

[51] W. Hacke *et al.*, "Thrombolysis with alteplase 3 to 4.5 hours after acute ischemic stroke," N. Engl. J. Med., 2008, doi: 10.1056/NEJMoa0804656.

[52] W. J. Powers *et al.*, "Guidelines for the early management of patients with acute ischemic stroke: 2019 update to the 2018 guidelines for the early management of acute ischemic stroke a guideline for healthcare professionals from the American Heart Association/ American Stroke A," *Stroke*. 2019, doi: 10.1161/STR.0000000000000211.

[53] C. J. Przybylowski, "Evolution of endovascular mechanical thrombectomy for acute ischemic stroke," World J. Clin. Cases, 2014, doi: 10.12998/wjcc.v2.i11.614.

[54] A. Furlan *et al.*, "Intra-arterial prourokinase for acute ischemic stroke. The PROACT II study: A randomized controlled trial," J. Am. Med. Assoc., 1999, doi: 10.1001/jama.282.21.2003.

[55] S. M. et al., "Safety of tirofiban in acute ischemic stroke: The SaTIS trial," Stroke, 2011.

[56] W. S. Smith *et al.*, "Safety and efficacy of mechanical embolectomy in acute ischemic stroke: Results of the MERCI trial," Stroke, 2005, doi: 10.1161/01.STR.0000171066.25248.1d.

[57] S. Po Sit, "The penumbra pivotal stroke trial: Safety and effectiveness of a new generation of mechanical devices for clot removal in intracranial large vessel occlusive disease," Stroke, 2009, doi: 10.1161/STROKEAHA.108.544957.

[58] J. L. Saver *et al.*, "Solitaire flow restoration device versus the Merci Retriever in patients with acute ischaemic stroke (SWIFT): A randomised, parallel-group, non-inferiority trial," Lancet, 2012, doi: 10.1016/S0140-6736(12)61384-1.

[59] R. G. Nogueira *et al.*, "Safety and efficacy of a 3-dimensional stent retriever with aspiration-based thrombectomy vs aspiration-based thrombectomy alone in acute ischemic stroke intervention a randomized clinical trial," JAMA Neurol., 2018, doi: 10.1001/jamaneurol.2017.3967.

[60] M. Goyal *et al.*, "Endovascular thrombectomy after large-vessel ischaemic stroke: A meta-analysis of individual patient data from five randomised trials," Lancet, 2016, doi: 10.1016/S0140-6736(16)00163-X.

[61] O. A. Berkhemer *et al.*, "A Randomized Trial of Intraarterial Treatment for Acute Ischemic Stroke," N. Engl. J. Med., 2015, doi: 10.1056/ nejmoa1411587.

[62] M. Goyal *et al.*, "Randomized Assessment of Rapid Endovascular Treatment of Ischemic Stroke," N. Engl. J. Med., 2015, doi: 10.1056/ nejmoa1414905.

[63] T. G. Jovin *et al.*, "Thrombectomy within 8 Hours after Symptom Onset in Ischemic Stroke," N. Engl. J. Med., 2015, doi: 10.1056/nejmoa1503780.

[64] J. L. Saver *et al.*, "Stent-Retriever Thrombectomy after Intravenous t-PA vs. t-PA Alone in Stroke," N. Engl. J. Med., 2015, doi: 10.1056/ nejmoa1415061.

[65] B. C. V. Campbell *et al.*, "Endovascular Therapy for Ischemic Stroke with Perfusion-Imaging Selection," N. Engl. J. Med., 2015, doi: 10.1056/nejmoa1414792.

[66] R. G. Nogueira *et al.*, "Thrombectomy 6 to 24 hours after stroke with a mismatch between deficit and infarct," N. Engl. J. Med., 2018, doi: 10.1056/NEJMoa1706442.

[67] G. W. Albers *et al.*, "Thrombectomy for Stroke at 6 to 16 Hours with Selection by Perfusion Imaging," N. Engl. J. Med., 2018, doi: 10.1056/ nejmoa1713973.

[68] E. I. Levy *et al.*, "First food and drug administration-approved prospective

trial of primary intracranial stenting for acute stroke: SARIS (Stent-Assisted Recanalization in Acute Ischemic Stroke)," Stroke, 2009, doi: 10.1161/STROKEAHA.109.561274.

[69] J. Gralla, C. Brekenfeld, P. Mordasini, and G. Schroth, "Mechanical thrombolysis and stenting in acute ischemic stroke," Stroke. 2012, doi: 10.1161/STROKEAHA.111.626903.

[70] E. Jüttler *et al.*, "Decompressive surgery for the treatment of malignant infarction of the middle cerebral artery (DESTINY): A randomized, controlled trial," Stroke, 2007, doi: 10.1161/STROKEAHA.107.485649.

[71] K. Vahedi *et al.*, "Sequential-design, multicenter, randomized, controlled trial of early decompressive craniectomy in malignant middle cerebral artery infarction (DECIMAL Trial)," Stroke, 2007, doi: 10.1161/STROKEAHA.107.485235.

[72] J. Hofmeijer, L. J. Kappelle, A. Algra, G. J. Amelink, J. van Gijn, and H. B. van der Worp, "Surgical decompression for space-occupying cerebral infarction (the Hemicraniectomy After Middle Cerebral Artery infarction with Life-threatening Edema Trial [HAMLET]): a multicentre, open, randomised trial," Lancet Neurol., 2009, doi: 10.1016/S1474-4422(09)70047-X.

[73] K. Vahedi *et al.*, "Early decompressive surgery in malignant infarction of the middle cerebral artery: a pooled analysis of three randomised controlled trials," Lancet Neurol., 2007, doi: 10.1016/S1474-4422(07)70036-4.

Chapter 9

The History and Development of Endovascular Neurosurgery

Xianli Lv

Abstract

Endovasuclar neurosurgery, neuroendovascular surgery and neurointervention are all defined as endovascular diagnosis and treatment of vascular lesions involving the brain and spinal cord using catheters in the DSA (digital subtraction angiography) unite. Based on literature evidences, the field of endovascular neurosurgery has evolved rapidly and successfully over the past half century and has resulted in effective endovascular therapies for carotid-cavernous fistulas (CCFs), intracranial aneurysms, arteriovenous malformations (AVMs), dural arteriovenous fistulas, atherosclerosis of cerebral arteries, acute stroke, carotid artery disease, and vascular tumors of the head, neck, and spinal vascular malformations and tumors. The scope of practice of neurovascular endovascular surgery has become complex, requiring training in specific skill sets and techniques. The evolution of the neuroendovascular field has resulted in the development of program requirements for residency or fellowship education in endovascular neurosurgery.

Keywords: cerebral aneurysm, arteriovenous malformation, stroke, endovascular technique

1. Introduction

Endovascular neurosurgery is now the most commonly practiced therapeutic approach for most vascular lesions involving the brain and spinal cord [1]. At the beginning, balloons are the only available techniques; latter coils, embolic agents, and stents are introduced [2]. With expansion of the endovascular devices and techniques, the treatment strategies for cerebrospinal vascular diseases has been refined [3]. Neurosurgeons must have the mindset to embrace and nurture the progress and technologic advances. The pioneers of endovascular neurosurgery considered the impossible and tenaciously stood by their dreams [4]. Their revolutionary ideas and inventions truly reflected their courage, faith, and determination. The shift away from open surgical approaches has had far-reaching implications for how we train neurosurgical residents and fellows and how we certify these individuals once their training is completed [5]. With the maturity of endovascular neurosurgery technology, we need to re-examine the resident and fellow training for neurovascular surgery. This chapter traces the evolution of endovascular neurosurgery and its current role as the dominant and frequently standard therapy for cerebral and spinal vascular diseases.

2. Cerebral angiography

Endovascular neurosurgery is based on cerebral angiography. It is well known that Portuguese neurologist Antonio Egas Moniz, the recipient of the Nobel Prize in Physiology and Medicine in 1949, developed and described cerebral angiography firstly in 1927 [6]. Before using cadaveric specimens of human to develop the technique, he had successfully obtained cerebral angiograms in dogs. His first cerebral angiography was performed in a 48-year-old patient with Parkinson's disease. The internal carotid artery (ICA) was ligated temporarily for 2 minutes and a 70% solution of strontium bromide was injected into the ICA at a dose of 13 to 14 ml. The middle and posterior cerebral arteries were demonstrated on his first film. Unfortunately, the patient died from thrombophlebitis 8 hours later. This invention ushered in the age of diagnostic and therapeutic angiography.

Cerebral angiography had a prominent role in defining neurosurgery as a specialty distinct from surgery. The cerebral angiography is based on X-ray imaging [7]. Contrast injection plus X-ray exposure combined with mask subtraction generates images of high resolution of the cerebral vasculature. In early angiogram systems, cut film and film cassettes were used, which required a technologist to exchange multiple cassettes to obtain series and angiography "runs". At that time, angiography generated radiopaque images of the cerebral vasculature and could be used to identify vessel occlusions and eventually identify vascular lesions [8]. Distortion and displacement of the vascular anatomy could be used for hematoma or tumor localization.

There has been an ongoing evolution of the cerebral angiography, first as a diagnostic tool but then the potential for intervening in vascular pathology became possible. Subsequently, the eventual introduction of braided catheters and hydrophilic wires, which allowed quick and safe catheterizations, set the foundation for intervention. Modern digital subtraction angiography (DSA) machines consist of an image intensifier and digital subtraction flat panel detectors that utilize a fraction of the radiation dosage for the acquisition of images of the finest detail [9]. The ability to rotate the image intensifier around the patient allowed the development of 3D rotational images [10].

Although cerebral angiography remains a mainstay in the diagnosis and endovascular treatment of cerebrospinal vascular disorders [11], several limitations of this technique are evident. X-ray based cerebral angiography cannot view neurovascular structures clearly in complex vascular lesions, lack resolution necessary to visualize small vessels and critical perforating vessels, which are essential to the treatment of many cerebrovascular disorders. As a real-time guide during therapy, intraluminal imaging with ultrasonography, maybe a resolution in the future. This technique will provide not only therapeutic guidance but also real-time documentation of the completeness of therapy.

3. Cerebral aneurysms

Endovascular treatment of cerebral aneurysms had its start in neurosurgery. Werner et al. firstly reported successful electrothermic thrombosis of an intracranial aneurysm in 1941 [12]. With a transorbital puncture, "thirty feet of No. 34 gauge coin silver enameled wire was introduced into the aneurysm through a special needle" and "the wire was heated to an average temperature of 80°C for a total of 40 seconds. The aneurysm no longer bled when the needle was cleared at the conclusion of the operation" [12].

After these early attempts, particularly in the 1960s and early 1970s, several neurosurgeons and neuroradiologists sought therapeutic alternatives to conventional surgery [2]. Lacking devices suitable for safe navigation in the intracranial vasculature, their efforts originally concentrated on the extravascular route. Under radiographic guidance, thrombosis was initiated by passing electrical current to an electrode needle introduced within the aneurysm sac through a burr hole [13]. Mullan et al. described the treatment of intracranial aneurysms in a series of 12 patients, 10 of whom had presented with aneurysmal subarachnoid hemorrhage, by inducing electrothrombosis [13].

Until 1964, Luessenhop and Velasquez made the first endovascular attempt to treat a cerebral aneurysm [14]. They attempt to occlude a supraclinoid aneurysm with a silicone balloon. Subsequently, Serbinenko developed a balloon-mounted microcatheter with flow-directional capabilities for more effective intracranial catheterization [15]. He further developed detachable and nondetachable balloon catheters to make parent artery sacrifice or direct aneurysmal obliteration and to allow temporary balloon occlusion safe and reliable in the 1970s. His contributions gave birth to endovascular neurosurgery [15]. Balloon occlusion techniques were further used with a vast amount of clinical experience during the 1970s and 1980s [16–18].

Several major limitations of balloon occlusion technique are apparent. Aneurysmal catheterization was difficult without help of guidewire. The balloon shape often could not adequately filling an irregular aneurysm with leaving the fundus unprotected or creating a ball-valve effect of aneurysmal refilling. Therefore, the endovascular therapy of cerebral aneurysms shifted from balloon occlusion to free (pushable) platinum coil occlusion [2]. At this time, coil embolization for cerebral aneurysms is a dangerous procedure because of the inability to retrieve the pushed coils that migrated into the distal intracranial vasculature.

The innovation of electrolytic detachable coils by the Italian neurosurgeon Guido Guglielmi in the early 1990s updated the endovascular treatment of cerebral aneurysms [19, 20]. In the early 1980s, Guglielmi found accidental electrolytic detachment of the electrode tip while applying current to a stainless steel electrode inserted into an experimental aneurysm to promote electrothrombosis. After several years, he worked with Ivan Sepetka, an engineer at Target Therapeutics, Inc., to combine the two processes of endovascular electrolysis and electrothrombosis, which eventually resulted in the development of the present-day Guglielmi detachable coil (GDC; Boston Scientific/Target Therapeutics, Fremont CA) [21]. The Guglielmi detachable coil (GDC) can be re-positioned and examined before the coil was released electrolytically from its tether. On the other hand, the flexibility and softness of the coil enabled the safe filling of an irregular aneurysm with a low risk of rupture. The first intracranial aneurysm was treated using this new technology on April 12, 1990 [19]. The first multicenter GDC clinical trial result was published by Guglielmi et al. in 1992 [20]. Immediate complete occlusion was obtained in 81% of small-necked and 15% of wide-necked aneurysms with low procedure-related morbidity and mortality rates less than 5%. The GDC system was immediately accepted worldwide and became the focus of most published works on cerebral aneurysm management (**Figure 1**).

Despite the advantages of the GDC system, wide-necked and large aneurysms remained difficult to treat. New techniques were performed to keep the detached coils within the aneurysmal sac. Moret et al. was the pioneer of the "remodeling technique" using a balloon as a mechanical barrier to keep coils within the aneurysmal sac during its delivery (**Figure 2**) [22]. Moret et al. [22] published their results with use of the "balloon-remodeling technique" for the treatment of 56 cases of previously untreatable wide-necked cerebral aneurysms in 1997 with low morbidity and mortality rates.

An alternative approach to introduce a stent to maintain a patent lumen and provid a buttress to prevent coil herniation. After some early attempts of Wakhloo

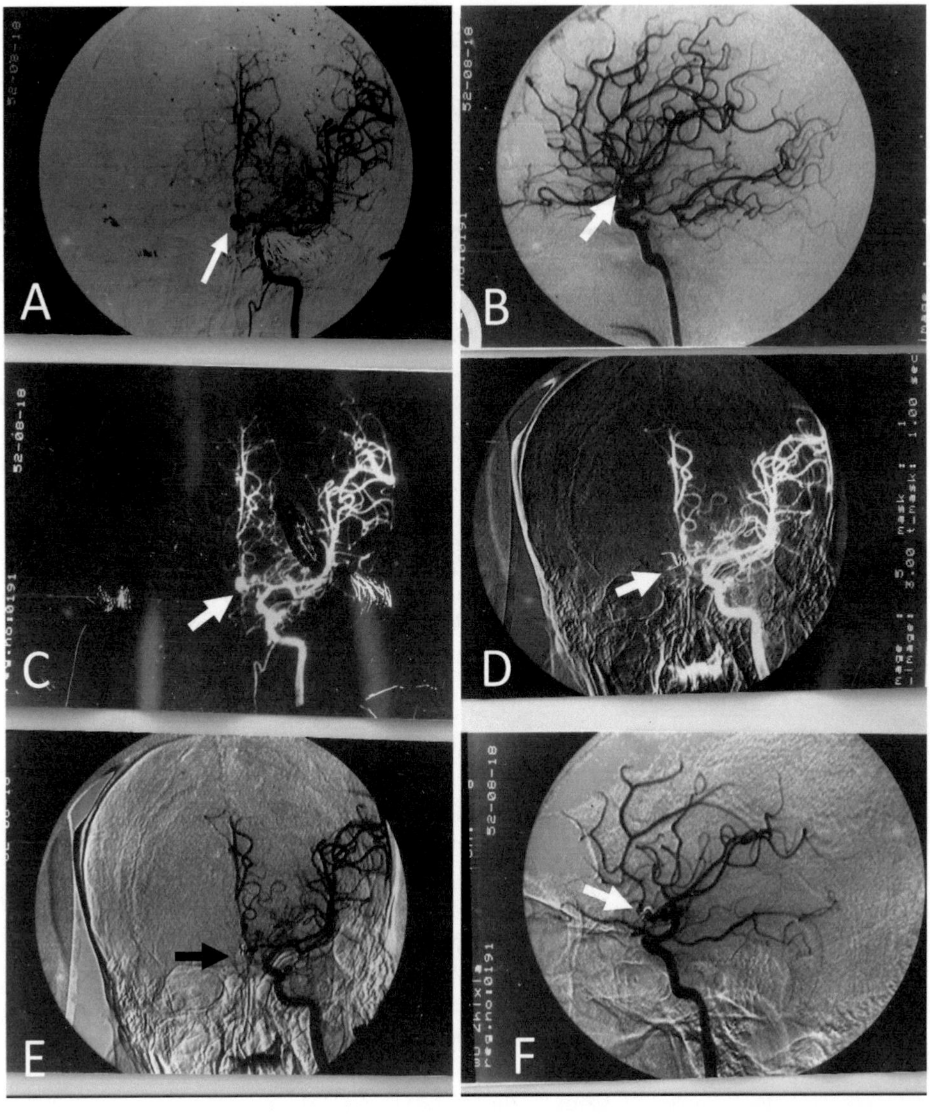

Figure 1.
A 46-year-old woman with a ruptured anterior communicating artery aneurysm was coiled with GDCs (Boston Scientific, USA) in 1998. A, frontal view of the left internal carotid artery injection. B, lateral view of the left internal carotid artery injection. Showing the aneurysm of the left anterior communicating artery (arrows). C, frontal view of the roadmap image of the left internal carotid artery injection showing the aneurysm (arrow). D, frontal view of the roadmap image after aneurysm coiling showing the disappearance of the aneurysm (arrow). E, frontal view of the left internal carotid artery injection after aneurysm coil embolization. F, lateral view of the left internal carotid artery injection after aneurysm coil embolization. Showing the aneurysm was completely occluded (arrows).

et al. [23] and Geremia et al. [24], this stent-assisting technique has been further explored and expanded by an increasing number of neurosurgeons [25]. Neurosurgeons and neurointerventional radiologists at several centers began to borrow stents from the interventional cardiology at the same time and publish their case reports about treating wide-necked aneurysms with a combination of stents and coils (**Figure 3**). These stents were designed specifically for cardiac usage and were stiffer and more difficult to use in the tortuous neurovascular anatomy.

With the introduction of neurovascular stents, specifically designed for intracranial use (Neuroform stent, Boston Scientific Target), borrowing cardiac stents soon became unnecessary [26]. Although the use of stents required a regimen of

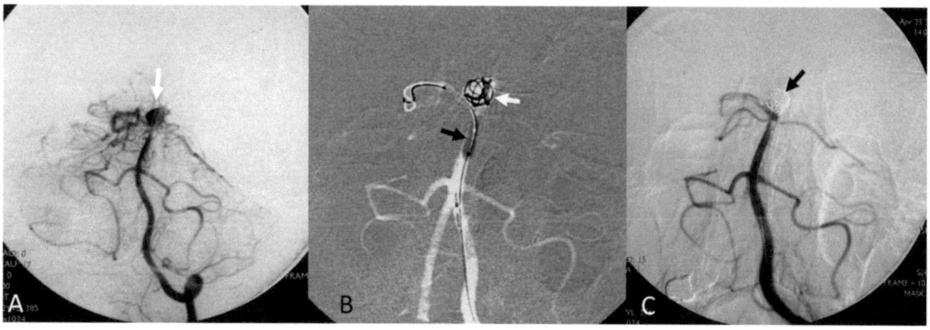

Figure 2.
A 37-year-old man presented with subarachnoid hemorrhage. A, frontal view of the left vertebral artery injection showing a basilar tip aneurysm (arrow). B, roadmap of the left vertebral artery injection showing the first orbit 3-D 7 mm × 13 cm coil and a 4 mm × 20 mm Hyperglide balloon catheter (Medtronic ev3, USA) (arrow). C, the left vertebral artery injection showing the aneurysm was completely occluded after subsequent coils (Microplex 6 mm × 15 cm,6 mm × 10 cm, 5 mm × 10 cm, orbit 5 mm × 15 cm, HydroCiol 3 mm × 7 cm, 2 mm × 4 cm, helix standard fiber 2 mm × 4 cm).

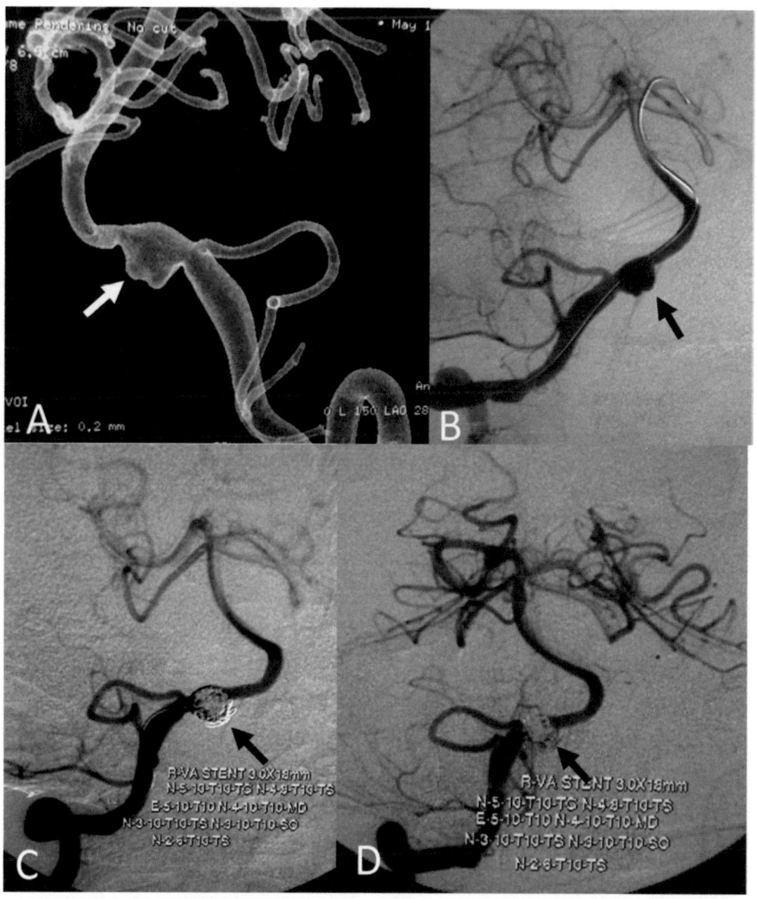

Figure 3.
A vertebral artery aneurysm treated with coronary artery stent and coiling in 1990s. A, 3-D angiogram of the right vertebral artery injection showing a dissecting aneurysm of vertebral artery-inferior posterior cerebellar artery (arrow). B, angiogram of the right vertebral artery injection showing a microwire was passed through the aneurysm for navigation of a BX coronary artery stent (Medtronic, USA). C, angiogram of the right vertebral artery injection showing the aneurysm was coiled with assistance of a 3.0 mm × 18 mm BX coronary artery stent (Medtronic, USA) (arrow). D, angiogram of the right vertebral artery injection showing the aneurysm was completely occluded (arrow).

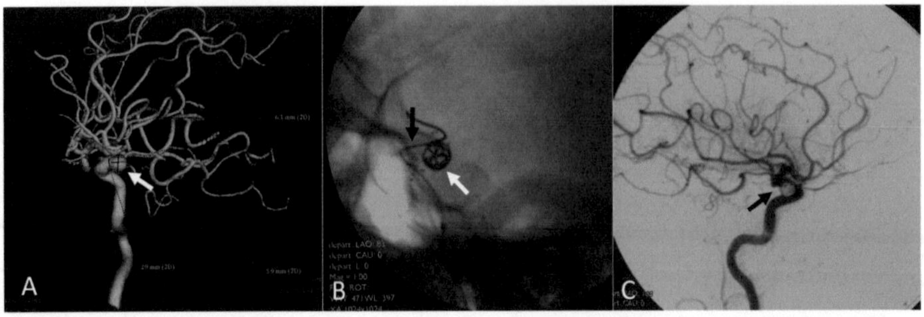

Figure 4.
A 62-year-old woman presented with an incidental paraclinoid aneurysm of the internal carotid artery. A, 3-D reconstruction of the right internal carotid artery injection showing the 6 mm × 6 mm paraclinoid aneurysm of the internal carotid artery (arrow), which was treated with 4 mm × 30 mm Neuroform stent and coils. B, the unsubtracted image showing the Neuroform stent (black arrow) and the first 3-D coil (white arrow). C, oblique view of the right internal carotid artery injection after treatment showing the aneurysm was occluded completely (arrow).

antiplatelet medication adding to the risk of the procedure itself as well as risks associated with the recovery period, these risks were quickly accommodated by interventionalists and improved overall occlusion rates as decreased the aneurysm recurrence (**Figure 4**) [27].

Bioactive coils were explored by some manufacturers to promote thrombus formation and endothelialization. However, these modified coils were shown to have limited efficacy and no clear advantage over pure platinum coils when used alone [28]. The use of polymers was also explored by some authors to treat cerebral aneurysms, but the increased risk and patient morbidity derailed this strategy and prevented its widespread acceptance [29].

It was firstly confirmed by the International Subarachnoid Aneurysm Trial (ISAT) that more and more aneurysm patients were being treated worldwide with the introduction of detachable coils and various intracranial stents [30]. An overall decreased risk of death and morbidity in the endovascular group treated with detachable coils when compared to those treated with open surgery were found [30]. The worldwide treatment of both ruptured and unruptured aneurysms by detachable coils quickly has surpassed open surgery as the primary treatment modality. Covered stents already are used successfully in the treatment of cerebral aneurysms, iatrogenic pseudoaneurysms, and carotid-cavernous fistulas (CCF) [31, 32].

4. Flow diverter

The introduction of flow diverter had a dramatic effect on the management of cerebral aneurysms. The concept of flow diverter was initially explored by Wakhloo in 2014, but Nelson and colleagues developed the first commercially available flow diverter [33]. Flow diverter introduced the concept of a more physiological therapy for aneurysms, focusing on treating the parent vessel without the requirement of entering the aneurysm dome [34]. With data that indicated complete occlusion rates that approached 90% at follow-up in systematic review, treatment recommendations for selected intracranial aneurysms was made [35]. Even giant aneurysms, in the past managed with balloon test occlusion and vessel sacrifice or complex bypasses, can now be managed with flow diverter with great efficacy and considerably lower morbidity [36, 37] (**Figure 5**). Moreover, the indications for flow diversion have been extended to smaller aneurysms that are usually treated with coiling, stent-coiling, or clipping [38].

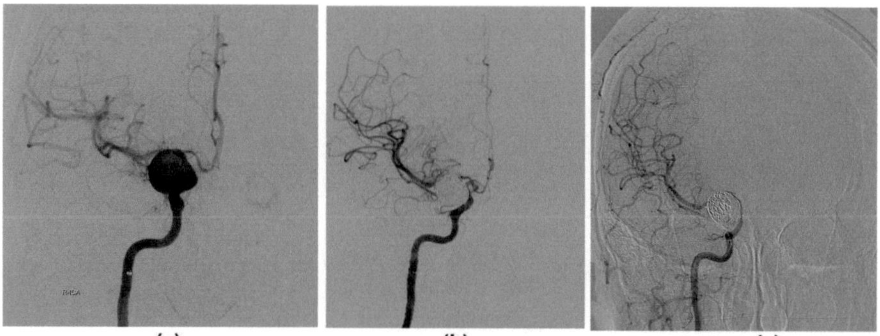

Figure 5.
A 58-year-old woman presented with visual deficit caused by a giant supraclinoid aneurysm of the internal carotid artery, which was treated by flow diverter. a, right internal carotid artery (ICA) angiogram (anteroposterior) demonstrating a giant aneurysm of the supraclinoid internal carotid artery. b, right ICA angiogram (anteroposterior) after pipeline flex flow diverter and coil embolization showing nearly complete occlusion of the aneurysm. c, right ICA angiogram (anteroposterior) at 1-year follow-up showing complete occlusion of the aneurysm.

Cerebral aneurysms, both ruptured and unruptured, can be treated with flow diverters [3]. Research into surface modification of devices to mitigate or negate the need for anticoagulation or antiplatelet medications is actively being pursued [3]. However, careful must be always taken in evaluating benefits and risks. In a recent paper by Gory et al., a total of 21.8% of interventions experienced at least 1 morbidity during the 12-month follow-up [39]. Among the serious events, 5.9% were considered permanent and related to the procedure. Moreover sixty-six (16%) of the 412 interventions had a complication, and 10 of them caused a neurological deficit [40].

5. Carotid-cavernous fistulas

Carotid-cavernous fistulas (CCF) are usually treated endovascularly by interventional neuroradiologists or neurosurgeons. The endovascular treatment strategies of CCF has dramatically changed with the evolution of endovascular neurosurgery. A series of treatment modalities have been traditionally attempted, including the carotid artery ligation or trapping, muscle embolization via cervical exposure of the carotid artery, and balloon embolization with or without carotid artery sacrifice [41]. Brooks reported successful closure of a CCF with a muscle embolus introduced surgically into the carotid artery in 1930 [42]. Serbinenko revolutionized the therapy for CCF in the 1970s by introducing detachable intravascular balloons [43]. Though these lesions were often treated with balloon test occlusion and vessel sacrifice in the early stage (**Figure 6**), CCFs are now almost exclusively treated by an endovascular strategy with preservation of the internal carotid artery. Balloon embolization of CCF through a transfemoral access with preservation of the distal ICA has reduced the morbidity related to the treatment. This method is the primary therapy in most cases of CCF [44]. In addition to the balloon embolization, several other modalities have been deemed useful in the treatment of CCF in recent years [45], such as detachable coils, covered stents, ethylene vinyl alcohol copolymer (EVOH) and flow diverter placement [45, 46] (**Figure 7**). Transvenous embolization via the inferior petrosal sinus, superior ophthalmic vein and EVOH embolization modalities have been used with success [46]. Spontaneous resolution and/or thrombosis of CCF has also been reported, especially in indirect CCF, but

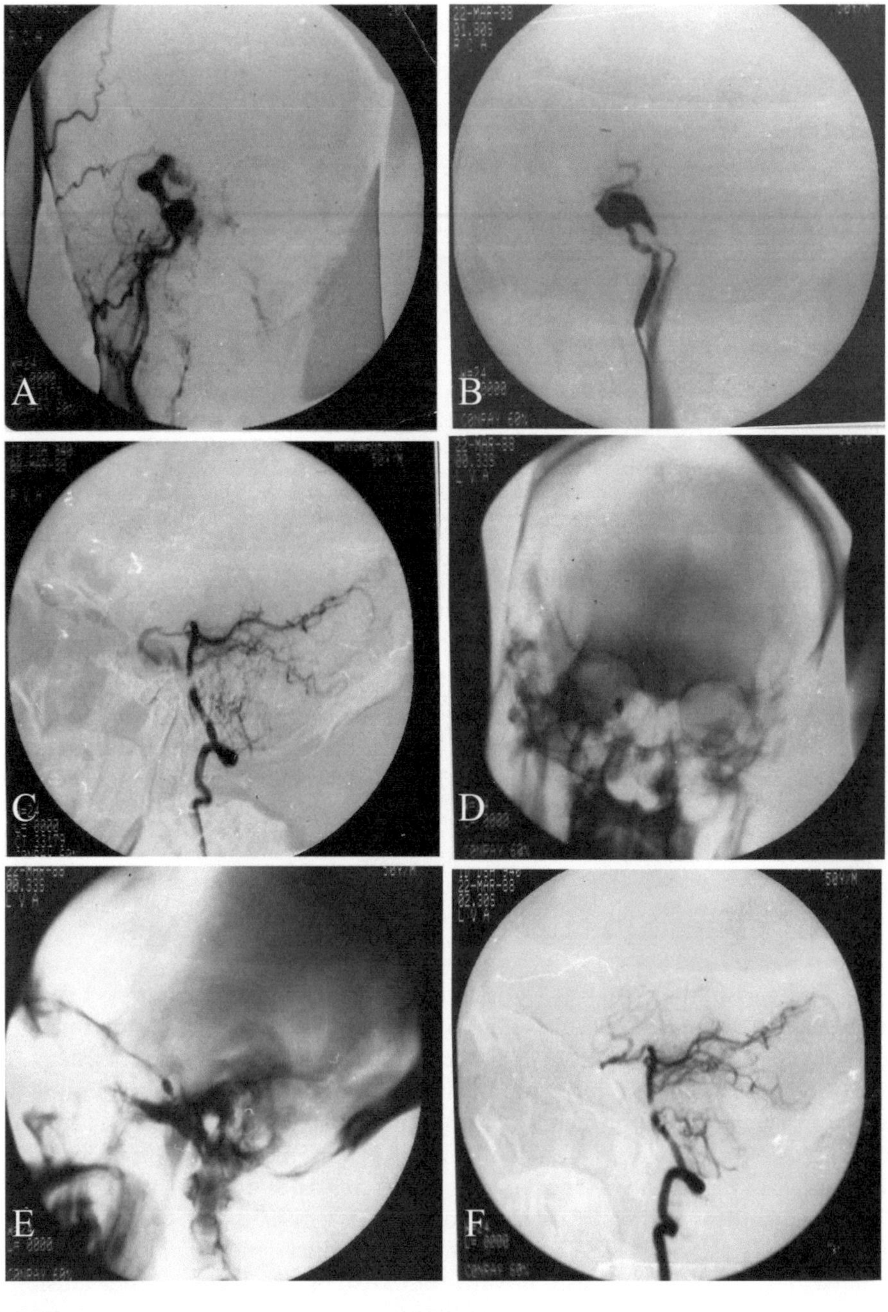

Figure 6.
A 50-year-old male patient of carotid-cavernous fistula was treated with detachable balloon in 1985. A, right internal carotid artery (ICA) angiogram (anteroposterior) and lateral (B) showing a direct carotid cavernous fistula and early opacification of right cavernous sinus with no antegrade flow beyond the cavernous sinus. C, left vertebral artery angiogram (lateral) showing opacification of right cavernous sinus. Because the patient had no neurological symptoms with no contribution from the right ICA, no balloon test occlusion was performed before sacrifice of the ICA. D, fluoroscopic view of the head (anteroposterior) and lateral (E) showing the placement of one detachable balloon in the ICA of fistula site. F, left vertebral artery angiogram confirming complete occlusion of the fistula with reconstitution of the distal ICA blood flow from the vertebral artery. No retrograde filling of the fistula is seen.

it is really rare. For less directly accessible lesions, superior ophthalmic vein access or direct puncture of the cavernous sinus and catheterization as an alternative approach to the cavernous sinus as well as transvenous routes can all be used [47].

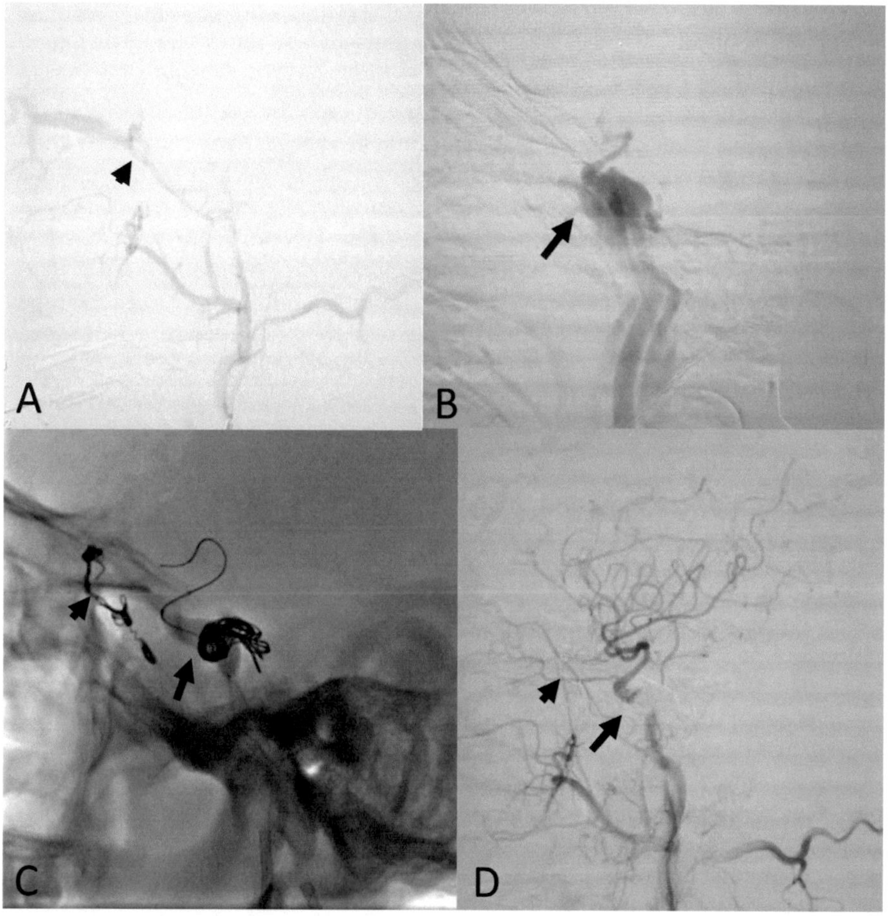

Figure 7.
A 33-year-old male patient of traumatic carotid-cavernous fistula was treated with preservation of the internal carotid artery. A, lateral view of the right external carotid artery showed an arteriovenous shunt between the anterior meningeal branch of the middle meningeal artery and the right superior ophthalmic vein (arrowhead). B, lateral view of the right carotid artery showed the high-flow carotid-cavernous fistula drained by the right superior ophthalmic vein and the right inferior petrosal sinus (arrow). C lateral view of unsubtracted image showed the inflated scepter C balloon (4 mm × 20 mm, Microvention, USA) in the right internal carotid artery (arrow) and the coils. Note the external carotid artery fistula was occluded with coils (arrowhead). D, lateral view of the left carotid artery angiogram after balloon-assisted onyx injection showed complete obliteration of the both fistulas and the intact left internal carotid artery.

6. Arteriovenous malformation

Exponential advances in catheter technology and refinements of embolic agents have greatly facilitated the rapid evolution of AVM embolization. In 1960's, Luessenhop and Spence performed the first embolization procedure on a cerebral AVM by surgically introducing silastic spheres made of methyl methacrylate into the ICA [48]. At that time, silk sutures, porcelain beads, Gelfoam, steel balls, Teflon-coated spheres, and polyvinyl alcohol were explored for AVM embolization with varying degrees of efficacy [49]. The use of these particle emboli was associated with a high complication rate secondary to inadvertent embolization of a normal cerebral vessel because the technologies and devices were not for direct nidus embolization.

Kerber developed the first calibrated-leak balloon, which allowed the direct embolization of an AVM nidus with the use of a rapidly solidifying polymer in

1976 [50]. This new system in combination with advances in imaging techniques and liquid embolic materials ushered in the modern era of AVM embolization. However, the use of calibrated-leak balloon catheters was associated with a high risk of arterial rupture. The introduction of liquid embolic agents, initially in the form of n-BCA, an acrylic adhesive [51], and advances in microcatheter and microwire design facilitated the distal catheterization of vascular malformations so that embolization of AVMs has evolved immensely over the last few decades to become a highly valuable therapy, and even an alternative in some cases, to surgery or stereotactic radiosurgery [52, 53]. The introduction of polymer non-adhesives (EVOH) allowed deep and extensive nidal penetration without the need for repeat distal catheterization and could be performed over long embolization procedure time periods [52].

Cerebral angiography detailed morphology study of the arteriovenous malformation involves evaluating the hemodynamic and anatomic characteristics of the lesion, including examination of the feeding arteries, the nidus itself, venous drainage of the lesion, coexisting aneurysms and arteriovenous fistulas [54]. A variety of strategies emerged, including multiple pedicle embolizations of the nidus. This was used by Lv et al. to "embolize AVM for cure" with low morbidity and mortality [55] (**Figures 8** and **9**). Endovascular surgery has specific indications in the treatment of AVMs, such as ruptured AVM, AVM of small size or deep locations, AVM with coexisting aneurysm and high flow fistula. Theoretically discussed and considered in the past, transvenous embolization is now being extensively explored, but its initial reports documented higher procedure-related hemorrhage rates [56].

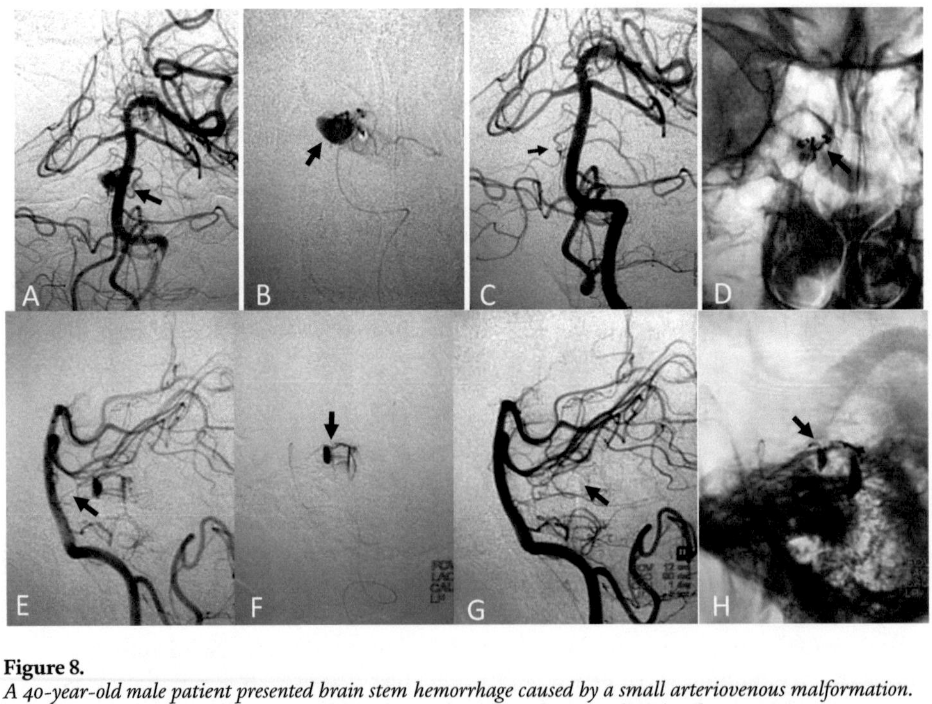

Figure 8.
A 40-year-old male patient presented brain stem hemorrhage caused by a small arteriovenous malformation. Anteroposterior angiography views (A-D) and lateral angiography views (E-H) . Showing a posterior pons arteriovenous malformation (AVM) fed by the left perforating artery of the basilar trunk (arrows in panels of a, E). Superselective angiogram demonstrating the ectasia of draining vein (arrows in panels of B, F). Angiograms after superselective onyx embolization showing complete disappearance of the AVM (arrows in panels of C, G). Postoperative images demonstrating onyx cast (arrows in panels of D, H).

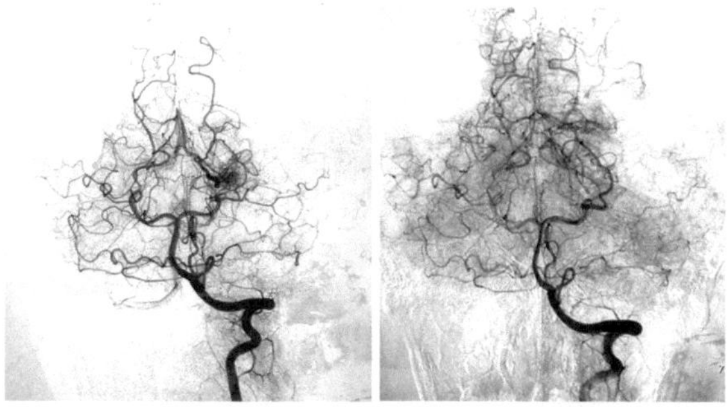

Figure 9.
A 5-year-old boy presented with intracranial hemorrhage caused by a small arteriovenous malformation. a, anteroposterior angiography of the left vertebral artery showing a small arteriovenous malformation (AVM) fed by the left posterior cerebral artery. b, anteroposterior angiography of the left vertebral artery after superselective onyx embolization showing complete disappearance of the AVM.

7. Vein of Galen malformations

Vein of Galen malformations are extremely rare lesions occurring in one out of a million live births [57]. They are treated almost exclusively with endovascular surgery. The lesions are amenable to endovascular embolization in the newborn presenting with heart failure or diagnosed in utero. An initial treatment stage is necessary and followed by additional staged embolization when the child is large enough to undergo more extensive embolization. Embolization strategies include closing the individual arteriovenous shunts or the initial venous side of the malformation.

8. Dural arteriovenous fistulas

Dural arteriovenous fistulas (DAVFs) represent a specific vascular lesion that incorporates the dural suppliers of the cranium or spine, contributing direct arterial shunting toward venous structures. Venous hypertension can lead to cortical

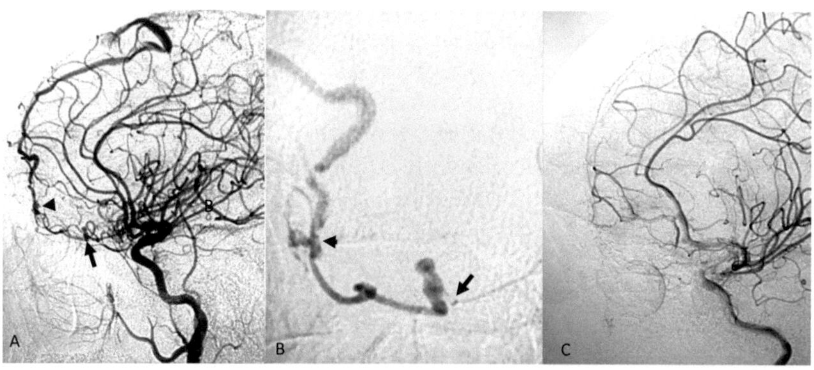

Figure 10.
A dural fistula fed by pial branches of the frontobasal artery was cured with onyx emblization. A, later internal carotid artery (ICA) angiogram showing a dural fistula fed by pial branches of the frontobasal artery and early opacification of frontal polar vein (arrowhead). Note the pseudoaneurysm on the feeding artery (arrow). B, superselective angiography by the microcatheter showing the pseudoaneurysm (arrow) and the fistula point (arrowhead). C, lateral internal carotid artery angiogram confirming complete occlusion of the aneurysm and the dural fistula.

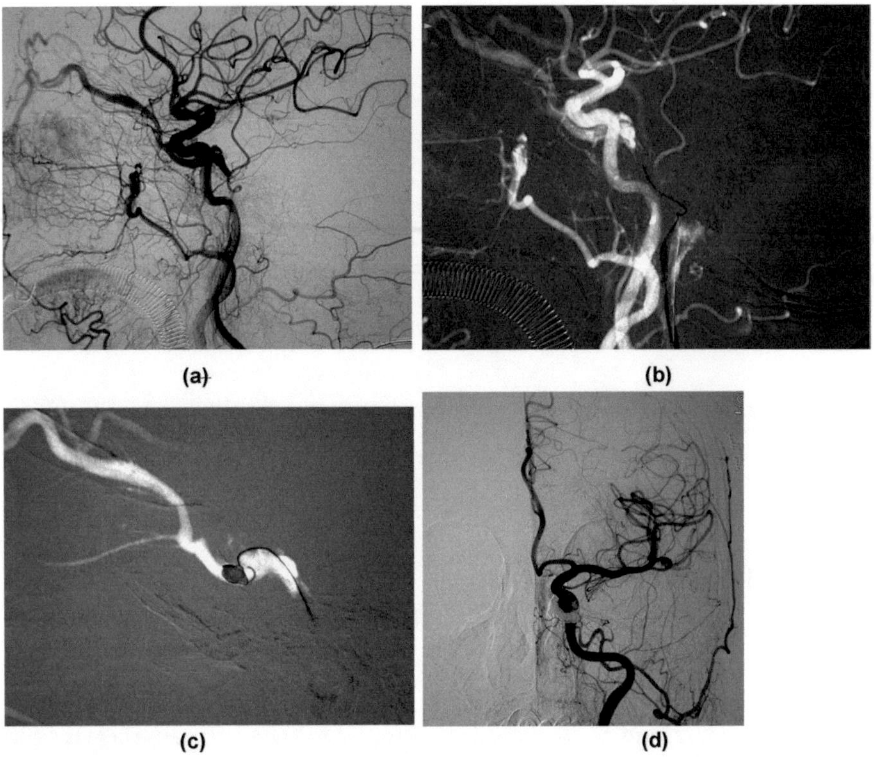

Figure 11.
A cavernous sinus dural fistula was cured with tranvenous access. a, lateral view of the left carotid artery showed the left indirect carotid-cavernous fistula drained by the left superior ophthalmic vein and the left inferior petrosal sinus was invisible. b, under roadmap image, the left inferior petrosal sinus was catheterized. c, under roadmap image, coils were delivered through the microcatheter in the left cavernous sinus through the left inferior petrosal sinus. d, frontal view of the left carotid artery showed complete obliteration of the carotid-cavernous fistula and the intact left internal carotid artery.

dysfunction, venous hypertension, and hemorrhage when DAVF occurs intracranially [58]. However, dilation of venous structures along the spinal cord can lead to myelopathy from tissue engorgement and venous hypertension as well as physical compression when DAVF occurs in the spine. The complex anatomy and points of arteriovenous shunting make their management complex. EVOH-based embolic materials have been proved to be useful in the endovascular obliteration of these lesions [59] (**Figure 10**). When these materials are combined with balloon catheters, a deep penetration to the point of arteriovenous shunts can be achieved [60]. Transvenous approaches are also routinely employed and highly successful when arterial access to the fistula point cannot be achieved (**Figure 11**) [61].

9. Spinal vascular malformations

Vascular lesions of the spine and spinal cord can be categorized into intramedullary and extramedullary lesions [62]. These lesions are rare and comprise a heterogeneous spectrum of diseases. They were first reported in the 19th century with the autopsy-based classification of Virchow and Picard [63]. However, it was in the 1970s, with the advent of selective spinal angiography, that they became better understood [64]. Their identification and localization have progressed significantly with the development of imaging techniques [65]. Several classification systems have been proposed over time to describe vascular lesions of the spine [66].

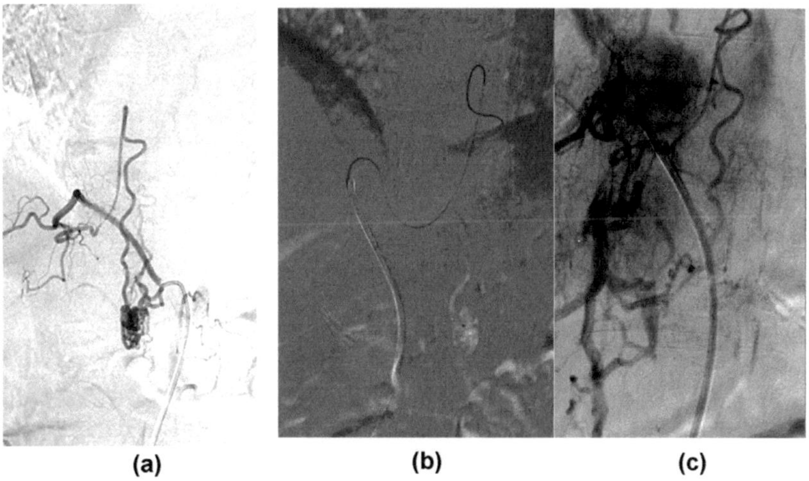

Figure 12.
A 49-year-old man presented weakness of two legs. a, left T-8 intercostal pedicle injection reveals the anterior spinal artery from above and below along the axis to supply the perimedullary fistula. b, under roadmap image a microcatheter was accessed to the fistulous point. c, control angiogram after onyx embolization reveals obliteration of the fistula with preservation of the anterior spinal axis.

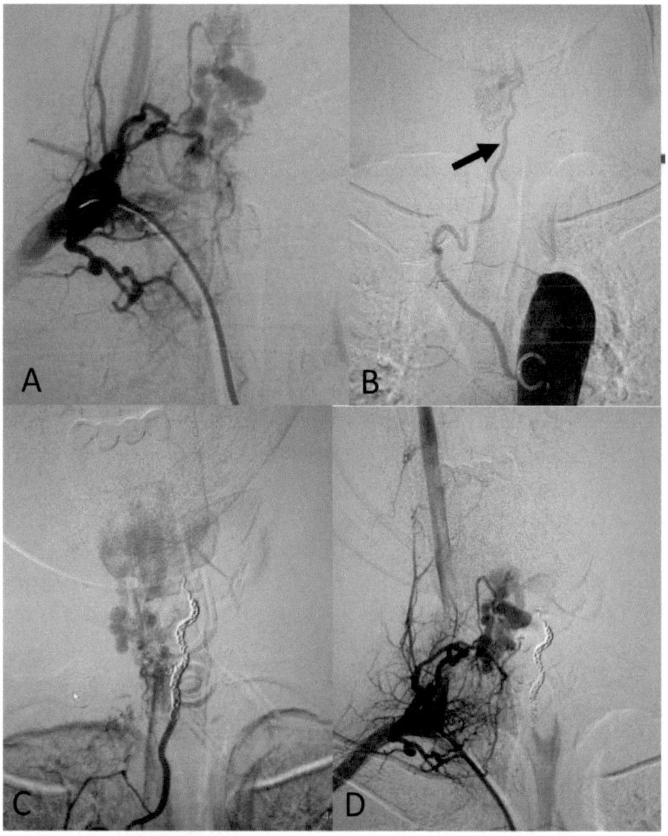

Figure 13.
A 37-year-old woman presented with SAH caused by a juvenile type spinal AVM. A, the right subclavian angiogram. B, aortic artery angiogram. Reveal supply to the AVM in the vertebra and the soft tissue around with feeders arising from right subclavian and intercostal arteries. After treatment, aortic artery angiogram (C) and the right subclavian angiogram (D), partial embolization with coils to reduce the venous congestion was performed through the left radiculomedullary artery (arrow).

The well known classification proposed by Anson and Spetzler in 1992 is type I, dural arteriovenous fistula (AVF); type II, glomus intramedullary AVM (**Figure 12**); type III, juvenile malformations (**Figure 13**); and type IV, perimedullary AVF [67]. With recent advances in embolic materials and devices in endovascular treatment, transarterial embolization plays an increasingly important role in the treatment of spinal AVMs. Complete angiographical obliteration of the nidus is not necessarily the goal of embolization, but rather, the treatment aims to reduce shunting volume and stabilize the symptoms [68].

10. Venous sinus stenting

Transvenous approaches have become quite useful in the treatment of dural sinus stenosis, often associated with a diverticulum of the sinus [69, 70]. With venous sinus stenting, promising results have been achieved in treating intracranial hypertension and venous stenosis–related pulsatile tinnitus. King et al. (1995) were the first to describe the venous stenosis through venography and manometry in intracranial hypertension but Higgins et al. became the first to stent the venous sinus in 2002 on a female with medically refractory intracranial hypertension [71]. Venography revealed bilateral transverse sinus stenosis and after stenting of one side, there was a significant improvement in trans-stenosis gradient and symptomatic control. Only in severe cases of cerebral sinus thrombosis that do not improve or deteriorate despite anticoagulant therapy, endovascular treatment would be considered.

11. Cerebral atherosclerotic stenoses

The development of angioplasty and stenting was influenced by the early work of endoluminal dilation of peripheral atherosclerotic disease. Until 1980, cerebral transluminal balloon catheter dilatation was reported to treat two patients with frequent, severe, progressive symptoms despite anticoagulation and high-grade intracranial atherosclerotic stenosis (ICAS) of the basilar artery [72]. The excellent angiographic and short-term clinical in these two patients and the prevalence of ICAS had favored further research of this approach. Unfortunately, frequent complications were reported in the next case series, including arterial dissection with consecutive thrombosis or rupture, residual stenosis due to sequestration or vessel recoiling and acute or subacute vascular occlusion due to the formation of a wall hematoma [72]. In order to reduce periprocedural complications of angioplasty alone, the rigid coronary Palmaz-Schatz stent was introduced for the first time in 1996 in a patient with recurrent TIA caused by severe ICAS of the right carotid artery despite antiplatelet and anticoagulant therapy [73]. The stent deployment led to a better angiographic result compared to angioplasty alone.

The first self-expanding, nitinol-composed Wingspan stent (Boston Scientific, Fremont, CA, USA) was approved by the US Food and Drug Administration (FDA) for patients with 50% or higher ICAS, symptomatic despite medical therapy in 2005 [74]. These patients might benefit from endovascular therapy since their plaques might not stabilize with best medical therapy alone and cause recurrent artery-to-artery embolic strokes. The development of new angioplasty balloon catheters and flexible stents has redefined the management strategy for symptomatic intracranial stenosis. A growing number of studies have reported a low complication profile and satisfactory rates of angiographic patency at follow-up [75].

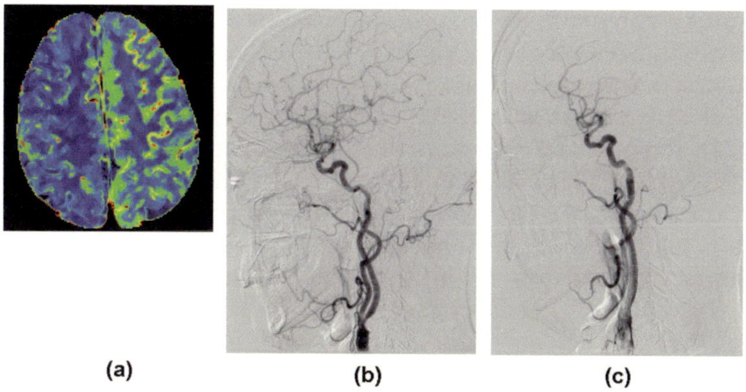

Figure 14.
A 79-year-old man presented with dizziness. a, CT perfusion image showing the low perfusion of the right cerebral hemisphere. b, right carotid artery angiogram showing the severe stenosis of the internal carotid artery. c, right carotid artery angiogram showing the stenosis was treated with angioplasty and stenting.

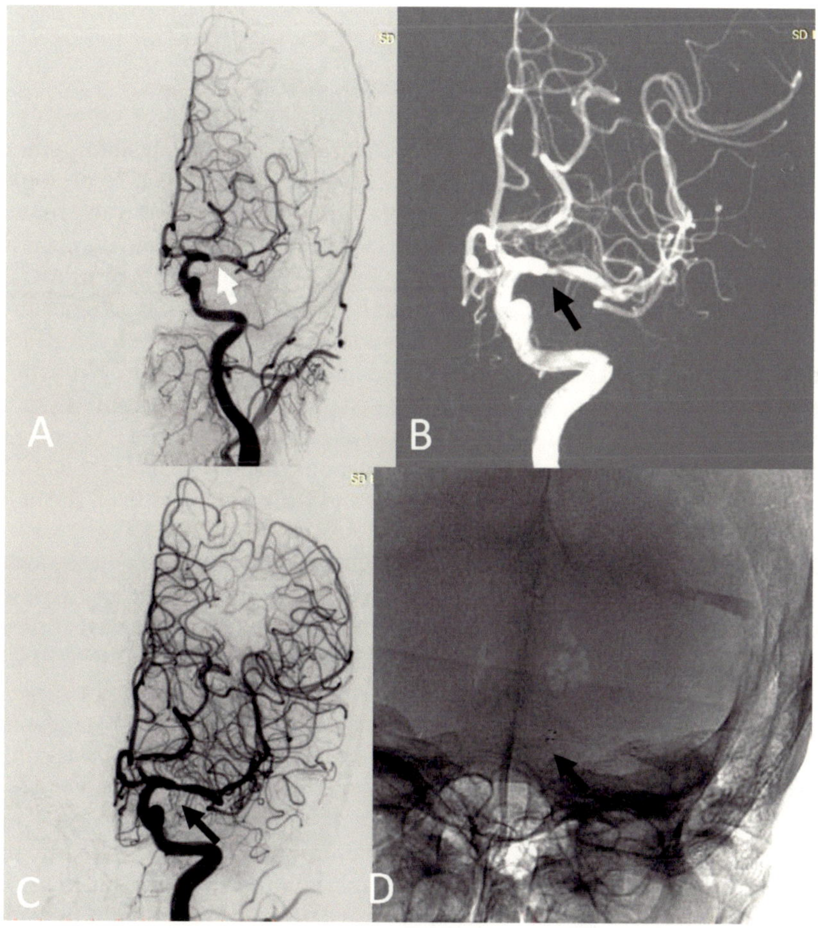

Figure 15.
A 64-year-old man presented with transient ischemic attack. A, left internal carotid artery (ICA) angiogram (anteroposterior) showing a severe stenosis of the M1 segment of the middle cerebral artery (arrow). B, under roadmap image showing a XT27 catheter (Stryker, USA) was advanced to the distal middle cerebral artery after balloon angioplasty (arrow). C, left internal carotid artery angiogram confirming the reconstitution of the middle cerebral artery (arrow). D, fluoroscopic view of the head showing the placement of a Neuroform EZ stent (arrow).

Angioplasty with stenting of carotid stenosis does not require general anesthesia and requires only a few seconds of carotid artery occlusion. Endoluminal revascularization has been proposed for the treatment of carotid stenosis in high-risk patients such as those with contralateral carotid occlusion [76], postendarterectomy stenosis [77], and/or severe coronary and other systemic diseases [78]. In a meta-analysis by Texakalidis et al. in 2018 including 13 comparative studies, compared to carotid artery endarterectomy carotid artery stenting had a lower incidence of cranial nerve injury, the two treatment approaches were similarly safe in terms of periprocedural stroke, myocardial infarction and death rates and carotid artery stent was associated with decreased restenosis risk (defined as either 60% or 70% stenosis) in the follow-up; however, without a significant difference in the risk of target lesion revascularization [79].

At present, we suggest that endovascular therapy may be considered as a treatment option for patients with recurrent ischaemic stroke despite best medical therapy and especially if pathophysiologically attributed to hypoperfusion with/without bad collaterals [80] (**Figures 14** and **15**). In future, better experience of interventionalists and improved features of stents deployed are also expected to boost outcome of endovascular therapy in ICAS.

12. Thrombolysis and mechanical thrombectomy

Before 1995, stroke therapy consisted exclusively of supportive management and efforts to prevent recurrence [81]. In 1995, the National Institute of Neurological Disorders and Stroke reported that early intravenous thrombolysis using tissue plasminogen activator was more effective than placebo [81]. The use of Alteplase for acute ischemic strokes was approved by The Food and Drug Administration (FDA) in 1996 [82]. Thrombolytic therapy was initially offered to eligible patients up to 4.5 hours from symptom onset. IV Alteplase was determined not to be as effective a therapy for patients with large vessel occlusions although it was proved to be an effective treatment. The concept of intraarterial pharmacologic thrombolysis was further expanded and solidified in 1999 with the completion of the Prolyse in Acute Cerebral Thromboembolism study [83]. Intravenous thrombolysis and intra-arterial thrombolysis received widespread acceptance and truly revolutionized the management of acute stroke.

Mechanical thrombectomy has transformed our field, leading to an explosion in intervention for large vessel occlusion. Endovascular thrombectomy became the standard of care of the large vessel occlusion as a result of 5 randomized control trials (RCTs) in 2015 [84]. These 5 trials, MR CLEAN, ESCAPE, SWIFT PRIME, EXTEND-IA, and REVASCAT, extended the field of endovascular neurosurgery. These RCTs proved that patients who had improved functional outcome scores at 90 days after thrombectomy with successful recanalization [84]. This was compared with patients who received IV thrombolytic therapy alone or were unable to receive IV thrombolytic therapy. Improved functional outcomes were also demonstrated by two additional landmark trials, DAWN and DEFUSE [85]. Endovascular thrombectomy for large vessel occlusion beyond the window of 3 to 4.5 hours has provided new treatment options and supportive data demonstrating improved functional outcome scores. Patients meeting eligibility criteria for mechanical thrombectomy had no additional risks in the extended window of 16 to 24 hours. The second generation of devices, including stent retrievers and aspiration catheters, has demonstrated a significantly improved safety, revascularization, and patient outcome. Therefore, the criteria for mechanical thrombectomy, including time limit and physiological preconditions should be re-examined. Not only were time limits extended, but also discussions on the ability to preserve additional tissue at risk, even in the setting of an established stroke, have made stroke intervention a significant part of the foundation of endovascular practice. "Stroke center," "mechanical thrombectomy ready," and "comprehensive stroke center" designations have all been applied.

13. Tumor embolization and intra-arterial chemotherapy

Direct vascular access to brain tumors both benign and malignant has been exploited since the 1970s [86]. Preoperative embolization can facilitate resection and decrease intraoperative blood loss in the treatment of meningiomas. As with all endovascular strategies, keen understanding of the vascular anatomy is required to prevent unnecessary risk. Over the past few years, intra-arterial chemotherapy for more malignant tumors, such as gliomas, has had a resurgence. In future, the new neuro-pharmaceutical/chemotherapy/immunotherapy drugs, which could be delivered intra-arterially, will be developed [87].

14. Subdural hematoma embolization

Chronic subdural hematoma may be one of the most common neurological conditions requiring treatment in the future because of an aging population and the regular use of antiplatelet and anticoagulation medications. Chronic subdural hematoma has been managed with craniotomy and/or drainage both operatively and at the bedside. Embolization of the middle meningeal artery supply to the dura and subdural membranes as a renewed treatment of chronic subdural hematoma has been originally described by Japanese neurosurgeons almost 20 years ago [88]. The technique can be used as a rescue technique in patients who have undergone previous craniotomy as well as a primary treatment in patients with significant comorbidities. Particle embolization and liquid embolic agents have demonstrated excellent results in recent publications [89]. These encouraging results suggested the need for a large prospective randomized trial to investigate the true role of middle meningeal artery embolization as a stand-alone treatment for chronic subdural hematoma.

15. Resident and fellowship training

The expansion of endovascular techniques has led to a need to train neurosurgical residents in the application of endovascular therapies, just as they would learn newer techniques in spine or tumor neurosurgery. The Neurosurgery Residency Review Committee and American Board of Neurological Surgeons (ABNS) have correctly made regular adjustments in the area of endovascular case minimums for neurosurgery residents not only to include cerebral angiography, but now also to include more complex intervention experience, such as aneurysm coiling [90].

The future of endovascular neurosurgery would be inseparable from the future of neurosurgery. Residents interested in the vascular disease processes that affect the central nervous system must understand the application of neuroendovascular techniques and if they want to treat these pathologies must be adequately trained in their implementation. In Japan and China, most endovascular surgery is carried out by neurosurgeons who carry out cerebral and spinal cord angiography and interpret the images obtained. This experience not only increases their knowledge of vascular anatomy, but also improves their surgical acumen.

We do not believe that the vascular neurosurgeon of the future must carry out both surgical and endovascular treatments. Precisely in order to reach the required excellence, there must be two figures, a vascular neurosurgeon who deals with the traditional surgical management knows the strengths and weaknesses of endovascular treatment, and an endovascular neurosurgeon knows the strengths and weaknesses of surgical treatment. To remain at the forefront of evaluating, caring for, and treating patients with cerebrovascular disease, vascular neurosurgery must evolve toward a specialty, mastering the knife as well as the catheter. We think it is time for neurosurgeons to start training residents in endovascular neurosurgery in the same way we train neurosurgeons in every other neurosurgical discipline.

16. Conclusion

Endovascular neurosurgery provides management of neurovascular conditions encountered in clinical practice, such as aneurysms (with or without subarachnoid hemorrhage), AVMs, dural AVFs, and carotid disease. The success of endovascular thrombectomy for large vessel occlusion is now irrefutable, making it an accepted standard of care. Endovascular treatment of cerebral aneurysms is no longer limited to primary coiling but now includes options such as stent or balloon assistance, flow diversion, intrasaccular and bifurcation-specific devices. Balloons, liquid embolic agents, and distal access catheters have updated the treatment of arteriovenous malformations and fistulae. The evolution of the neuroendovascular field has resulted in the development of program requirements for residency or fellowship education in endovascular neurosurgery.

Author details

Xianli Lv, MD
Neurosurgery Department, Beijing Tsinghua Changgung Hospital, School of Clinical Medicine, Tsinghua University, Beijing, China

*Address all correspondence to: lvxianli000@163.com

References

[1] Boulos AS, Levy EI, Bendok BR, Kim SH, Qureshi AI, Guterman LR, Hopkins LN. Evolution of neuroendovascular intervention: a review of advancement in device technology. Neurosurgery. 2004 Feb;54(2):438-53.

[2] Hopkins LN, Lanzino G, Guterman LR. Treating complex nervous system vascular disorders through a "needle stick": origins, evolution, and future of neuroendovascular therapy. Neurosurgery. 2001 Mar;48(3): 463-75.

[3] Iosif C. Neurovascular devices for the treatment of intracranial aneurysms: emerging and future technologies. Expert Rev Med Devices. 2020 Mar;17(3):173-188.

[4] Wang H, Fraser K, Wang D, Lanzino G. The evolution of endovascular therapy for neurosurgical disease. Neurosurg Clin N Am. 2005 Apr;16(2):223-9.

[5] Day AL, Siddiqui AH, Meyers PM, Jovin TG, Derdeyn CP, Hoh BL, et al: Training standards in neuroendovascular surgery: program accreditation and practitioner certification. Stroke 48:2318-2325, 2017

[6] Lobo-Antunes J. Egas Moniz and cerebral angiography. J Neurosurg 1974;40:427-32.

[7] Artico M, Spoletini M, Fumagalli L, Biagioni F, Ryskalin L, Fornai F, et al: Egas Moniz: 90 years (1927-2017) from cerebral angiography. Front Neuroanat 11:81, 2017

[8] Wolpert SM, Caplan LR. Current role of cerebral angiography in the diagnosis of cerebrovascular diseases. AJR Am J Roentgenol. 1992 Jul;159(1):191-7.

[9] Zhu XL, Chan MS, Poon WS. Spontaneous intracranial hemorrhage: which patients need diagnostic cerebral angiography? A prospective study of 206 cases and review of the literature. Stroke. 1997 Jul;28(7):1406-9.

[10] Cardinale F, Pero G, Quilici L, Piano M, Colombo P, Moscato A, Castana L, Casaceli G, Fuschillo D, Gennari L, Cenzato M, Lo Russo G, Cossu M. Cerebral Angiography for Multimodal Surgical Planning in Epilepsy Surgery: Description of a New Three-Dimensional Technique and Literature Review. World Neurosurg. 2015 Aug;84(2):358-67.

[11] Lv X, Li W, Li Y. Training residents and fellows in the procedure of diagnostic cervicocerebral angiography: Techniques to avoid complications. Neurol India. 2018 May-Jun;66(3):652-656.

[12] Werner SC, Blakemore AH, King BG. Aneurysm of the internal carotid artery within the skull: wiring and electrothermic coagulation. JAMA 1941;116: 578-82.

[13] Mullan S, Raimondi AJ, Dobben G, Vailati G, Hekmatpanah J. Electrically induced thrombosis in intracranial aneurysms. J Neurosurg 1965;22:539-47.

[14] Luessenhop AJ, Velasquez AC. Observations on the tolerance of intracranial arteries to catheterization. J Neurosurg 1964;21:85-91.

[15] Teitelbaum GP, Larsen DW, Zelman V, Lysachev AG, Likhterman LB. A tribute to Dr. Fedor A. Serbinenko, founder of endovascular neurosurgery. Neurosurgery 2000;46(2):462-70.

[16] HorowitzMB, Levy E, Kassam A, Purdy PD. Endovascular therapy for intracranial aneurysms: a historical

and present status review. Surg Neurol 2002;57:147-59.

[17] Higashida RT, Halbach VV, Dowd C, Barnwell SL, Dormandy B, Bell J, et al. Endovascular detachable balloon embolization therapy of cavernous carotid artery aneurysms: results in 87 cases. J Neurosurg 1990;72:857-63.

[18] Moret J, Boulin A, Mawad M, Castaings L. Endovascular treatment of berry aneurysms by endosaccular balloon occlusion. Neuroradiology 1991; 33(Suppl):135-6.

[19] Guglielmi G, Vinuela F, Dion J, Duckwiler G. Electrothrombosis of saccular aneurysms via endovascular approach. Part 2: preliminary clinical experience. J Neurosurg 1991;75:8-14.

[20] Guglielmi G, Vinuela F, Duckwiler G. Endovascular treatment of posterior circulation aneurysms by electrothrombosis using electrically detachable coils. J Neurosurg 1992;77:515-24.

[21] Target Therapeutics: Target Therapeutics: History of the GDC. Fremont, Target Therapeutics.

[22] Moret J, Cognard C, Weill A, Castaings L, Rey A. The "remodeling technique" in the treatment of wide neck intracranial aneurysms: angiographic results and clinical follow-up in 56 cases. Intervent Neuroradiol 1997;21:838-45.

[23] Wakhloo AK, Schellhammer F, de Vries J, Haberstroh J, Schumacher M. Self-expanding and balloon-expandable stents in the treatment of carotid aneurysms: an experimental study in a canine model. AJNR Am J Neuroradiol 1994;15(3):493-502.

[24] Geremia G, Haklin M, Brennecke L. Embolization of experimentally created aneurysms with intravascular stent devices. AJNR Am J Neuroradiol 1994; 15(3):1223-31.

[25] Wakhloo AK, Lanzino G, Lieber BB, Hopkins LN: Stents for intracranial aneurysms: The beginning of a new endovascular era? Neurosurgery 43:377-379, 1998.

[26] Henkes H, Bose A, Felber S, Miloslavski E, Berg-Dammer E, Kühne D. Endovascular coil occlusion of intracranial aneurysms assisted by a novel self-expandable nitinol microstent (neuroform). Interv Neuroradiol. 2002 Jun 30;8(2):107-19.

[27] Zhang J, Lv M, Lv X, Jiang C, Li Y, Wu Z. Endovascular treatment using stents for cerebral aneurysms. Neuroradiol J. 2010;23:730-736

[28] McDougall CG, Johnston SC, Gholkar A, Barnwell SL, Vazquez Suarez JC, Massó Romero J, Chaloupka JC, Bonafe A, Wakhloo AK, Tampieri D, Dowd CF, Fox AJ, Imm SJ, Carroll K, Turk AS; MAPS Investigators. Bioactive versus bare platinum coils in the treatment of intracranial aneurysms: the MAPS (Matrix and Platinum Science) trial. AJNR Am J Neuroradiol. 2014 May;35(5):935-42.

[29] Simon SD, Eskioglu E, Reig A, Mericle RA. Endovascular treatment of side wall aneurysms using a liquid embolic agent: a US single-center prospective trial. Neurosurgery. 2010 Sep;67(3):855-60.

[30] van Donkelaar CE, Bakker NA, Birks J, Clarke A, Sneade M, Kerr RSC, Veeger NJGM, van Dijk JMC, Molyneux AJ. Impact of Treatment Delay on Outcome in the International Subarachnoid Aneurysm Trial. Stroke. 2020 May;51(5):1600-1603.

[31] Lv X, Jiang C, Li Y, Lv M, Zhang J, Wu Z. Intracranial pseudoaneurysms, dissections and carotid-cavernous

fistulas: repair with percutaneous implantation of endovascular covered stents. Interv Neuroradiol 2008;14:435-440

[32] Liu Y, Yang HF, Xiong ZY, Zheng J, Liu CY, Zhao HY, Hu XB. Efficacy and Safety of Willis Covered Stent for Treatment of Complex Vascular Diseases of the Internal Carotid Artery. Ann Vasc Surg. 2019 Nov;61:203-211.

[33] Pierot L. Flow diverter stents in the treatment of intracranial aneurysms: Where are we? J Neuroradiol. 2011 Mar;38(1):40-6.

[34] D'Urso PI, Lanzino G, Cloft HJ, Kallmes DF. Flow diversion for intracranial aneurysms: a review. Stroke. 2011 Aug;42(8):2363-8.

[35] Lv X, Yang H, Liu P, Li Y. Flow-diverter devices in treatment of intracranial aneurysms: A Meta-analysis and systematic review. Neuroradiol J. 2016;29(1):66-71.

[36] Lv X, Yu J, Liao T, Wang J, Wang G. Unruptured giant intracavernous aneurysms untolerate internal carotid artery occlusion test: Untreated and treated with flow-diversion. Neuroradiol J. 2020;33(2):105-111.

[37] Liang S, Yuan R, Lv X. A novel treatment of a patient with a giant ruptured middle cerebral artery aneurysm by acute coiling followed by scheduled Pipeline flex placement. Neuroradiol J. 2020 Dec;33(6):517-519.

[38] Lv X, Jiang C, Wu Z, Jiang W, Wang G. Complex cerebral aneurysms: intra-luminal reconstruction using Pipeline flow-diverting stent and the obliteration mechanism. Neuroradiol J. 2020;33(2):91-97.

[39] Gory B, Berge J, Bonafé A, Pierot L, Spelle L, Piotin M, et al.; DIVERSION Investigators. Flow diverters for intracranial aneurysms: the DIVERSION National Prospective Cohort Study. Stroke. 2019; 50:3471-3480.

[40] Rustemi O, Raneri F, Scerrati A. Letter by Rustemi et al. Regarding Article "Flow Diverters for Intracranial Aneurysms: The DIVERSION National Prospective Cohort Study". Stroke. 2020 Feb;51(2):e35.

[41] Lang M, Habboub G, Mullin JP, Rasmussen PA. A brief history of carotid-cavernous fistula. J Neurosurg. 2017 Jun;126(6):1995-2001.

[42] Vitek JJ, Smith MJ. The myth of the Brooks method of embolization: a brief history of the endovascular treatment of carotid-cavernous sinus fistula. J Neurointerv Surg. 2009 Dec;1(2):108-11.

[43] Serbinenko FA. Balloon catheterization and occlusion of major cerebral vessels. J Neurosurg 1974;41:125-45.

[44] Lv X, Li Y, Yang X, Jiang C, Wu Z. Endovascular management of direct carotid-cavernous sinus fistulas. Neuroradiol J. 2012 Mar;25(1):130-4.

[45] Lv X, Jiang C, Li Y, Lv M, Zhang J, Wu Z. Intracranial pseudoaneurysms, dissections and carotid-cavernous fistulas: repair with percutaneous implantation of endovascular covered stents. Interv Neuroradiol 2008;14:435-440

[46] Zhang J, Lv X, Jiang C, Li Y, Yang X, Wu Z. Transarterial and transvenous embolization for cavernous sinus dural arteriovenous fistulae. Interv Neuroradiol 2010;16:269-277

[47] Jiang C, Lv X, Li Y, Wu Z, Shi J. Surgical access on the superior ophthalmic vein to the cavernous sinus dural fistula for embolization. J Neurointerv Surg. 2013;5(3):e13.

[48] Luessenhop AJ, Spence WT. Artificial embolization of cerebral arteries: report of use in a case of arteriovenous malformation. JAMA 1960;172:1153-5.

[49] Sorkin GC, Dumont TM, Eller JL, Mokin M, Snyder KV, Levy EI, Siddiqui AH, Hopkins LN. Cerebrovascular neurosurgery in evolution: the endovascular paradigm. Neurosurgery. 2014 Feb;74 Suppl 1:S191-7.

[50] Kerber C. Balloon catheter with a calibrated leak: a new system for superselective angiography and occlusive catheter therapy. Radiology 1976;120: 547-50.

[51] Triano MJ, Lara-Reyna J, Schupper AJ, Yaeger KA. Embolic Agents and Microcatheters for Endovascular Treatment of Cerebral Arteriovenous Malformations. World Neurosurg. 2020 Sep;141:383-388.

[52] Lv X, Wu Z, Li Y. Arteriovenous Malformation in the Brain: a Theoretical Study Explaining the Behavior of Liquid Embolic Agents during Endovascular Treatment. Neuroradiol J. 2013;26:661-668

[53] Lv X, Liang S. Update Onyx embolization for plexiform arteriovenous malformation: Ante-grade drifting technique. Neuroradiol J. 2020;33(5):386-392.

[54] Lv X, Wu Z, Jiang C, Yang X, Li Y, Sun Y, Zhang N. Angioarchitectural characteristics of brain arteriovenous malformations presenting with and without hemorrhage. World Neurosurgery 2011; 76:95-99

[55] Lv X, Hu X, Li W, He H, Jiang C, Li Y. Curative and adjunctive AVM Onyx embolization of AVMs through the choroidal arteries. Interv Neuroradiol. 2017;23:392-398.

[56] Lv X, Song C, He H, Jiang C, Li Y. Transvenous retrograde AVM embolization: Indications, techniques, complications and outcomes. Interv Neuroradiol. 2017 Oct;23(5):504-509

[57] Lv X, Jiang C, Wang J. Pediatric intracranial arteriovenous shunts: Advances in diagnosis and treatment. Eur J Paediatr Neurol. 2020;25:29-39.

[58] Liu P, Chen X, You W, Li Y, Lv M, Lv X. Hemorrhagic risk factors of endovascular onyx embolization of intracranial dural arteriovenous fistulas. Interv Neuroradiol. 2020 Oct;26(5):643-650.

[59] Baharvahdat H, Ooi YC, Kim WJ, Mowla A, Coon AL, Colby GP. Updates in the management of cranial dural arteriovenous fistula. Stroke Vasc Neurol. 2019 Nov 21;5(1):50-58.

[60] Zamponi JO Jr, Trivelato FP, Rezende MTS, Freitas RK, de Castro-Afonso LH, Nakiri GS, Abud TG, Ulhôa AC, Abud DG. Transarterial Treatment of Cranial Dural Arteriovenous Fistulas: The Role of Transarterial and Transvenous Balloon-Assisted Embolization. AJNR Am J Neuroradiol. 2020 Nov;41(11):2100-2106.

[61] Lv X, Jiang C, Li Y, Yang X, Wu Z. Recovery of opthalmoplegia associated with cavernous sinus dural arteriovenous fistulas after transvenous cavernous sinus packing. Eur J Radiol 2010 ;75 :139-142

[62] Lv X, Li Y, Yang X, Jiang C, Wu Z. Endovascular embolization for symptomatic perimedullary AVF and intramedullary AVM: a series and literature review. Neuroradiology. 2012;54:349-359

[63] Virchow R, Picard PDeMddW. La pathologie cellulaire base\0301e sur l'e\0301tude physiologique et

pathologique des tissus. Traduit de l'allemand sur la seconde edition par p. Picard. E\0301dition revue et corrige\0301e par l'auteur. Avec 144 figures. Paris: Saint-Germain [printed]; 1864

[64] Djindjian R, Kricheff II. Angiography of the Spinal Cord. Baltimore: University Park Press; 1970.

[65] Gailloud P. Introduction to Diagnostic and Therapeutic Spinal Angiography. Neuroimaging Clin N Am. 2019 Nov;29(4):595-614.

[66] Lenck S, Nicholson P, Tymianski R, Hilditch C, Nouet A, Patel K, Krings T, Tymianski M, Radovanovic I, Mendes Pereira V. Spinal and Paraspinal Arteriovenous Lesions. Stroke. 2019 Aug;50(8):2259-2269.

[67] Anson JA, Spetzler RF. Interventional neuroradiology for spinal pathology. Clin Neurosurg. 1992;39:388-417.

[68] Endo T, Endo H, Sato K, Matsumoto Y, Tominaga T. Surgical and Endovascular Treatment for Spinal Arteriovenous Malformations. Neurol Med Chir (Tokyo). 2016 Aug 15;56(8):457-64.

[69] Li B, Lv X, Wu Z, et al. Stent-Assisted Coil Embolization of a Transverse-Sigmoid Sinus Diverticulum Presenting with Pulsatile Tinnitus. Turk Neurosurg. 2016;26(4):632-634.

[70] Li B, Lv X, Wu Z, et al. Occult Pulsatile Tinnitus in Association with a Prominent Vein of Hypoglossal Canal: Two Case Reports. Turk Neurosurg. 2016;26(6):953-956.

[71] Daggubati LC, Liu KC. Intracranial Venous Sinus Stenting: A Review of Idiopathic Intracranial Hypertension and Expanding Indications. Cureus. 2019 Feb 4;11(2):e4008.

[72] Brown MM. Balloon angioplasty for cerebrovascular disease. Neurol Res. 1992;14(2 Suppl):159-63.

[73] Lylyk P, Cohen JE, Ceratto R, et al. Angioplasty and stent placement in intracranial atherosclerotic stenosis and dissections. AJNR Am J Neuroradiol 2002;23:430-6.

[74] Bose A, Hartmann M, Henkes H, et al. A novel, self- expanding, nitinol stent in medically refractory intracranial atherosclerotic stenoses. Stroke 2007;38:1531-7.

[75] Yu W, Jiang W- J. Stenting for intracranial stenosis: potential future for the prevention of disabling or fatal stroke. Stroke Vasc Neurol 2018;3:140-6.

[76] Hopkins LN. Carotid artery angioplasty and use of stents in high-risk patients with contralateral occlusions. J Neurosurg. 1999 Jun;90(6):1031-6.

[77] Wangqin R, Krafft PR, Piper K, Kumar J, Xu K, Mokin M, Ren Z. Management of De Novo Carotid Stenosis and Postintervention Restenosis-Carotid Endarterectomy Versus Carotid Artery Stenting-a Review of Literature. Transl Stroke Res. 2019 Oct;10(5):460-474.

[78] Xiong J, Wang L, Tian J, Li Y, Gong C, Lv X. Stent-Assisted Coiling of Brain Aneurysms Under Conscious Sedation and Simultaneous Coronary Heart Disease Stenting: A New Concept. Ann Indian Acad Neurol. 2020 Jul-Aug;23(4):572-574.

[79] Texakalidis P, Giannopoulos S, Jonnalagadda AK, Kokkinidis DG, Machinis T, Reavey-Cantwell J, Armstrong EJ, Jabbour P. Carotid Artery Endarterectomy versus Carotid Artery Stenting for Restenosis After Carotid Artery Endarterectomy: A Systematic Review and Meta-Analysis. World Neurosurg. 2018 Jul;115:421-429.e1.

[80] Krasteva MP, Lau KK, Mordasini P, Tsang ACO, Heldner MR. Intracranial Atherosclerotic Stenoses: Pathophysiology, Epidemiology, Risk Factors and Current Therapy Options. Adv Ther. 2020 May;37(5):1829-1865.

[81] Tissue plasminogen activator for acute ischemic stroke. The National Institute of Neurological Disorders and Stroke rtPA Stroke Study Group. N Engl J Med 1995;333:1581-1587

[82] Sweid A, Hammoud B, Ramesh S, Wong D, Alexander TD, Weinberg JH, Deprince M, Dougherty J, Maamari DJ, Tjoumakaris S, Zarzour H, Gooch MR, Herial N, Romo V, Hasan DM, Rosenwasser RH, Jabbour P. Acute ischaemic stroke interventions: large vessel occlusion and beyond. Stroke Vasc Neurol. 2019 Nov 28;5(1):80-85.

[83] Furlan A, Higashida R, Wechsler L, Gent M, Rowley H, Kase C, Pessin M, Ahuja A, Callahan F, Clark WM, Silver F, Rivera F. Intra-arterial prourokinase for acute ischemic stroke. The PROACT II study: a randomized controlled trial. Prolyse in Acute Cerebral Thromboembolism. JAMA. 1999 Dec 1;282(21):2003-11.

[84] Goyal M, Menon BK, van Zwam WH, et al. Endovascular thrombectomy after large vessel ischaemic stroke: a meta-analysis of individual patient data from five randomised trials. Lancet 2018;387(10029):1723-31.

[85] Keigher KM. Large Vessel Occlusion in the Acute Stroke Patient: Identification, Treatment, and Management. Crit Care Nurs Clin North Am. 2020 Mar;32(1):21-36.

[86] Guterman LR, Standard SC, Ahuja A, Hopkins LN. Vascular and endovascular neurosurgery. Curr Opin Neurol. 1993 Dec;6(6):854-9.

[87] Haumann R, Videira JC, Kaspers GJL, van Vuurden DG, Hulleman E. Overview of Current Drug Delivery Methods Across the Blood-Brain Barrier for the Treatment of Primary Brain Tumors. CNS Drugs. 2020 Nov;34(11):1121-1131.

[88] Mandai S, Sakurai M, Matsumoto Y. Middle meningeal artery embolization for refractory chronic subdural hematoma. Case report. J Neurosurg. 2000 Oct;93(4):686-8.

[89] Waqas M, Vakhari K, Weimer PV, Hashmi E, Davies JM, Siddiqui AH. Safety and Effectiveness of Embolization for Chronic Subdural Hematoma: Systematic Review and Case Series. World Neurosurg. 2019 Jun;126:228-236.

[90] Harbaugh RE, Agarwal A. Training residents in endovascular neurosurgery. Neurosurgery. 2006 Nov;59(5 Suppl 3):S277-281.

Section 4

Spinal Surgery

Chapter 10

Neurosurgical Spasticity Treatment: From Lesion to Neuromodulation Procedures

José Damián Carrillo-Ruíz, Jesús Quetzalcoatl Beltran, José Rodrigo Carrillo-Márquez, José Luis Navarro-Olvera, Luis García, Francisco Villegas-López and Francisco Velasco

Abstract

Spasticity is one of the most important and residual signs after pyramidal and para-pyramidal catastrophic lesions after diverse neurological insults, including stroke, brain and spine trauma and post-radiation; infection and immunological diseases affecting nervous system, between others. Spasticity is normally a compensatory motor mechanism that could ameliorate the patients´ disability. Nevertheless, disastrous spasticity is described when the extremities force is diminished in the affected limbs, or when is impossible to wake o to take objects, maximum when hand or foot deformity is exposed. The objective of this chapter is centered in the neurosurgical treatment of spasticity, including brain lesions with specific targets and the spine with its different modalities. This review shows not only the basic aspects in these techniques, but also the option of infusion pumps and deep brain stimulation. To close, a proposal is stablished to determinate the possible path to treat the spasticity in the future.

Keywords: spasticity, neuroablation, neuromodulation, lesioning neurosurgery, motor disorders

1. Introduction

Spasticity is a motor disorder characterized by muscular hypertonia with resistance to passive movement, in a context of hyperexcitability of the stretch reflex. This disorder is a component of the upper motor neuron syndrome, an alteration where the inhibitory influence of supraspinal structures is lost. Spasticity is an important clinical problem frequently found in neurological patients. This condition is estimated to occur in 17–39% of patients with stroke [1], 37–78% of patients with multiple sclerosis [2], 65–78% of patients with spinal cord injury [3], and 90% of patients with cerebral palsy [4]. Spasticity could be very disabling for patients and its management requires several specialists and different therapeutic options.

If acceptable control of spasticity is not achieved with pharmacological treatment, physical therapy and rehabilitation, surgical procedures are the next treatment option. The goal of surgery in these patients is to decrease the excess muscle tone and rebalance agonist and antagonist muscle groups to improve function and limit deformities. To promote a better restoration of function in patients with spasticity, it is important to know the functional alterations of this disorder. Furthermore, in order to measure the effects on the pathology after some treatment, it is necessary to use classifications and scales. In the following sections, the first topic to be addressed is the neurophysiological alterations of spasticity and then it will be mentioned the scales with which the degree of affection is classified. Later, it is going to be described the neurosurgical procedures, both ablative and neuromodulatory, available to compensate for the physiological alterations of this disorder.

2. Spasticity: pathophysiology and classification

2.1 Pathophysiology of spasticity

Muscle tone depends on the intrinsic elasticity/stiffness of the muscle, and this in turn is modulated by the nervous system. In physiological conditions, the neural circuits in the spinal cord mediate muscle stretch reflexes. These local circuits also provide a mechanism to adjust muscle tone from supraspinal structures according to physiological requirements. Due to this configuration, lesions in these supraspinal structures or in the descending motor pathways are frequently associated with alterations in muscle tone. These alterations may involve an abnormal increase or decrease in tone. The most common form of hypertonia is spasticity, which is characterized by a velocity-dependent resistance to passive movement of a joint and its associated musculature. A slowly applied stretch in a patient with spasticity causes little resistance, but as the speed of the stretch increases, the stretch resistance also increases progressively. Thus, spasticity is primarily a phasic phenomenon. An active reflex contraction that occurs only during a rapid stretch; when the muscle is held in an elongated position, the reflex contraction decreases. However, in some cases hypertonia also has a tonic component, for example if reflex contractions persist even after the muscle is no longer stretched [5].

In the last years, the pathophysiology of spasticity has been increasingly understood. Stretch reflex hyperactivity was long thought to be caused by overactive gamma motor neurons. However, although gamma motor neurons may be overactive in some cases, changes in the background activity of alpha motor neurons and interneurons are probably more important. Particularly relevant seem to be modifications in the intrinsic properties of motor neurons that generate a sustained firing in response to a brief excitatory input. Another mechanism that produces spasticity is the strong facilitation of synaptic transmission in the sensory fiber of the monosynaptic reflex pathway. In fact, this provides a mechanism for treating this disorder. Currently, a relatively common therapeutic procedure favors presynaptic inhibition in the *Ia* fiber terminals by the intrathecal infusion of baclofen, a GABA-B receptor agonist, that blocks neurotransmitter release [5, 6].

2.2 Classification of spasticity

Classifying the severity and distribution of spasticity in each patient is an essential element to achieve effective treatment and to observe its response over time. The severity of this disorder can range from a focal problem with mild muscle stiffness to a severe and painful diffuse spasticity.

Based on its location, spasticity can be classified into Focal, Regional, and Generalized. In the first case, a single muscle group or part of the body is affected, in regional spasticity, adjacent muscle groups are affected in a region of the body. In the patients with generalized spasticity, all or almost all areas of the body are affected [6].

3. Spasticity assessment

The degree of affection, its evolution over time, and the response to the therapeutic options can be evaluated with the use of some scales. There are several widely used scales: Ashworth Scale (AS), Modified Ashworth Scale (MAS) and Gross Motor Function Classification System (GMFCS). They are formed of different points to construct ordinal scale that assess muscle tone. A higher score indicates a more intense spasticity [7].

Moreover, to comprehend correctly the information said before it is necessary to understand the meaning of two important concepts: spasticity and spasms. Spasticity is "hypertonia that is associated with one or both of the following signs: resistance to passive movement that increases with speed of stretch, or when the resistance to externally imposed movement rises rapidly above a threshold speed or joint angle" [8]. On the other hand, spasms can be defined as "episodes of involuntary motor contractions that occur following a lesion of the ascending motor pathway" [9]. It is important to mention that spasticity is detrimental to human health due to the miscommunication between the brain and the muscles, as a consequence those patients have a diminished quality of life. Spasms can be presented in long periods of time that is why problems in the musculoskeletal system can appear, affecting mobility and tone of posture.

Bryan Ashworth, in 1964, created a classification in which patients with multiple sclerosis could be graded in order of their clinical manifestations, starting to objectivize the knowledge of the pathology mentioned before [10]. Between the decades of 1960's to late 1980's the scale was used by doctors all over the world to help get a more accurate diagnose of spasticity, contributing to the progress of science in the field of neurology.

Table 1 shows the classic Ashworth Scale that consist in five different types of categories that describe clinical manifestations of spasticity [11].

Furthermore, in 1987 Richard Bohannon's group added to the scale a category "1+" for a more accurate classification regarding clinical manifestations in patients with spasticity. Since then, the scientific community has been using this scale of measure to add a more specific diagnose in patients that present rigid upper limb due to its extension [12]. It is important to mention that both scales, Ashworth and Modified Ashworth, are useful in the detection of spasticity and can be helpful to objectivize the manifestations of spasticity.

In this image, it can be seen the modifications that Richard Bohannon added to the Ashworth Scale (**Table 2**) [13].

Richard Penn has published several articles concerning spasticity, and also is attributed as the creator of a scale that measures the frequency of spasms "Penn Spasm Frequency Scale (PSFS)".

Table 3 shows the different categories of spasms over time to identify characteristics according to the clinical manifestations [14].

Scale	Description
0	No increase in muscle tone.
1	Slight increase in muscle tone, manifested by a catch and release.
2	Marked increase in muscle tone throughout most of the range of motion, but affected part(s) easily move.
3	Considerable increase in muscle tone; passive movement difficult.
4	Affected part(s) rigid in flexion or extension.

Table 1.
Ashworth scale.

Scale	Description
0	No increase in muscle tone.
1	Slight increase in muscle tone, manifested by a catch and release.
1+	Slight increase in muscle tone, manifested as a catch, followed through the remainder of the range of motion.
2	Marked increase in muscle tone throughout most of the range of motion, but affected part(s) easily move.
3	Considerable increase in muscle tone; passive movement difficult.
4	Affected part(s) rigid in flexion or extension.

Table 2.
Modified Ashworth scale (MAS).

Scale	Description
0	None
1	Lack of spontaneous spasms; vigorous sensory and motor stimulation outcome in spasms.
2	Occasional spontaneous spasms occurring es than once per hour.
3	Greater than 1, but less than 10 spontaneous spasms per hour.
4	Greater than 10 spontaneous spasms per hour

Table 3.
Penn spasm frequency score (PSFS).

4. Treatment

The objective of the different pharmacological and surgical treatment options is to compensate the excitation/inhibition imbalance that occurs in the motoneurons of the ventral horn, the common final pathway for motor control. When possible, the underlying cause (e.g., tumor, abscess) that could be generated this imbalance should be eliminated. It is important to say that spasticity does not always require specific treatment. In many cases, spasticity can be helpful in maintaining balance and compensate for loss of motor power. Thus, spasticity should be treated when excess muscle tone leads to further functional disability, impaired locomotion, causes deformities, or induces chronic pain [5].

The different treatment options can be classified according to the location (focal vs. general) and duration (temporary vs. permanent) of their therapeutic effect. The choice of a treatment is made according to the severity and extent of spasticity and is adjusted according to the response and evolution of each patient. In general, surgical treatment is considered a second-line option, for patients with non-satisfactory response with drugs and physical therapy. Neurosurgical treatment options are divided into neuroablative and neuromodulatory procedures. The latter allow chemical or electrical regulation in the functioning of the neural circuits involved in spasticity. Importantly, such neuromodulation is characteristically adjustable and reversible. Ablative procedures are fixed and non-reversible. However, they still constitute a viable option for many patients, especially in those circumstances in which the use of neuromodulation equipment is not available. **Figure 1** shows a general algorithm for the treatment of a patient with spasticity from its initial assessment to management with lesioning procedures. This algorithm is only a general guide, and in each patient the treatment should be individualized in the context of a multidisciplinary management.

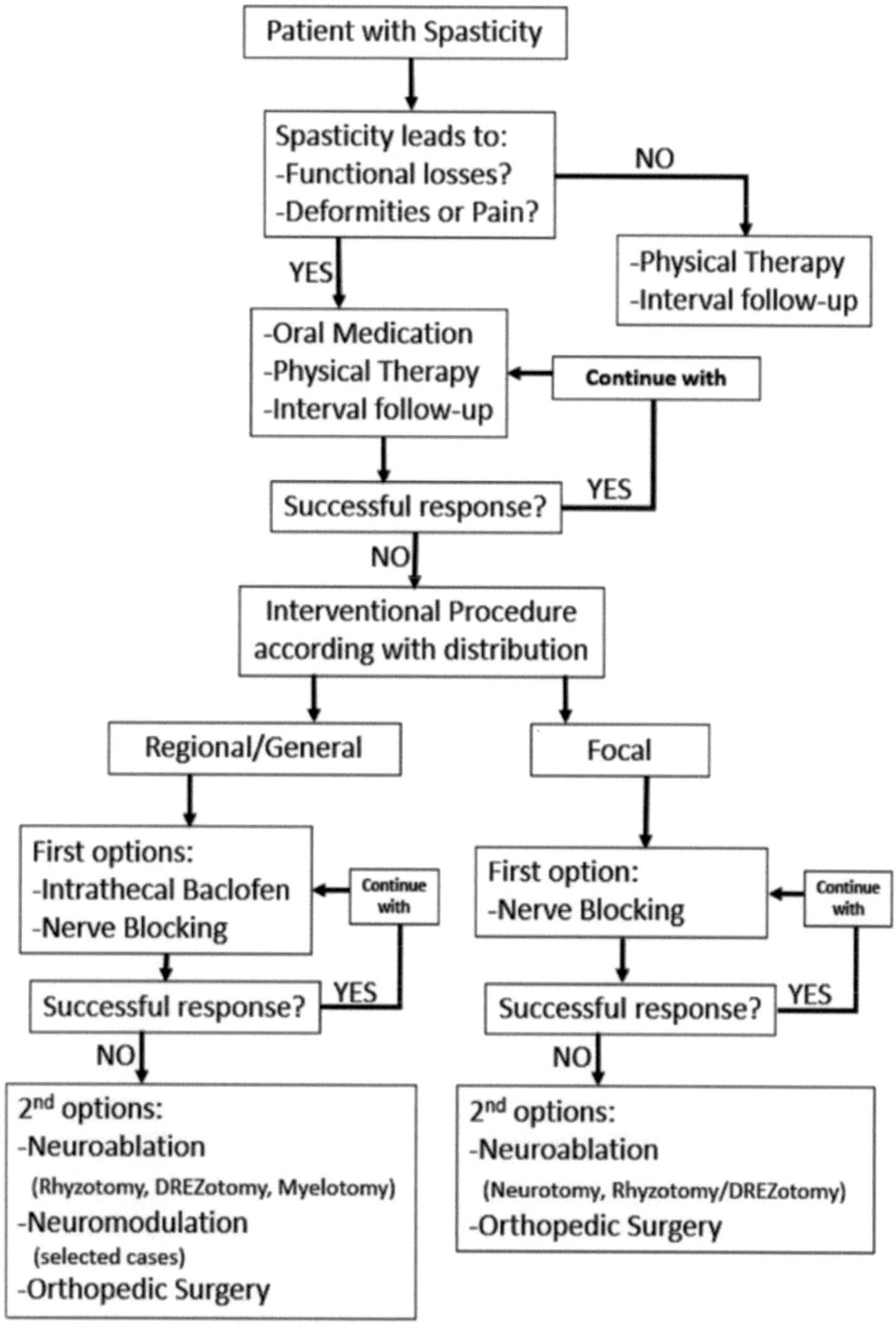

Figure 1.
General purpose algorithm for the treatment of spastic patients.

4.1 Ablative treatment

This treatment modality implies the realization of some injury in certain levels of the nervous system that participate in the motor function in order to counteract spasticity. These lesions include selective neurotomies, rhizotomies, DREZotomies, myelotomies, and supramedular lesions. These procedures should be performed in such a way as to reduce excess muscle tone, but preserving residual sensorimotor functions and useful muscle tone. In cases of refractory spasticity, including paraplegic, hemiplegic or tetraplegic patients, the evolution and severity of the spasticity may require neuroablative management. In these cases, the injury procedure must be selective, and will be chosen considering the location of the spasticity (**Figure 1**). The characteristics of the most important and useful injuries will be reviewed below.

4.1.1 Selective neurotomy

Peripheral neurotomy was first introduced by Lorenz in 1887 for hip spasticity and by Stoffel in 1912 for spasticity in the foot [15]. This procedure consists of selectively identifying and injuring one motor nerve bundle that supply the spastic muscles. The goal of selective neurotomy is to inhibit the segmental reflex arc and thus limit the level of muscle spasticity. Selective neurotomy is indicated in cases of localized spasticity in a single or a few muscle groups, both in cases of focal or multifocal spasticity. The target nerves are selected according to the spastic region affected. Examples include lower subscapular nerve injury for spastic shoulder, median nerve injury for pronation spasticity of the upper limb, ulnar neurotomy for spastic wrist flexion with ulnar deviation, obturator nerve lesion in case of hip adduction spasticity, sciatic nerve for knee flexion spasticity and tibial neurotomy for equinus or equinovarus spastic foot [16].

The evaluation prior to neurotomy should include nerve blocks with a reversible agent such as botulinum toxin. These blocks allow us to observe a therapeutic effect previous to neurotomy and to evaluate its usefulness and acceptance. The injury must be performed with intraoperative electrophysiological monitoring of the nerve to be injured and must include 50–80% of the spastic muscle fibers to expect an effective result [5]. The most relevant long-term complications of the neurotomies are allodynia and neuropathic pain. To reduce the probability of the appearance of these adverse effects, it is important to identify and try to avoid sensory fibers during the procedure [17].

4.1.2 Selective dorsal rhizotomy

Sir Charles Sherrington, in 1898, showed that stiffness could be abolished by dorsal rhizotomy in a feline model with midbrain transection [18]. With this background, Otfrid Foerester, in 1913, reported the first dorsal rhizotomy for the management of lower limb spasticity in patients with cerebral palsy [19]. Rhizotomy consists of the selective section of the dorsal roots of the spinal nerve at a specific medullary level. It is thought that its effect is due to the reduction of the afferent information of the *Ia* fibers of the spastic muscle, which would produce a decrease in the excitatory input, and an increase in the inhibitory activity of the interneurons, to the alpha motoneurons [18, 19]. Dorsal rhizotomy is indicated in patients with diffuse or regional spasticity, in patients with spasticity in one or two limbs. There is no consensus on the precise selection criteria, but it is most frequently performed in paraplegic patients with spasticity in the lower extremities, however, it has also been performed successfully in the cervical region in patients with spasticity in the upper extremities [20, 21].

The procedure for the lower extremities is usually performed on the posterior roots of L1-S2 levels, exposed with a laminectomy or laminoplasty. For spasticity of the upper extremities, rhizotomy has been described from C1-C3 levels, not sectioning dorsal root of C4 to avoid affecting the diagrammatic function [20, 21]. Similar to neurotomies, it is important to perform intraoperative electrophysiological mapping to identify the roots that contribute to spasticity. In cases of pediatric cerebral palsy, it has been observed that the patients with the greatest improvement are those between 4 and 7 years old and have a preoperative gross motor function measure test (GMFM-88) between 65–85% [22]. The most important side effects of this procedure are impaired sensation, sphincter dysfunction, cerebrospinal fluid fistula, and chronic low back pain [17]. Techniques with more limited and selective lesions have been tried to improve the results and reduce the probability of the appearance of side effects [7].

4.1.3 DREZotomy

This procedure was initially performed by Sindou, in 1972, for the surgical treatment of pain. He observed that this technique also produced important hypotonia in the muscles corresponding to the severed medullary segment, and suggested its application in cases of spasticity [23, 24]. This surgery is similar to rhizotomy, but the injury here is made in the spinal cord, at the Dorsal Root Entry Zone (DREZ). The underlying mechanism in this case, is a disruption of *Ia* afferent inputs to the dorsal horn and a disruption of local circuits that contribute to muscle tone [6]. This procedure is indicated in cases of severe regional spasticity, especially those associated with pain and poor or no regional function, such as in paraplegic or hemiplegic patients with painful hyperspasticity or severe spasms [25, 26]. The surgery, which requires an intradural approach and adequate visualization of the posterior surface of the spinal cord, consists of 3-mm deep incision at the dorsolateral sulcus, down to the dorsal horn, following its axis. When spasticity is associated with focal dystonia, DREZotomy should be more deeply down to the base of the ventral horn [5]. DREZotomy can be performed at the C5-C8 medullary levels (at 35° angle) for the management of spasticity in the upper extremities or at L1-S2 levels (at 45° angle) for the lower extremity affection. The most important complications of this technique are damage to the pyramidal pathway with loss of strength and severe hypotonia, so it should be considered in patients with severe refractory spasticity who have little residual function in the limb.

4.1.4 Longitudinal myelotomy

Bischof originally described the longitudinal myelotomy in 1951, and it was subsequently performed more selectively by Pourpre in 1960, and by Laitinen & Singounas in 1971 [8, 27, 28]. This procedure consists of a frontal separation between the ventral and dorsal horns at the level of the lumbosacral enlargement. The goal of surgery is to interrupt the spinal reflex arc by severing the connection between the posterior and anterior horns of the spinal cord. Through a T9-L1 laminectomy or laminoplasty, the procedure is performed at the T11-S2 medullary levels. Once the spinal cord is exposed, a posterior longitudinal sagittal incision is made deep to the central canal prior to performing a transverse cut using a stylet with a right-angled extremity, to separate the ventral and dorsal horns [7]. This surgery has been used in the treatment of patients with paraplegia, especially in cases with triple flexion and loss of sphincter function [6].

4.1.5 Other procedures

Some stereotaxic procedures in the thalamus and cerebellum have been performed for the treatment of spasticity in selected cases. These lesioning procedures include ventrolateral thalamotomy, pulvinarotomy, dentatotomy, and lesion of nucleus fastigii [29]. Due to the complexity, risks and lack of better effectiveness compared to the surgical options for spinal cord and peripheral nerve, these procedures were abandoned [6].

On the other hand, orthopedic surgery is another lesioning option. Neurosurgical procedures are the first choice for the management of spasticity and dystonia, but orthopedic surgery is a complementary surgical option for cases in which spasticity persists after neurosurgical treatment. Orthopedic surgery can reduce spasticity by releasing or lengthening tendons in the affected region. Orthopedic procedures may be indicated primarily when contractures and ankyloses are predominant or like the last option when the deformity is so strong [6].

4.2 Neuromodulation treatment

The classic procedures to treat spasticity are focused to perform lesions or ablative brain, spinal or nerve surgeries, but in recent times it exists the opportunity of neuromodulation. This term involved the use of chemical or electric pulses to increase or decrease neuron threshold with the main goal to diminish or abolish neurological or/and psychiatry symptoms. Neuromodulation is widespread to treat neuropathic and phantom pain, movement disorders abnormalities like Parkinson's disease, essential tremor and dystonia; partial and generalized epilepsy; obsessive–compulsive disorder, depression or anorexia; motor problems of neurogenic bladder, and neurologic deafness and blindness.

In this sense, neuromodulation in spasticity is concerned mainly to the use of infusion pumps, treatment acknowledged all over the world. Nevertheless, it exists the possibility to utilize electric stimulation in two targets: spinal cord and cerebellar sites to ameliorate the stiffness limb, but is not spread like infusion pumps.

4.2.1 Infusion pumps in spasticity

The next lines are dedicated to resume the infusion pump in the treatment of spasticity. It should be said that there is no cure to spasticity, but different methods and treatments can be useful. Infusion pumps are generally described as: "Complicated electromechanical systems that are used to deliver anesthetic drugs with moderate precision" [30]. Regarding neurosciences, different drugs are used in order to help patients with spasticity and other similar illnesses, mainly baclofen. Since 1984, the usage of infusion pumps with baclofen was proposed by Richard Penn due to prior scientific evidence that this chemical could work as an analogue of "γ-aminobutyric acid" (GABA) in its B receptor, how it is mentioned [31].

Humans can be treated effectively with intrathecal baclofen to decrease drastically the symptoms, and the burden that this illness means. Baclofen is a GABAergic drug that is transmitted intrathecally by infusion to the subarachnoid space. Although baclofen can be taken orally, the quickness and effectiveness of the chemical is decreased in comparison with the utilization of pumps to treat patients with spasticity. When taken orally, baclofen can have as a maximum dosage approximately 360 mg per day, but when infused intrathecally the dosage reduces to approximately 250–500 μg per day. Although, Baclofen is a very effective chemical it also has some repercussions like muscle weakness and slowness in walking speed due to the effects that induces, but they can be controlled if the dose is adequate for the patient (**Table 4**) [32].

Overall, the experience of scientists and neurosurgeons using intrathecal baclofen can be described as a positive one, but most important good results have been shown for patients with spasticity. In **Table 4**, it can be seen how several authors have been using this technique to improve the development of the pathology. The former table contains twelve different categories in which all the authors present the results obtained by the research. In the "year" column it can be seen when the paper was published, and in the "number of patients" the amount of people that took participation in the research. In general, the "follow-up" period

Number	Author	Year	No. patients	Follow-up "months"	% improvement	Ashworth PRE	Ashworth POP	Other Scale PRE	Other scale POP	Baclophen's Dose	Other Dose
1	R D Penn	1989	n = 20	19.2(10–33)	70%	4(1)	1.2(0.4)	NS	NS	100–150 μg/day	NS
2	P. G. Loubser	1991	n = 9	3–22	69.31%	3.78(1.34)	1.16(0.48)	Reflex: 3.57(1.05)	Reflex: 0.64(0.87)	535.8(269) μg/day	NS
3	R. Becker	1996	n = 18	13–54	48%	4.5	2.33	PSFS: 2.16	PSFS: 0.94	265 μg/day	NS
4	Alexei I. Korenkov	2002	n = 12	12	48%	4.2	2.2	NS	NS	180(65–280) μg/day	NS
5	Daniel Guillaume	2005	n = 138	12	51.24%	4.02(0.92)	1.96(0.78)	NS	NS	288 μg/d	NS
6	Giulia Stampacchia	2016	n = 14	12	86%	3.5	0.5	NS	NS	250.5(187.5) μg/day	NS
7	Tanja Kraus	2017	n = 13	60 (12–100)	55.26%	3.8	1.7	NS	NS	According patients' needs: pediatrics	NS
8	Mithra B Maneyapanda	2017	n = 42	36	NS	NS	NS	NS	Functional Independence: 13 (33%)	605.89(333.1) μg/day	NS
9	Elke Pucks-Faes	2018	n = 116	64.4(40.7)	50%	4	2	NS	NS	152.7(76.8) μg/day	NS
10	Pedro Videira Reis	2019	n = 155	96 (9–132)	75%	4(3–4)	1(1–2)	PSFS: 4(3–4)	PSFS: 1(0–1)	230(95 to 400) μg/day	NS

Table 4.
Comparison between authors according to baclofen treatment in this table it has been merged information from different articles that inform about intrathecal baclofen usage [14]; [33–41].
NS = not specified.

was variant, but the tendency as years pass is determined to give the patient a longer period between the follow-up in comparison with the older papers. It should be said, that when analyzing the Ashworth Scale comparing the preoperatory and the post-operatory, results show that using intrathecal baclofen can help reduce drastically the stiffness to a slight increased muscle tone in the majority of the patients.

Regarding the "dose", the difference between pediatric and adult treatment should be addressed to understand how to apply intrathecal pumps. Some factors in children may affect the treatment, that is why there should be a pediatrician involved in the process of treating infants in order to apply the correct dosage and time to realize the pump implantation, and do not interfere with their development. In adults, it can be said that covering a good dosage is easier because developed organisms can receive intrathecal treatments better with doses from 200–600 μg/day. Moreover, due to biological variability different patients need more baclofen if they are still showing symptoms of spasticity, and less in the case of having problems with movement and also muscle weakness; that is why the doctor should be ready to evaluate when to adjust the dose of the drug according to patients' requirements.

Authors with long number of participants tend to have similar results, that is why it is important to have a correct number of participants and dose to generate a more accurate investigation. The dose of those investigations with more than a hundred participants express that the amount of baclofen needed to help a patient can approximately be 220 μg/day as a good reference to start the drug's usage. Although, none of the authors used another drug in their papers it should be said that baclofen is an effective chemical that can help patients with spasticity infused intrathecally. Also, it is important that doctors have to analyze correctly the dose for a better performance of the pump in each individual, and avoid toxicity problems (**Figures 2–6**).

In the following years, neurosurgeons and their teams have been adding information to the methods and the correct usage of this technique, gathering approximately 35 years of experience in the field of infusion pumps and the usage of baclofen in order to treat spasticity.

4.2.2 Spinal cord stimulation

The first person who used SCS in the treatment of an illness was Shealy when he was neurosurgery resident in the 60's decade. In the 50's, the original idea was emerged after the use of battery connected to cardiac electrodes located in the animal's atrium and modified the myocardial electricity in the treatment of arrhythmias. After an experimental period, the use of a voltaic pile and heart electrodes brings the first pacemaker in man, and stablished one of the most important medical knowledge about implants in the human being until now.

Shealy thought this principle of pacemakers, first in dogs and after in humans, could be used in neurologic patients. He took the first patients with uncontrolled pain cancer, and he implanted in the spinal cord, a system similar to the cardiac patients. The results are the amelioration of pain. Indeed, in this moment Shealy was opened the door to Neuromodulation at the neurologic patients [42, 43].

With respect to spasticity, based in the experience of Shealy with SCS for pain treatment in 1973, Cook and Wenstein reported one Multiple Sclerosis (MS) patient with pain alleviation but with the fortuitous finding that also limb spasticity amelioration was presented [44]. In 1976, Illis in UK introduced percutaneous electrodes in two MS patients and peridural space was stimulated and improved spasticity [45]. In 1979, Richardson and cols wrote an article with six spastic patients, in which spasticity was measure by a scale similar to Ashworth, with 36.11% of improvement, and also for first time the article described SCS

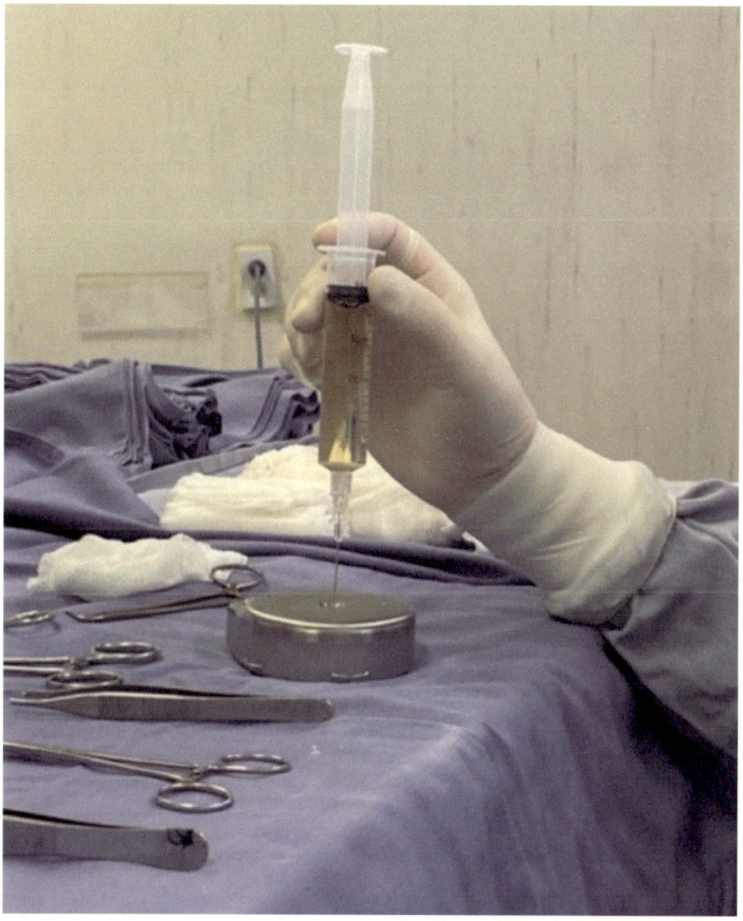

Figure 2.
It is shown how baclofen should be injected into the pump's reserve.

electric parameters of stimulation (Voltage from 0.5 to 2 V, frequency 33 to 75 HZ, and pulse width of 100 to 200 μsec) [46]. In 1980, Read and cols reported 16 MS patients: 9 had spasticity amelioration, 3 without change and 2 had worst evolution with increase in spasticity; the total alleviation was 56.25% in the group [47]. In the same year, Siegfried showed his experience with originally 26 patients using test stimulation before definitive implantation, consisting in percutaneous electrodes and depending if the test was positive, they implanted a definitive one. Only 11 patients were operated and followed 3 years with amelioration of the spasticity. Best results depending of spinal and partial damage more than cerebral site of spasticity. They also used electrophysiological measures like H-reflex to contrast the amelioration [48]. Also, in this year, Dimitrijevic showed the results of 11 patients with spasticity that improved 56.56% after SCS, mainly clonus and EMG patterns. In 1985, Barolat-Romana reported 6 spasticity patients with spasms and the immediate alleviation after SCS [49]. In 1986, Dimitrijevic and cols studied 59 patients in which spasticity was reduced in 63% of the group. They found spasticity was controlled better if the electrode was located below the spinal lesion more than above, also patients had better results with partial lesion that with complete ones [50]. In 1986, the same group with Campos (like the first author) described 8 patients with minimal function of posterior columns, 90% responded to the

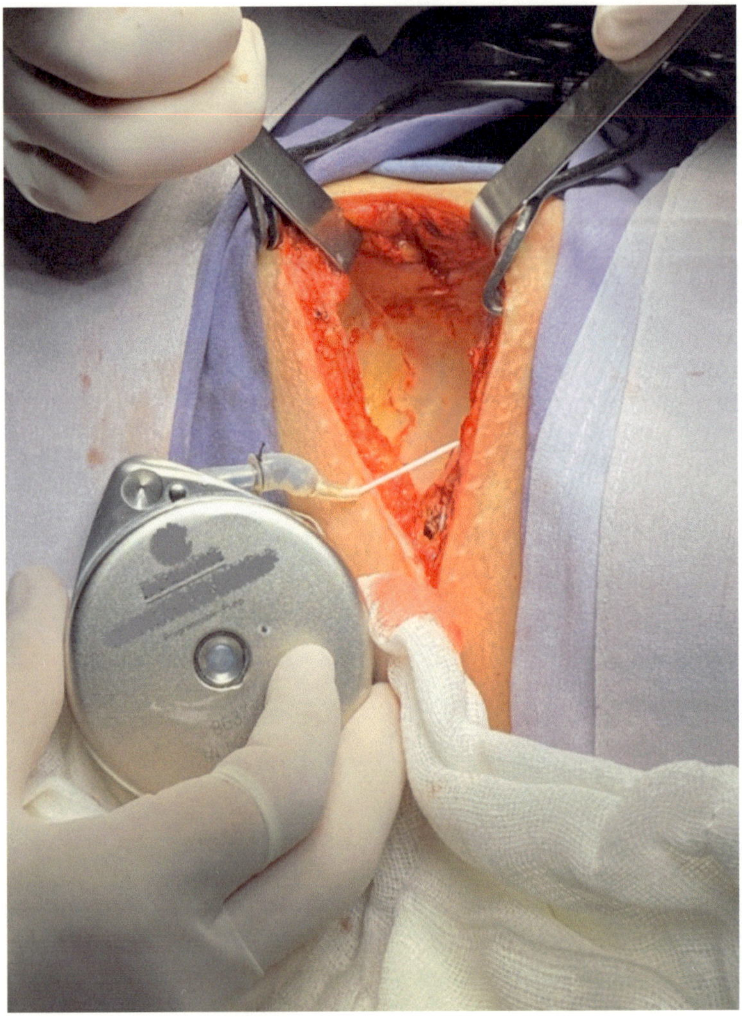

Figure 3.
It is demonstrated how the pump should be implanted, so as the stitch used in order to seal the neck of the gadget with the catheter.

epidural stimulation [51]. In 1988, Barolat made a clinical trial expanded the initial experience to 16 myelopathic subjects with amelioration of spasm and clonus, inclusive from one year of follow-up [52]. In 1993, the same group was amplified the experience of 509 plates implanted in patients suffered pain and spasticity: 350 in the whole group, 227 for pain, 105 for motor disturbances (spasms/spasticity following spinal cord or cranial trauma, multiple sclerosis, cerebral palsy, spasmodic torticollis and other motor problems) and 18 patients with both condition: pain and spasticity. From these, 3.4% had infection, 1.1% with electrode migration and less of 1%, breakage [53]. In the decade of 1990's it existed poorly advanced in this area. In 2000, Pinter and Dimitrijevic discovered that severe spasticity in paraplegic patients could improve with the electrode's position upper to the spinal lesion, with frequency of 50–100 Hz, 2–7 Volts and 210 μsec and adapted depended of the case [54]. In 2015, Dekopov and Russian team evaluated two groups of spasticity patients: Cerebral palsy and spinal cord lesion. SCS ameliorated Ashworth scale (58.8%) in cerebral palsy group, but it did not for the spinal cord lesion [55].

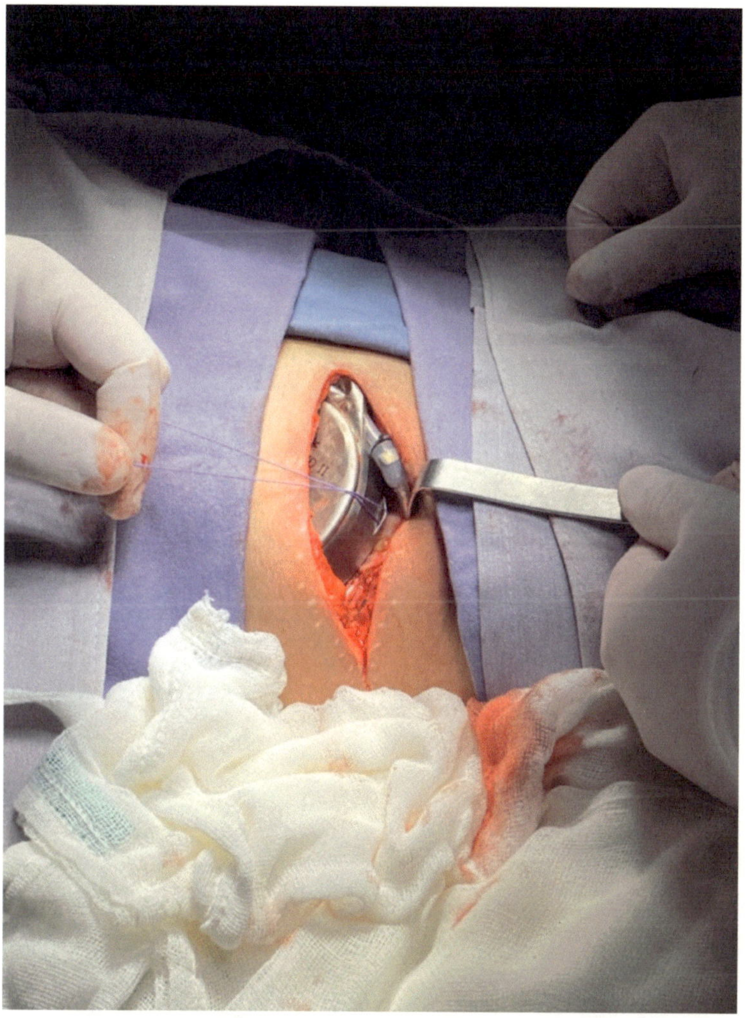

Figure 4.
In the implantation process is important to attach the pump handles to the tissue surrounding the equipment in order to stabilize the device and prevent future complications.

4.2.3 Cerebellar stimulation

The understanding of cerebellar human stimulation began in the experiments developed in rats, cats, dogs and monkeys. It was based in these antecedent that Cooper and cols in 1973 located electrodes on the anterior and posterior surface of cerebellum to treat not only spasticity, but seizures also [56–58]. After these reports, Cooper and his group contribute significantly to this neuromodulation area with different types of articles including implantation technique, clinic evolution, surgical complications, neurophysiological changes, psychological reactions, between other issues [59–64]. Other groups started to perform CS. In 1977, Manrique and cols implanted 4 patients with good results to diminished spasticity [65], Penn found in some patients diminished spasticity and, in other, no changes [66, 67]. Cooper's work was continued by Davis [68–73] spreading the experience in this field. In 2003 and 2007, respectively, Galanda & Horvath proposed new insights about CS [74, 75]. In the last decade there has been no progress in this area.

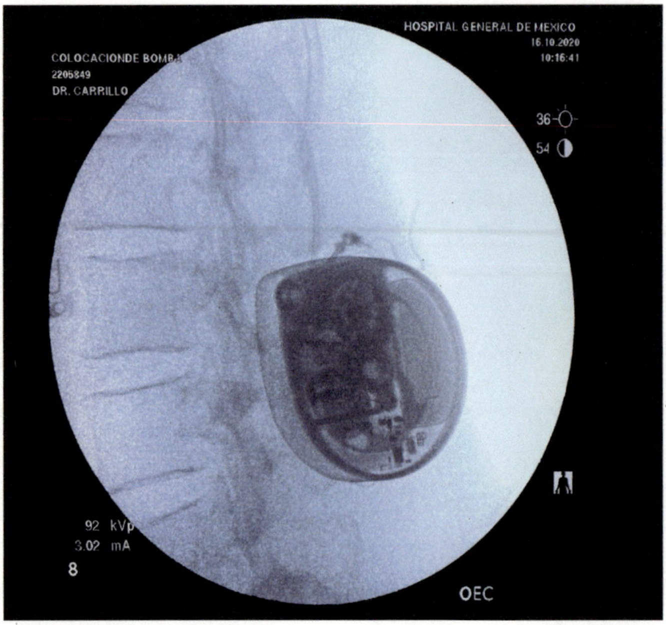

Figure 5.
Post-operatory picture of the pump immediately after the implantation surgery. X-ray image must be taken to verify the correct placement of the equipment.

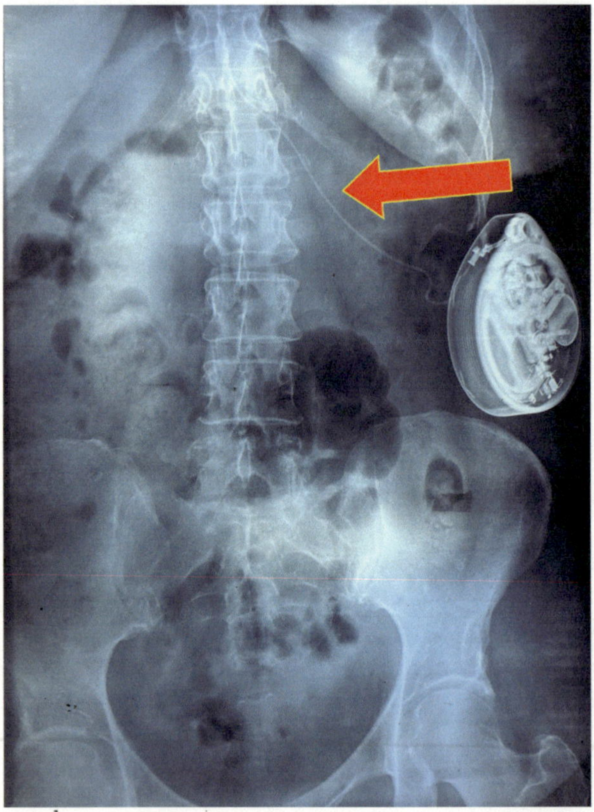

Figure 6.
X-ray image shows the infusion pump implanted in the lower part of the left hypochondria. The red arrow indicates the catheter connected to the infusion pump, and the tip goes to T-10 level into the subarachnoid space.

5. Post-surgery considerations

After any surgical procedure, physical therapy and recovery are very important. There is no consensus on the duration and specific type of rehabilitation that should be followed. There is great variability in the literature, but some authors recommend close follow-up to 3 months after hospital convalescence [16]. The physical therapy and rehabilitation protocols must be adapted to each patient, and so should be empathized that is crucial to promote functional improvement after surgical management. The results and their functional impact on patients can be seen in variable times, and the follow-up should be at least for 6 months. All management and follow-up of the patient with spasticity should be carried out, whenever possible, by a multidisciplinary team to promote the best results, as well as avoid possible problems [5].

6. Other techniques and targets

Recently, it exists other possibilities to treat spasticity. It is only mentioned to avoid extend this review. For one side, magnetic transcranial or spinal stimulation. These techniques mean the performance of a coil connected to an electric source to produce electromagnetic waves modifying the brain's plasticity: primary motor cortex or cerebellar cortex are the selected targets; or in an experimental manner in spinal circuitry.

On the other hand, electrical transcutaneous stimulation over the limb or spinal cord try to ameliorate also spasticity. It is remarkable that neurosurgical procedures in spasticity are the second line of treatment, when rehabilitation maneuvers were excluded. After the surgery has been performed the use of physical exercises is mandatory. To finish, it should be said that orthopedic procedures must be done when the extremities are deformed.

Conflict of interest

The authors declare no conflict of interest.

Author details

José Damián Carrillo-Ruíz[1,2]*, Jesús Quetzalcoatl Beltran[1],
José Rodrigo Carrillo-Márquez[2], José Luis Navarro-Olvera[1], Luis García[1],
Francisco Villegas-López[1] and Francisco Velasco[1]

1 Stereotactic and Functional Neurosurgery Unit, Mexico General Hospital, Mexico City, Mexico

2 Faculty of Health Sciences, Anahuac Mexico University, Mexico City, Mexico

*Address all correspondence to: josecarrilloruiz@yahoo.com

References

[1] Brainin M, *et al.* "Poststroke chronic disease management: towards improved identification and interventions for poststroke spasticity-related complications," Int J Stroke 2011; 6 (1):42-46.

[2] Barnes M P, Kent R M, Semlyen J K, McMullen K M. "Spasticity in multiple sclerosis," Neurorehab Neural Repair 2003; 17 (1): 66-70.

[3] Adams M M, Hicks A L."Spasticity after spinal cord injury," Spinal Cord 2005; 43 (10): 577-586.

[4] Yeargin-Allsopp M, Braun K V N, Doernberg N S, Benedict R E, Kirby R S, Durkin M S. "Prevalence of cerebral palsy in 8-year-old children in three areas of the United States in 2002: a multisite collaboration," *Pediatrics* 2008; 121(3): 547-554.

[5] Sindou M, Georgoulis G, Mertens P. "Lesioning surgery for spasticity," in *Youmans and Winn Neurological Surgery*, 7th ed., M. H. Richard Winn, Ed. Phi. Elsevier 2017: 716-728.

[6] Sindou M, Georgoulis G, Mertens P. *Neurosurgery for Spasticity: A Practical Guide for Treating Children and Adults*. Springer 2014.

[7] Sindou M, Mertens P. "Destructive neurosurgical procedures for spasticity," in *Textbook of Stereotactic and Functional Neurosurgery*, R. Lozano, Andres M. Gildenberg, Philip. Tasker, Ed 2009.

[8] Laitinen L, Singounas E. "Longitudinal myelotomy in the treatment of spasticity of the legs". J Neurosurg 1971; 35(5): 536-540.

[9] Sanger TD, Delgado MR, Gaebler-Spira D, Hallett M, Mink JW. Classification and definition of disorders causing hypertonia in childhood. Pediatrics 2003; 111(1): 89-97.

[10] Khurana SR, Garg DS. Spasticity and the use of intrathecal baclofen in patients with spinal cord injury. Phys Med Rehab Clin 2014; 25(3):655-669.

[11] Ashworth B. Preliminary Trial of Carisoprodol in Multiple Sclerosis. Practitioner 1964; 192: 540-542. PMID: 14143329.

[12] Harb A, Kishner S. Modified Ashworth Scale. StatPearls. Treasure Island (FL): StatPearls Pub 2020; https://www.ncbi.nlm.nih.gov/books/NBK554572/

[13] Bohannon R W, Smith M B. Interrater Reliability of a Modified Ashworth Scale of Muscle Spasticity, Phys Tx 1987; 67 (2):206-207, https://doi.org/10.1093/ptj/67.2.206

[14] Penn RD, Savoy SM, Corcos D, Latash M, Gottlieb G, Parke B, Kroin JS. Intrathecal baclofen for severe spinal spasticity. NEJM 1989; 320 (23): 1517-1521.

[15] Stoffel A. "The treatment of spastic contractures". Am J Orthop Surg 1912; 10: 611-644.

[16] Madsen P J, Chen H-C I, Lang S-S "Neurosurgical Approaches". Phys Med Rehabil Clin 2018; 29(3): 553-565.

[17] Sitthinamsuwan B, Nunta-Aree S. "Ablative neurosurgery for movement disorders related to cerebral palsy". J Neurosurg Sci 2015; 59(4): 393-404.

[18] Sherrington CS. "Decerebrate rigidity, and reflex coordination of movements". *J Physiol* 1898; 22(4): 319.

[19] Foerster O. "On the indications and results of the excision of posterior spinal nerve roots in men". Surg Gynecol Obs 1913; 16: 463-475.

[20] Kottke FJ. "Modification of athetosis by denervation of the tonic neck

reflexes," *Dev Med Child Neurol* 1970; 12(2); 236.

[21] Heimburger R F, Slominski A, Griswold P. "Cervical posterior rhizotomy for reducing spasticity in cerebral palsy". J Neurosurg 1973; 39(1): 30-34.

[22] Funk J F, *et al.* "Predictors for the benefit of selective dorsal rhizotomy". Res Dev Disabil 2015; 37: 127-134.

[23] Sindou M. "Étude de la jonction radiculo-médullaire postérieure, la radicellotomie postérieure sélective dans la chirurgie de la douleur". Impr HM 1972.

[24] Sindou M, G Fischer, R Goutelle, B Schott, Mansuy, "La radicellotomie posterieure selective dans le traitement des spasticites". Rev Neurol 1974; 30: 201-215.

[25] Sindou M, Mifsud J J, Boisson D, A. Goutelle. "Selective posterior rhizotomy in the dorsal root entry zone for treatment of hyperspasticity and pain in the hemiplegic upper limb". Neurosurgery 1986; 18(5): 587-595.

[26] Sindou M, Jeanmonod D. "Microsurgical DREZ-otomy for the treatment of spasticity and pain in the lower limbs". Neurosurgery 1989; 24(5): 655-670.

[27] Pourpre M H. "Traitement neurochirurgical des contractures chez les paraplégiques post-traumatiques". Neurochirurgie 1960; 6: 229-236.

[28] W. Bischof, "Die longitudinale myelotomie," Zentralbl Neurochir 1951; 11: 79-88.

[29] Siegfried J. "Destructive stereotatic procedures for spasticity directed to the brain and the cerebellum". Ed Springer. *Neurosurgery for Spasticity* 1991; 187-190.

[30] Mandel JE. Understanding Infusion Pumps. Anesthesia & Analgesia 2018; 1, 126(4): 1186-9.

[31] Penn R, Kroin J. Intrathecal baclofen alleviates spinal cord spasticity. Lancet 1984; 1(8385): 1078.

[32] Ghai A, Garg N, Hooda S, Gupta T. Spasticity–Pathogenesis, prevention and treatment strategies. Saudi journal of anaesthesia 2013; 7(4):453-460.

[33] Loubser PG, Narayan RK, Sandin KJ, Donovan WH, Russell KD. Continuous infusion of intrathecal baclofen: long-term effects on spasticity in spinal cord injury. Spinal Cord 1991; 29(1):48-64.

[34] Becker R, Alberti O, Bauer BL. Continuous intrathecal baclofen infusion in severe spasticity after traumatic or hypoxic brain injury. J Neurol 1997; 244(3):160-166.

[35] Korenkov AI, Niendorf WR, Darwish N, Glaeser E, Gaab MR. Continuous intrathecal infusion of baclofen in patients with spasticity caused by spinal cord injuries. Neurosurgical rev 2002; 25(4):228-230.

[36] Guillaume D, Van Havenbergh A, Vloeberghs M, Vidal J, Roeste G. A clinical study of intrathecal baclofen using a programmable pump for intractable spasticity. Archives of physical medicine and rehabilitation 2005; 86(11): 2165-2171.

[37] Stampacchia G, Gerini A, Mazzoleni S. Effects of severe spasticity treatment with intrathecal Baclofen in multiple sclerosis patients: Long term follow-up. Neuro Rehabilitation 2016; 38(4): 385-393.

[38] Kraus T, Gegenleitner K, Svehlik M, Novak M, Steinwender G, Singer G. Long-term therapy with intrathecal baclofen improves quality of life in children with severe spastic cerebral palsy. Eu J Paediatr Neurol 2017; 21(3): 565-569.

[39] Maneyapanda MB, McCormick ZL, Marciniak C, Reger C. Long-term dosing

of intrathecal baclofen in the treatment of spasticity after acquired brain injury. PM&R 2017; 9(6): 556-562.

[40] Pucks-Faes E, Matzak H, Hitzenberger G, Genelin E, Halbmayer LM, Fava E, Fritz J, Saltuari L. Intrathecal Baclofen Trial Before Device Implantation: 12-Year Experience with Continuous Administration. Arch Phys Med Rehabil 2019; 100(5): 837-843.

[41] Reis PV, Vieira CR, Midões AC, Rebelo V, Barbosa P, Gomes A. Intrathecal Baclofen Infusion Pumps in the Treatment of Spasticity: A Retrospective Cohort Study in a Portuguese Centre. Acta Médica Portuguesa 2019; 32(12):754-759.

[42] Shealy CN, Mortimer JT, Reswick JB. Electrical inhibition of pain by stimulation of the dorsal columns: preliminary clinical report. Anesth Analg 1967; 46(4): 489-491.

[43] Shealy CN, Taslitz N, Mortimer JT, Becker DP Electrical inhibition of pain: experimental evaluation. Anesth Analg 1967; 46(3): 299-305.

[44] Cook AW, Weinstein SP. Chronic dorsal column stimulation in multiple sclerosis. Preliminary report. N Y State J Med 1973; 73(24): 2868-2872.

[45] Illis LS, Oygar AE, Sedgwick EM, Awadalla MA. Dorsal-column stimulation in the rehabilitation of patients with multiple sclerosis. Lancet 1976; 1 (7974):1383-1386. doi: 10.1016/s0140-6736(76)93030-0

[46] Richardson RR, Cerullo LJ, McLone DG, Gutierrez FA, Lewis V. Percutaneous epidural neurostimulation in modulation of paraplegic spasticity. Six case reports. Acta Neurochir (Wien) 1979; 49(3-4): 235-243. doi: 10.1007/BF01808963.

[47] Read DJ, Matthews WB, Higson RH. The effect of spinal cord stimulation on function in patients with multiple sclerosis. Brain 1980; 103(4): 803-833. doi: 10.1093/brain/103.4.803.

[48] Siegfried J. Treatment of spasticity by dorsal cord stimulation. Int Rehabil Med 1980; 2(1): 31-34. doi: 10.3109/09638288009163952.

[49] Barolat-Romana G, Myklebust JB, Hemmy DC, Myklebust B, Wenninger W Immediate effects of spinal cord stimulation in spinal spasticity. JNS 1985; 62(4): 558-562. doi: 10.3171/jns.1985.62.4.0558.

[50] Dimitrijevic MM, Dimitrijevic MR, Illis LS, Nakajima K, Sharkey PC, Sherwood AM. Spinal cord stimulation for the control of spasticity in patients with chronic spinal cord injury: I. Clinical observations. Springer. Cent Nerv Syst Trauma 1986; 3(2): 129-144. doi: 10.1089/cns.1986.3.129.

[51] Campos RJ, Dimitrijevic MR, Sharkey PC, Sherwood AM. Epidural spinal cord stimulation in spastic spinal cord injury patients. Appl Neurophysiol 1987; 50(1-6): 453-454. doi: 10.1159/000100763.

[52] Barolat G, Myklebust JB, Wenninger W. Effects of spinal cord stimulation on spasticity and spasms secondary to myelopathy. Appl Neurophysiol 1988; 51(1): 29-44. doi: 10.1159/000099381.

[53] Barolat G. Experience with 509 plate electrodes implanted epidurally from C1 to L1.Stereotact Funct Neurosurg 1993; 61(2): 60-79. doi: 10.1159/000100624.

[54] Pinter MM, Gerstenbrand F, Dimitrijevic MR. Epidural electrical stimulation of posterior structures of the human lumbosacral cord: 3. Control Of spasticity. Cord 2000; 38(9): 524-531. doi: 10.1038/sj.sc.3101040.

[55] Dekopov AV, Shabalov VA, Tomsky AA, Hit MV, Salova EM. Chronic

Spinal Cord Stimulation in the Treatment of Cerebral and Spinal Spasticity. Stereotact Funct Neurosurg 2015; 93(2):133-139. doi: 10.1159/000368905.

[56] Cooper IS. Effect of chronic stimulation of anterior cerebellum on neurological disease. Lancet 1973; 1(7796): 206. doi: 10.1016/s0140-6736(73)90042-1.

[57] Cooper IS. Effect of stimulation of posterior cerebellum on neurological disease. Lancet. 1973; 1(7815): 1321. doi: 10.1016/s0140-6736(73)91338-x.

[58] Cooper IS, Crighel E, Amin I. Clinical and physiological effects of stimulation of the paleocerebellum in humans. J Am Geriatr Soc. 1973; 21(1): 40-43. doi: 10.1111/j.1532-5415.1973.tb00849.x.

[59] Upton AR, Cooper IS. Some neurophysiological effects of cerebellar stimulation in man. Can J Neurol Sci. 1976; 3(4): 237-254. doi: 10.1017/s031716710002535x.

[60] Riklan M, Cullinan T, Shulman M, Cooper IS. A psychometric study of chronic cerebellar stimulation in man. Biol Psychiatry 1976; 11(5): 543-574.

[61] Cooper IS, Amin I, Upton A, Riklan M, Watkins S, McLellan L. Safety and efficacy of chronic stimulation. Neurosurgery 1977; 1(2): 203-205. doi: 10.1097/00006123-197709000-00019.

[62] Riklan M, Cullinan T, Cooper IS. Tension reduction and alerting in man following chronic cerebellar stimulation for the relief of spasticity or intractable seizures.J Nerv Ment Dis 1977; 164(3): 176-181. doi: 10.1097/00005053-197703000-00003.

[63] McLellan DL, Selwyn M, Cooper IS. Time course of clinical and physiological effects of stimulation of the cerebellar surface in patients with spasticity. Neurol Neurosurg Psychiatry 1978; 41(2): 150-160. doi: 10.1136/jnnp.41.2.150.

[64] Cooper IS, Upton AR, Amin I. Chronic cerebellar stimulation (CCS) and deep brain stimulation (DBS) in involuntary movement disorders.Appl Neurophysiol 1982; 45(3): 209-217. doi: 10.1159/000101601.

[65] Manrique M, Oya S, Vaquero J, Lozano AP, Herrero J, Bravo G. Chronic paleocerebellar stimulation for the treatment of neuromuscular disorders. Four case report.Appl Neurophysiol 1978; 41(1-4): 237-247. doi: 10.1159/000102423.

[66] Penn RD, Gottlieb GL, Agarwal GC. Cerebellar stimulation in man. Quantitative changes in spasticity. J Neurosurg 1978; 48(5): 779-786. doi: 10.3171/jns.1978.48.5.0779.

[67] Fisher MA, Penn RD. Evidence for changes in segmental motoneurone pools by chronic cerebellar stimulation and its clinical significance.J Neurol Neurosurg Psychiatry 1978; 41(7): 630-635. doi: 10.1136/jnnp.41.7.630.

[68] Davis R, Flitter MA. Cerebellar stimulation. Surg Neurol 1978; 9(2): 115.

[69] Davis R, Barolat-Romana G, Engle H. Chronic cerebellar stimulation for cerebral palsy-five-year study. Acta Neurochir Suppl (Wien) 1980; 30:317-332. doi: 10.1007/978-3-7091-8592-6_39.

[70] Davis R, Engle H, Kudzma J, Gray E, Ryan T, Dusnak A. Update of chronic cerebellar stimulation for spasticity and epilepsy. Appl Neurophysiol 1982; 45(1-2): 44-50. doi: 10.1159/000101577.

[71] Davis R, Schulman J, Nanes M, Delehanty A. Cerebellar stimulation for spastic cerebral palsy--double-blind quantitative study. Appl Neurophysiol 1987; 50(1-6): 451-452. doi: 10.1159/000100762.

[72] Davis R. Cerebellar stimulation for cerebral palsy spasticity, function, and seizures. Arch Med Res 2000; 31(3): 290-9. doi: 10.1016/s0188-4409(00)00065-5.

[73] Davis R. Twenty-eight years of clinical experience with implantable neuroprostheses for various applications. Artif Organs 2002; 26(3):280-283. doi: 10.1046/j.1525-1594.2002.06937.x.

[74] Galanda M, Horvath S. Effect of stereotactic high-frequency stimulation in the anterior lobe of the cerebellum in cerebral palsy: a new suboccipital approach. Stereotact Funct Neurosurg 2003; 80(1-4): 102-107. doi: 10.1159/000075168.

[75] Galanda M, Horvath S. Stereotactic stimulation of the anterior lobe of the cerebellum in cerebral palsy from a suboccipital approach. Acta Neurochir Suppl 2007; 97(2): 239-243. doi: 10.1007/978-3-211-33081-4_27.

Chapter 11

Planning Cervical Deformity Surgery Including DJK Prevention Strategies

Themistocles Protopsaltis and Ethan Sissman

Abstract

Distal junctional kyphosis (DJK) is a major concern following cervical deformity (CD) correction, leading to failed realignment and revision surgery. In this chapter, we describe our approach to the treatment of cervical deformity and the steps taken to minimize the risk of DJK post-operatively by tailoring the construction to the individual patient. In this chapter, we describe our approach to the treatment of cervical deformity and the steps taken to minimize the risk of DJK post-operatively by tailoring the construction to the individual patient. First we focus on characterization of the baseline deformity. Secondly, we assess our patients clinically. Thirdly, we simulate the correction with the use of novel in-construct measurements. The fourth step is to develop a DJK prevention strategy tailored to the individual. The last step is to perform surgery and check correction during the operation.

Keywords: cervical deformity, DJK, distal junctional kyphosis, DJK prevention, in-construct measurements, cervical deformity correction

1. Introduction

Recent studies have focused on how sagittal malalignment of the cervical spine influences outcomes and promotes impairment of quality of life. In order to further understand cervical movement, compensatory mechanisms and pathologies, there are basic biomechanical properties parameters that should be considered. These include mass (m), force (F), standard gravity (g), moment arm (L), bending moments (M) and instantaneous axis of rotation (IAR). In the upright position the head creates a gravitational force on the cervical spine with a magnitude, of $F = m \times g$. This gravitational force then creates a forward bending moment, M, around a fulcrum of rotation, also known as the IAR. The magnitude of the bending moment is calculated by $M = F \times L$, in which L is the distance between the IAR and the center of gravity line.

Yogadanan et al. [1–6] showed that for cadaver studies conducted in the last five decades the center of gravity (COG) or center of mass (COM) of the head is located approximately 1.8 cm anterior and 6.0 cm superior to the occipital condyle. The numbers vary from one cadaver study to the next [6–16]. The head to total body mass (TBM) ratio was 7.37% + − 0.6%. The mean head mass was 4.770.3 kg [17].

In a normally aligned lordotic cervical spine, the posterior tension band and paraspinal muscles counteract the forward bending movement created by the weight of the head, maintaining the natural cervical alignment. When cervical kyphotic deformity is present, the head COM moves anteriorly and the moment arm, L, increases relative to the IAR, creating a larger bending moment, M. This results in greater paraspinal muscle contraction to keep the head erect, ultimately followed by exertion and pain.

The weight-bearing features of the cervical spine have been grouped into an anterior column, including the vertebral bodies and intervertebral discs, and two posterior columns, consisting of the facet joints [6]. It has been estimated that the anterior column is responsible for bearing up to 82% of the weight of the head while the posterior column is responsible for up to 33% [18]. By creating a larger bending moment, M, the kyphotic cervical deformity shifts the axial load anteriorly, which probably accelerates cervical disc degeneration. Disc degeneration might cause further cervical kyphosis, leading to an apparent vicious cycle.

Likewise, junctional failures of fusion are clearly the result of an imbalance of anterior column compression forces and posterior column tension band strength [1]. Biomechanical studies investigating the effects of spinal fusion on adjacent levels have shown that adjacent unfused levels compensate for the loss of cervical range of motion (ROM) in fused levels [19]. Maiman et al. [20] described a finite-element model of the cervical spine to investigate the effect of cervical spine fusion on adjacent levels. There was increased flexion-extension rotational movement of the disc in the sagittal plane especially at the upper adjacent level of the fusion. And this may contribute further to the pathologic progress.

Individualized optimization of surgical alignment has been shown to improve outcome regarding PJK [21].

Adult cervical deformity (ACD) of the spine has been shown to have a substantial negative impact on health-related measurements [20]. Therefore surgery to correct ACD can have a profound effect on improving the patient's health status. A common complication following fusion surgery is excessive kyphosis at one end of the fused construct. For example, thoracolumbar deformity correction commonly results in proximal junctional kyphosis (PJK), with reported rates as high as 40% [22]. In ACD surgery, fusions are usually extended to the upper cervical spine, which increases the likelihood of stress at the caudal part of the fusion construct, potentially leading to distal junctional kyphosis (DJK) or failure (DJF). In 2019, Oren et al. [23] introduced the utility of measurements of spinopelvic angles on prone lateral radiographs as predictors of global post-operative alignment in thoraco-lumbar deformity surgery. Similar measures are now in development for cervical deformity correction.

In this chapter, we describe our approach to the treatment of cervical deformity and the steps taken to minimize the risk of DJK post-operatively by tailoring the construction to the individual patient.

First we focus on characterization of the baseline deformity. Secondly, we assess our patients clinically. Thirdly, we simulate the correction with the use of novel in-construct measurements. The fourth step is to develop a DJK prevention strategy tailored to the individual. The last step is to perform surgery and check correction during the operation.

2. Characterization of the deformity

Ames and colleagues [23] have developed a comprehensive system of classification for cervical deformity. It defines the deformity driver and assigns severity points for four cervical parameters, the cSVA, CBVA, TS-CL, and myelopathy.

The classic measure of sagittal alignment in the cervical spine is the **cervical sagittal vertical axis (cSVA)** which measures the distance between a plumb line dropped from the centroid of C2 to the posterior superior aspect of C7. Hardecker et al. defined normative values ranging from 0.5 to 2.5 cm [24]. Several studies, one of them Tang et al. [25] have shown that high post-operative cSVA correlated with poor post-operative outcomes in patients undergoing cervical fusion. A cSVA over 4 cm corresponds to a moderate disability threshold. cSVA correlates with outcome measures in patients with thoracolumbar deformity as well as myelopathy.

The **T1 slope (T1S)** has emerged as an important measurement for pre-operative planning. It is the angle formed by a line drawn along the superior endplate of T1 and a horizontal reference line at the median sagittal cervical vertebra from the CT radiographs. Knott et al. [26] predicted that when the T1 slope is higher than 25 degrees, patients had at least 10 cm of positive sagittal imbalance. Ayres et al. [27] showed that a T1 slope above 30 degrees, indicates the need to perform full-length spine radiographs to identify potential concurrent thoracolumbar (TL) deformity. The right technical conditions with the use of long X-ray cassette radiographs should be met from the beginning, as shown by Ramchandran [28, 29]. In his survey among spine surgeons, 58% opted for longer fusion constructs to the mid- or lower thoracic spine in cervical deformity, when presented with long cassette radiographs. A T1 Slope above 30 degrees was associated with worse sagittal balance and spino-pelvic parameters values after corrective surgery [30]. Kim et al. showed that a high T1 slope in myelopathy patients undergoing laminoplasty predicted postoperative kyphotic alignment after laminoplasty [31].

An important marker of cervical deformity is the **C2 slope (C2S)**, which correlates with **T1 Slope Minus Cervical Lordosis (TS-CL)**, one of the Ames parameters of CD. This correlation is explained by the fact that the C2 slope is a mathematical approximation of the TS-CL [32]. However, C2S is simpler and more efficient to measure since it is just one angle. A high C2S of over 20 degrees correlates with poor Health-Related Quality of Life scores [32]. These results have been further corroborated by other groups including Hyun et al. [32] who found that a TS-CL greater than 22.2 degrees corresponded to severe disability (NDI > 25) and positive cervical sagittal malalignment, defined as a C2-C7 SVA greater than 43.5 mm.

Finally, an efficient assessment of concurrent thoracolumbar deformity is necessary. A helpful singular measurement in this regard is the **T1 pelvic angle (TPA)**. It simultaneously combines the measurement of sagittal deformity (as measured by T1 spinopelvic inclination, analogous to SVA) and pelvic compensation (pelvic tilt). The TPA is the angle subtended by a line from the femoral heads to the center of the T1 vertebral body and a line from the femoral heads to the center of the superior sacral end plate. Protopsaltis et al. [33, 34] showed excellent intra- and inter-observer reliability of this measurement.

Moreover the TPA remains constant, regardless of pelvic compensatory retroversion.

To summarize, we may include these four parameters as our key alignment parameters. The cSVA correlates well with every outcome measure. The T1S gives us information about the underlying thoracolumbar deformity. TPA gives us a quick and compensatory mechanism-independent overview of global thoracolumbar deformity. C2S tells us if a patient can compensate for the cervical spine deformity.

3. Clinical assessment

In the second step we evaluate the patient's symptoms and spinal function. There is as yet no standard measure of disability in cervical deformity. It is important to determine the patient's disability status with respect to concrete, everyday activities. Existing HRQL do not adequately capture CD disability and do not correlate with cervical malalignment. Therefore Stekas et al. [35] introduced the cervical deformity patient generated index (CD-PGI) that is designed to describe the most important limitations in health status for patients with cervical deformity.

Assessment of the patient's symptoms and complaints, as well as standing alignment, gait, and muscle weaknesses is essential. With progressive cervical malalignment, additional impairments can occur, including problems with horizontal gaze, coughing, swallowing and respiration. In addition, the patient is allowed to lie supine for at least five minutes in order to observe any passive correction of the neck deformity.

A full neurologic exam is needed. More severe deformity can lead to myelopathy and/or radiculopathy. Correlation between cervical kyphosis and severity of myelopathy is still under debate. Smith et al. [36] demonstrated correlation between cervical sagittal balance to myelopathy based on the Modified Japanese Orthopedic Association (mJOA) score. Additionally, we determine whether the patient is medically fit to undergo an extensive operation.

This raises the question of supine imaging which is considered the most realistic assessment of deformity as it does not require active extension. Unfortunately, the landmarks of the lower cervical spine used to assess lordosis are often obscured on plain radiographs. However, supine advanced imaging in the form of MRI or CT offers the simultaneous advantages of allowing for a truer assessment of lordosis, and clear visualization of landmarks in the lower cervical spine. It is recommended to request extensive supine sagittal imaging that includes the cervicothoracic junction and planned lower instrumented vertebra (LIV). Furthermore, these modalities are often obtained during routine workup of cervical deformity and therefore do not require any additional cost and radiation. The use of supine imaging before

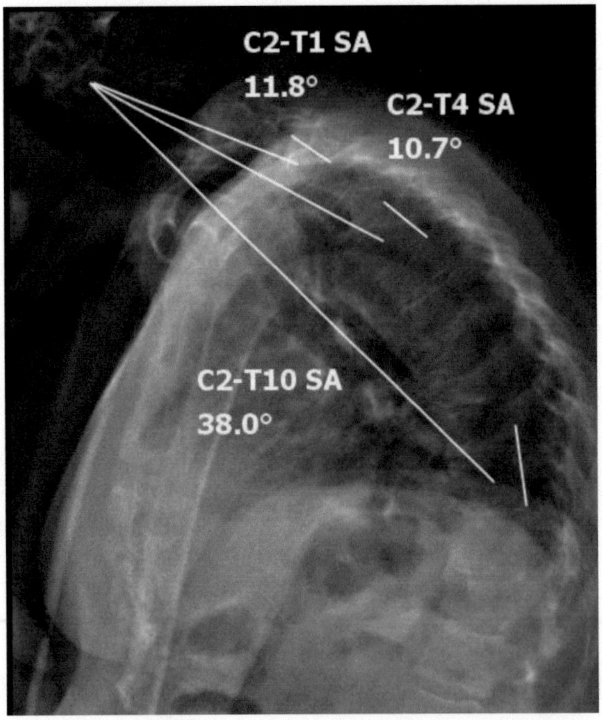

Figure 1.
Sagittal radiograph of a patient showing the measurement of C2-T1 SA, C2-T4 SA and C2-T10SA.

and during surgery has led to the development of new in-construct measurements, namely the C2-T1 sagittal angle (C2-T1 SA), C2-T4 sagittal angle (C2-T4 SA) and C2-T10 sagittal angle (C2-T10 SA) (**Figure 1**). These measurements have the advantage that they are independent of radiographic modality and patient position, as long as the fusion construct is stable. The **C2-T1 SA** is defined as the angle formed by a line from the centroid of C2 to the Centroid of T1, and a line parallel to the posterior body of T1. Similarly **C2-T4 SA** and **C2-T10 SA** are the angles formed by a line from the centroid of C2 to the Centroid of T4 and T10 respectively, and a line parallel to the posterior vertebral body of T4 and T10 respectively. Depending on the planned LIV, we further recommend adding one of these parameters to the other four main parameters, cSVA, T1S, C2S and TPA [28].

4. Classification

Currently there is ongoing focus on research to find a classification system that dictates treatment modality and predicts outcome. Ames et al. [37] (**Figure 2**) was built on basic deformity descriptors and five associated modifiers. Deformity descriptors differentiated deformity by type, ranging from sagittal to craniovertebral junction deformities, as well as regional location factoring thoracolumbar deformities. The selected modifiers accounted for various factors correlating with ACD and thoracolumbar deformity; Diebo et al. [38] described in his proposal of classification a two-step approach. Initially identifying the five most discriminate parameters are cSVA and T1 slope on lateral view, and maximum focal kyphosis, C2 slope and number of kyphotic levels on extension view. Those parameters were able to describe most of the deformity. On the second step his team proposed 3 distinct morphologies of sagittal cervical deformities based on lateral

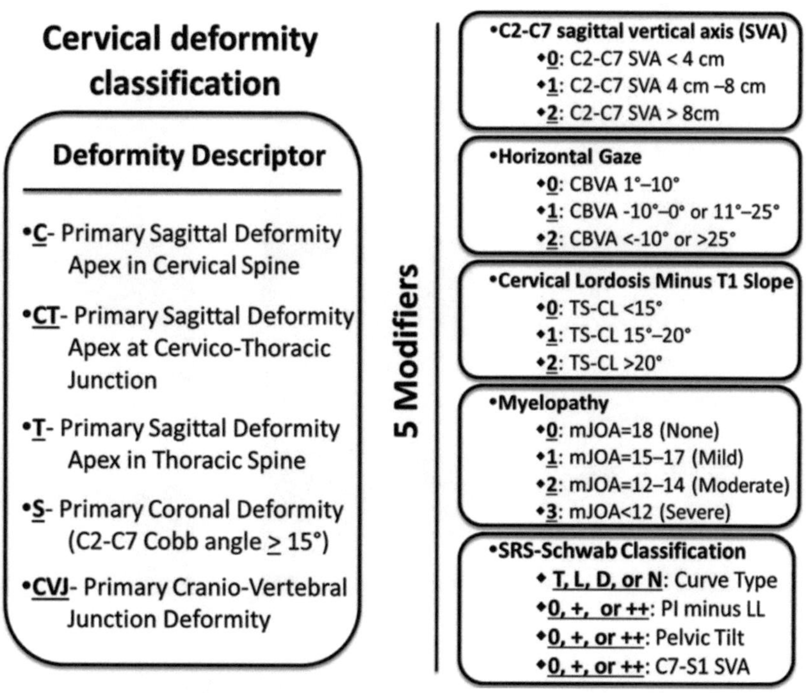

Figure 2.
Description of the CSD classification system, which includes a deformity descriptor and 5 modifiers. D = double; L = lordosis; N = none; T = thoracic.

and extension radiographs. Overall, the current classifications remain limited to radiographic or clinical description.

5. Surgical techniques

Ames et al. [39] proposed a cervical osteotomy classification scheme that ranges from least invasive to most invasive and includes: (I) partial facet joint resection, (II) complete facet joint/(Ponte) osteotomy, (III) partial or complete corpectomy, (IV) complete uncovertebral joint resection to the transverse foramen, (V) opening wedge osteotomy, (VI) closing wedge osteotomy, and (VII) complete vertebral column resection.

Osteotomies are the mainstay of treatment in deformity correction. In the thoracolumbar region, posterior osteotomies are well established, including opening wedge osteotomy and pedicle subtraction osteotomy (PSO). However, these techniques are limited in the cervical region due to the presence of the vertebral artery, the sensitivity of the cervical nerve roots to traction, and the small size of the cervical vertebrae. Pioneered by Simmons [40], a posterior column osteotomy with controlled osteoclasis of the anterior column of the cervical spine can result in significant improvement in cervical spine alignment and in the patients' ability to maintain forward gaze and adequately perform activities of daily living.

Osteotomies utilizing an anterior approach for cervical deformity corrections have been described by Riew [41] and Kim [41]. Common anterior techniques include anterior cervical discectomy and fusion (ACDF), cervical corpectomy, anterior osteotomy (ATO), and the Riew osteotomy [42, 43]. Anterior techniques can often be combined with posterior techniques to achieve circumferential spinal

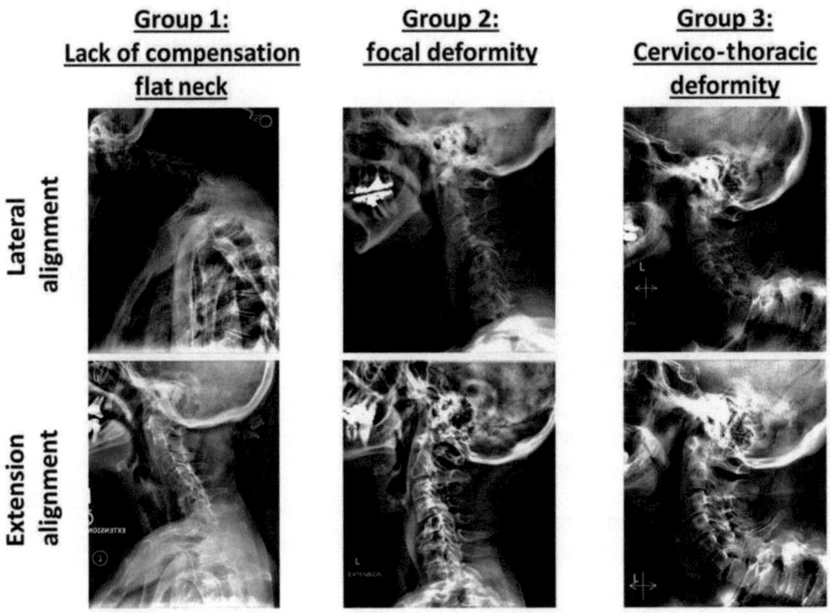

Figure 3.
New cervical deformity morphologies described by Diebo et al. [38]: Group 1 (46.1%): Flatneck with lack of compensation, largeT1S-CL, flexible CL; Group2 (30.8%): Focal deformity, large focal kyphosis between 2 segments, No large regional cervical kyphosis under the setting of a low T1S; group 3 (23.1%): Cervico-thoracic deformity, very large T1S, hyperlordosis of the cervical spine, no extension reserve left.

reconstruction. It remains inconclusive whether adding a posterior approach augments angular correction and improves stability [43]. As a general rule, the amount of lordosis obtained is about 3–5 degrees for single-level ACDF, 10 degrees for the Smith-Petersen osteotomy (SPO), 17 degrees for ATO, and up to 35 degrees for C7 PSO [44–46].

In severe cases, upper thoracic and cervical PSO's may not get the same correction as a Vertebral Column Resection (VCR). Hoh et al. [47] reported the use of two-stage (posterior–anterior) VCR for the treatment of ankylosing spondylitis. Garg et al. [48] reported the use of three-stage (anterior–posterior–anterior) VCR for a patient with kyphotic cervical deformity following tuberculosis infection. Funayama [49] reported a case of severe kyphotic deformity which showed an improvement from 75 degrees to 21 degrees with a three-stage VCR.

Several retrospective studies [23, 50, 51] presented a large potential of coronal and sagittal correction with posterior VCR. However this procedure can be associated with significant morbidity, particularly in the correction of kyphotic deformity.

Due to the complexity of the neurovascular anatomy in the cervicothoracic region, posteriorly based osteotomy techniques are challenging. Riew et al. [52] makes a case for combining ATO with SPO and posterior cervical fusion, which generated a mean angular correction of 28 degrees per level, providing equal or better corrections than isolated PSOs [9, 53–55] (**Figure 3**).

6. Planning the tailored strategy

In the pre-surgical planning, radiographic measurements of spinopelvic parameters are determined using validated software such as Surgimap (Nemaris Inc., New York, NY). The senior surgeon (TSP) maps out the correction with planning software.

Measuring Hounsfield units (HU) on clinical CT scans of the thorax, abdomen or pre-operative spine CTs demonstrated a reliable correlation between T values of the DEXA measurement and HU of the same vertebral body [56, 57].

Preoperative CT-scan determination of bone density can predict the risk of screw loosening and impact on the technical preferences [57] and has proven to be superior to a pre-operative DEXA scan in the assessment of screw loosening in degenerative spine disease [58].

The LIV is planned for an area with no kyphosis, that is, in an area of neutral alignment. Bone quality is evaluated with CT Hounsfield units, particularly at the LIV and LIV-1 level where failure tends to occur.

Subjacent reciprocal compensation is anticipated at the distal end of the instrumentation construct. The increase of thoracic kyphosis/(the DJK angle change) below the fusion is predicted with a mathematical formula, which includes the change in cervical lordosis (change in CL), and most importantly the actual change in construct alignment (change in C2-LIV SA) [59]:

$$\begin{aligned} \mathrm{DJKA}\left(\mathrm{DJKA}_{\mathrm{post}}\right).\mathrm{DJKA}_{\mathrm{post}} &= 9.365 + 0.315 * \left(\mathrm{C2} - \mathrm{LIV}_{\mathrm{post}}\right) \\ &\quad + 0.504 * \left(\mathrm{DJKA}_{\mathrm{pre}}\right) + 0.123 * (\Delta \mathrm{CL}) \end{aligned} \tag{1}$$

The formula also includes the preoperative DJK angle, underscoring the importance of planning the LIV in a region where there is no preoperative kyphotic alignment.

7. Intraoperative assessment of correction

Fluoroscopy can be used to measure the focal correction during surgery after performing an osteotomy procedure. Next a 36 inch X-ray cassette that captures the entire fusion construct is recommended. The in-construct measurement appropriate for the patient's instrumentation can be measured (for example, C2-T10 SA for a posterior fusion from C2 to T10) (see **Figure 4**).

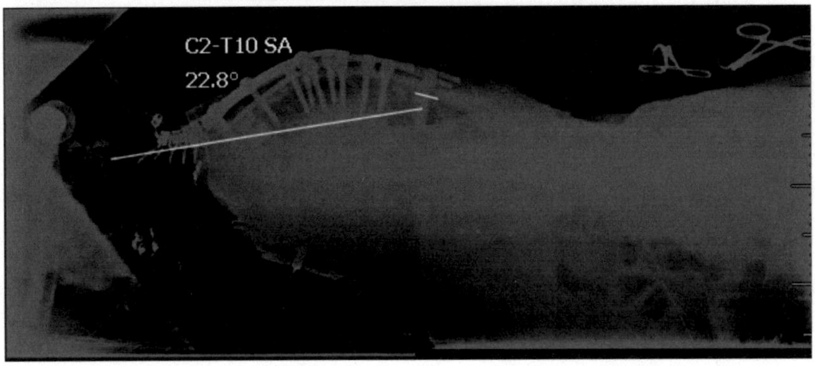

Figure 4.
The in-construct measurement appropriate for the patient's instrumentation can be measured during surgery (for example: C2-T10 SA for a posterior fusion from C2 to T10).

8. Intraoperative neuromonitoring

Intraoperative neuromonitoring is a tool with the goal of providing patients with limited morbidities and optimal outcomes during and after surgery. The aim of neuromonitoring during an operation is to provide the surgeon with a real-time analysis of spinal cord function at a time when there is still a possibility to correct any possibility of morbidity. Spine surgeons need to be aware of the low sensitivity and positive predictive value with neuromonitoring so that they rely more on their clinical and surgical judgment and interpret neuromonitoring with more scrutiny [60].

9. The DJK prevention strategy

Surgeons need to know when their intraoperative corrections are adequate to align CD patients optimally [61]. We propose a strategy of several steps that can be taken to minimize the risk of DJK. First is determination of the correct alignment to be achieved during surgery by utilizing the newly developed in-construct measurements. This involves anticipating the subjacent reciprocal changes to give a final result of a C2S of under 20 degrees and a cSVA of under 4 cm [62].

Secondly, the use of softer materials at the distal junction may protect against the development of Adjacent Segment Disease (ASD) and junctional kyphosis. In a retrospective case–control study by Han et al. [63] the use of cobalt chrome multiple-rod constructs (CoCr MRCs) versus titanium alloy two-rod constructs (Ti TRCs) were evaluated with a minimum of 1-year follow-up. They suggested that increasing the number of rods and their stiffness promotes proximal junctional kyphosis (PJK) in ASD surgery. PJK prevention strategies that should be considered for preventing DJK include minimizing the destruction of soft tissue at the Upper Instrumented Vertebra (UIV) (PJK) and therefore LIV (DJK) and using transition rods with softer metals [64].

Thirdly, optimization of bone health is critical. The role of pharmacotherapy in aiding implant fixation or fusion has been studied for bisphosphonates and teriparatide (Human recombinant PTH 1–34, Forteo, Ely Lilly, Indianapolis, IN). Zolendronate was found to make no statistically significant difference. Prospective trials [65] showed a significant advantage in prescribing teriparatide over bisphosphonate to aid fusion and lower the rate of pedicle screw loosening. However, the most recent published study by Oba et al. [66] must be evaluated carefully due to the short follow-up duration as well as the cost and the potential for serious side-effects with the use of teriparatide.

Teriparatide is very expensive, and due to the limited on-label indications it can be challenging to secure insurance coverage. However, in light of the costs associated with spinal fusion surgery and the importance of preventing osteoporosis-related complications as defined by Bjerke et al. [67], insurers are becoming more willing to consider off-label orthopedic indications for teriparatide. In addition, in most cases the patients do qualify based on their diagnosed level of osteoporosis. This emphasizes the importance of a pre-operative workup. The most commonly described and FDA-approved dosing schedule for teriparatide is 20 mcg/day. Yet, an effective [59] weekly dosing schedule of 56.5 mcg/week has been described for vertebral compression fracture (VCF) and spine fusion. Timing of treatment before and after spinal surgery is still evolving and may vary. Several studies suggest a benefit to initiating teriparatide 3 months before surgery, which is a challenge to insurance approval. Consequently, it has been suggested [60] that patients have at least 4–6 weeks of teriparatide therapy prior to surgical intervention. Following surgery, patients stay on teriparatide for at least 10 months, for a minimum of 12 months of total therapy.

Abaloparatide is a newer parathyroid hormone 1 receptor (PTH1R) agonist indicated for the treatment of osteoporosis in postmenopausal women with a high risk for fracture [61]. Because of its recent approval, abaloparatide is not mentioned in clinical guidelines for the treatment of postmenopausal osteoporosis, but its place in therapy is likely to be similar to that of teriparatide because the two drugs share a common mechanism of action. Use of either of these agents for more than two years is not recommended.

In a multi-center, multi-national, double-blind placebo-controlled clinical trial, Leder et al. [62] observed lumbar Bone Mineral Density (BMD) increases up to 6.7% over 24 weeks with abaloparatide versus only 5.5% and 1.6% in the teriparatide and placebo groups respectively ($p = <0.001$). Bilezikian et al. [63], in a Phase 2 randomized control trial of postmenopausal women aged 55–85 years, demonstrated consistently greater dose-dependent improvements in lumbar trabecular bone score by 12 weeks with abaloparatide when compared to teriparatide or a placebo. Trabecular bone score might correlate with subsequent improvement in pedicle screw strength [64]. Denosumab, a RANK-L inhibitor, has been approved by the FDA (Food and Drug Administration) and established in the treatment of osteoporosis, but its role in spine fusion has yet to be evaluated.

10. Conclusion

It has been estimated that the cost of healthcare in the United States is nearly twice as much as any other developed countries [65]. Therefore the prevention of complications and revision costs are becoming increasingly recognized and recent efforts have been made to qualify and quantify new prevention measures against failure. Passias et al. [66] have found that DJK is a significant predictor of surgical readmission after ASD operations. In Scheuerman patients DJK might be well tolerated without symptoms, loss of alignment or mechanical decompensation [67].

Our DJK prevention strategy has proved successful in providing tools for the surgeon to foresee the risks of failure and modify the treatment in order to prevent disability, complications and revision surgery in cervical deformity patients.

Author details

Themistocles Protopsaltis[1,2*] and Ethan Sissman[1,3]

1 Department of Orthopedic Surgery, NYU Langone Health, New York

2 Division of Spine Surgery, Department of Orthopedic Surgery, NYU Langone Health, New York, United States

3 Department of Orthopedic Surgery, Sheba Medical Center, Ramat Gan, Israel

*Address all correspondence to: themistocles.protopsaltis@nyulangone.org

References

[1] Tang JA, Scheer JK, Smith JS, et al. The impact of standing regional cervical sagittal alignment on outcomes in posterior cervical fusion surgery. *Neurosurgery*. 2012;71(3):662-669. doi:10.1227/NEU.0b013e31826100c9

[2] Smith JS, Line B, Bess S, et al. The health impact of adult cervical deformity in patients presenting for surgical treatment: Comparison to United States population norms and chronic disease states based on the EuroQuol-5 dimensions questionnaire. *Clinical Neurosurgery*. 2017;80(5):716-725. doi:10.1093/neuros/nyx028

[3] Lee JS, Youn MS, Shin JK, Goh TS, Kang SS. Relationship between cervical sagittal alignment and quality of life in ankylosing spondylitis. *European Spine Journal*. 2015;24(6):1199-1203. doi:10.1007/s00586-014-3491-8

[4] Albert TJ, Vacarro A. Postlaminectomy kyphosis. *Spine*. 1998;23(24):2738-2745. doi:10.1097/00007632-199812150-00014

[5] Scheer JK, Tang JA, Smith JS, et al. Cervical spine alignment, sagittal deformity, and clinical implications: A review. *Journal of Neurosurgery: Spine*. 2013;19(2):141-159. doi:10.3171/2013.4.SPINE12838

[6] Ames CP, Smith JS, Eastlack R, et al. Reliability assessment of a novel cervical spine deformity classification system. *Journal of Neurosurgery: Spine*. 2015;23(6):673-683. doi:10.3171/2014.12.SPINE14780

[7] Cho SK, Shin JI, Kim YJ. Proximal junctional kyphosis following adult spinal deformity surgery. *European Spine Journal*. 2014;23(12):2726-2736. doi:10.1007/s00586-014-3531-4

[8] Rubery PT, Molinari R, Menga EN. Proximal Junctional Kyphosis. 2019;7(4):1-11.

[9] Glattes RC, Bridwell KH, Lenke LG, Kim YJ, Rinella A, Edwards C. *Proximal Junctional Kyphosis in Adult Spinal Deformity Following Long Instrumented Posterior Spinal Fusion Incidence, Outcomes, and Risk Factor Analysis*. Vol 30.

[10] Yagi M, Akilah KB, Boachie-Adjei O. Incidence, risk factors and classification of proximal junctional kyphosis: Surgical outcomes review of adult idiopathic scoliosis. *Spine*. 2011;36(1). doi:10.1097/BRS.0b013e3181eeaee2

[11] Ha Y, Maruo K, Racine L, et al. Proximal junctional kyphosis and clinical outcomes in adult spinal deformity surgery with fusion from the thoracic spine to the sacrum: A comparison of proximal and distal upper instrumented vertebrae Clinical article. *Journal of Neurosurgery: Spine*. 2013;19(3):360-369. doi:10.3171/2013.5.SPINE12737

[12] Maruo K, Ha Y, Inoue S, et al. Predictive factors for proximal junctional kyphosis in long fusions to the sacrum in adult spinal deformity. *Spine*. 2013;38(23). doi:10.1097/BRS.0b013e3182a51d43

[13] Kim HJ, Bridwell KH, Lenke LG, et al. Proximal Junctional Kyphosis Results in Inferior SRS Pain Subscores in Adult Deformity Patients Level of Evidence: 3 Spine 2013;38:896-901. *SPINE*. 38(11):896-901. doi:10.1097/BRS.ObOI

[14] Watanabe K, Lenke LG, Bridwell KH, Kim YJ, Koester L, Hensley M. *Proximal Junctional Vertebral Fracture in Adults After Spinal Deformity Surgery Using Pedicle Screw Constructs Analysis of Morphological Features*. Vol 35.

[15] Hart RA, McCarthy I, Ames CP, Shaffrey CI, Hamilton DK, Hostin R. Proximal Junctional Kyphosis and Proximal Junctional Failure.

Neurosurgery Clinics of North America. 2013;24(2):213-218. doi:10.1016/j.nec.2013.01.001

[16] Hostin R, McCarthy I, O'Brien M, et al. Incidence, mode, and location of acute proximal junctional failures after surgical treatment of adult spinal deformity. *Spine*. 2013;38(12):1008-1015. doi:10.1097/BRS.0b013e318271319c

[17] Oren JH, Tishelman JC, Day LM, et al. Measurement of Spinopelvic Angles on Prone Intraoperative Long-Cassette Lateral Radiographs Predicts Postoperative Standing Global Alignment in Adult Spinal Deformity Surgery. *Spine Deformity*. 2019;7(2):325-330. doi:10.1016/j.jspd.2018.07.007

[18] Hardacker JW, Shuford RF, Capicotto PN, Pryor PW. Radiographic standing cervical segmental alignment in adult volunteers without neck symptoms. *Spine*. 1997;22(13):1472-1480; discussion 1480. doi:10.1097/00007632-199707010-00009

[19] Knott PT, Mardjetko SM, Techy F. The use of the T1 sagittal angle in predicting overall sagittal balance of the spine. *Spine Journal*. 2010;10(11):994-998. doi:10.1016/j.spinee.2010.08.031

[20] Ayres EW, Woo D, Vasquez-Montes D, et al. 71. High preoperative T1 slope is a marker for global sagittal malalignment. *The Spine Journal*. 2019;19(9):S35. doi:10.1016/j.spinee.2019.05.084

[21] Ramchandran S, Smith JS, Ailon T, et al. Assessment of impact of long-cassette standing X-rays on surgical planning for cervical pathology: An international survey of spine surgeons. Neurosurgery. 2016;78(5):717-724. doi:10.1227/NEU.0000000000001128

[22] Kim TH, Lee SY, Kim YC, Park MS, Kim SW. T1 slope as a predictor of kyphotic alignment change after laminoplasty in patients with cervical myelopathy. *Spine*. 2013;38(16). doi:10.1097/BRS.0b013e3182972e1b

[23] Protopsaltis TS, Ramchandran S, Tishelman JC, et al. The Importance of C2 Slope, a Singular Marker of Cervical Deformity, Correlates with Patient-reported Outcomes. *Spine*. 2020;45(3):184-192. doi:10.1097/BRS.0000000000003214

[24] Hyun SJ, Kim KJ, Jahng TA, Kim HJ. Clinical Impact of T1 Slope Minus Cervical Lordosis after Multilevel Posterior Cervical Fusion Surgery. *Spine*. 2017;42(24):1859-1864. doi:10.1097/BRS.0000000000002250

[25] Protopsaltis T, Schwab F, Bronsard N, et al. The T1 pelvic angle, a novel radiographic measure of global sagittal deformity, accounts for both spinal inclination and pelvic tilt and correlates with health-related quality of life. *Journal of Bone and Joint Surgery - American Volume*. 2014;96(19):1631-1640. doi:10.2106/JBJS.M.01459

[26] Stekas N, Ayres EW, Woo D, et al. P98. What drives disability in cervical deformity: novel patient generated outcome versus legacy HRQL. *The Spine Journal*. 2019;19(9):S203-S204. doi:10.1016/j.spinee.2019.05.523

[27] Smith JS, Lafage V, Ryan DJ, et al. Association of myelopathy scores with cervical sagittal balance and normalized spinal cord volume: analysis of 56 preoperative cases from the AOSpine North America Myelopathy study. *Spine*. 2013;38(22 Suppl 1). doi:10.1097/BRS.0b013e3182a7eb9e

[28] Ames CP, Smith JS, Eastlack R, et al. Reliability assessment of a novel cervical spine deformity classification system. *Journal of Neurosurgery: Spine*. 2015;23(6):673-683. doi:10.3171/2014.12.SPINE14780

[29] Ames CP, Smith JS, Scheer JK, et al. A standardized nomenclature zor cervical spine sozt-tissue release and osteotomy zor deformity correction. *Journal of Neurosurgery: Spine*. 2013;19(3):269-278. doi:10.3171/2013.5.SPINE121067

[30] Simmons ED, Distefano RJ, Zheng Y, Simmons EH. *Thirty-Six Years Experience of Cervical Extension Osteotomy in Ankylosing Spondylitis Techniques and Outcomes*. Vol 31.

[31] Safaee MM, Tan LA, Riew KD. Anterior osteotomy for rigid cervical deformity correction. *Journal of Spine Surgery*. 2020;6(1):210-216. doi:10.21037/jss.2019.12.10

[32] Kim HJ, Piyaskulkaew C, Riew KD. Anterior cervical osteotomy for fixed cervical deformities. *Spine*. 2014;39(21):1751-1757. doi:10.1097/BRS.0000000000000502

[33] Kim HJ, Piyaskulkaew C, Riew KD. Comparison of Smith-Petersen osteotomy versus pedicle subtraction osteotomy versus anterior–posterior osteotomy types for the correction of cervical spine deformities. *Spine*. 2015;40(3):143-146. doi:10.1097/BRS.0000000000000707

[34] Gillis CC, Kaszuba MC, Traynelis VC. Cervical radiographic parameters in 1- and 2-level anterior cervical discectomy and fusion. *Journal of Neurosurgery: Spine*. 2016;25(4):421-429. doi:10.3171/2016.2.SPINE151056

[35] Hoh DJ, Khoueir P, Wang MY. Management of cervical deformity in ankylosing spondylitis. *Neurosurgical Focus*. 2008;24(1). doi:10.3171/FOC/2008/24/1/E9

[36] Garg B, Mehta N, Vatsya P. Surgical strategy for correction of severe, rigid, post-tubercular cervical kyphosis: an experience of two cases. *Spine Deformity*. 2020;8(4):801-807. doi:10.1007/s43390-020-00104-6

[37] Ames CP, Smith JS, Eastlack R, et al. Reliability assessment of a novel cervical spine deformity classification system. *Journal of neurosurgery Spine*. 2015;23(6):673-683. doi:10.3171/2014.12.SPINE14780

[38] Diebo, B.G., Shah, N.V., Solow, M et al. Adult cervical deformity: radiographic and osteotomy classifications. Orthopäde 47, 496-504 (2018). https://doi.org/10.1007/s00132-018-3581-0

[39] Funayama T, Abe T, Noguchi H, et al. Severe, rigid cervical kyphotic deformity associated with SAPHO syndrome successfully treated with three-stage correction surgery combined with C7 vertebral column resection: a technical case report. *Spine Deformity*. Published online September 18, 2020. doi:10.1007/s43390-020-00203-4

[40] Saifi C, Laratta JL, Petridis P, Shillingford JN, Lehman RA, Lenke LG. Vertebral column resection for rigid spinal deformity. *Global Spine Journal*. 2017;7(3):280-290. doi:10.1177/2192568217699203

[41] Tan LA, Riew KD. Anterior cervical osteotomy: operative technique. *European Spine Journal*. 2018;27:39-47. doi:10.1007/s00586-017-5163-y

[42] Scheyerer MJ, Ullrich B, Osterhoff G, Spiegl UA, Schnake KJ. Hounsfield units as a measure of bone density—applications in spine surgery. *Unfallchirurg*. 2019;122(8):654-661. doi:10.1007/s00113-019-0658-0

[43] Bredow J, Boese CK, Werner CML, et al. Predictive validity of preoperative CT scans and the risk of pedicle screw loosening in spinal surgery. *Archives of Orthopaedic and Trauma Surgery*.

2016;136(8):1063-1067. doi:10.1007/s00402-016-2487-8

[44] Zou D, Li W, Deng C, Du G, Xu N. The use of CT Hounsfield unit values to identify the undiagnosed spinal osteoporosis in patients with lumbar degenerative diseases. *European Spine Journal*. 2019;28(8):1758-1766. doi:10.1007/s00586-018-5776-9

[45] Pickhardt PJ, Pooler; B Dustin, Lauder T, Muñ Oz Del Rio A, Bruce RJ, Binkley N. *Opportunistic Screening for Osteoporosis Using Abdominal Computed Tomography Scans Obtained for Other Indications*.; 2013. www.annals.org

[46] Zou D, Sun Z, Zhou S, Zhong W, Li W. Hounsfield units value is a better predictor of pedicle screw loosening than the T-score of DXA in patients with lumbar degenerative diseases. *European Spine Journal*. 2020;29(5):1105-1111. doi:10.1007/s00586-020-06386-8

[47] Ethan W. Ayres, MD; Themistocles S. Protopsaltis, MD; Renaud Lafage, MSc; Gregory M. Mundis Jr., MD; Justin S. Smith, MD, PhD; D. Kojo Hamilton, MD; Eric O. Klineberg, MD; Daniel M. Sciubba, MD; Robert A. Hart, MD; Shay Bess, MD; Christopher I. Shaffrey, M. Predicting the magnitude of DJK following cervical deformity correction. https://exhibit.nassannualmeeting.org/AM2019/Public/SessionDetails.aspx?FromPage=Speakers.aspx&SessionID=1263&nav=true&Role=U%27

[48] Ibrahim T, Mrowczynski O, Zalatimo O, et al. The Impact of Neurophysiological Intraoperative Monitoring during Spinal Cord and Spine Surgery: A Critical Analysis of 121 Cases. *Cureus*. Published online November 20, 2017. doi:10.7759/cureus.1861

[49] Schwab FJ, Patel A, Shaffrey CI, et al. Sagittal realignment failures following pedicle subtraction osteotomy surgery: are we doing enough?: Clinical article. *Journal of neurosurgery Spine*. 2012;16(6):539-546. doi:10.3171/2012.2.SPINE11120

[50] Jalai CM, Passias PG, Lafage V, et al. A comparative analysis of the prevalence and characteristics of cervical malalignment in adults presenting with thoracolumbar spine deformity based on variations in treatment approach over 2 years. *European spine journal: official publication of the European Spine Society, the European Spinal Deformity Society, and the European Section of the Cervical Spine Research Society*. 2016;25(8):2423-2432. doi:10.1007/s00586-016-4564-7

[51] Themistocles S. Protopsaltis, MD, Subaraman Ramchandran M, D. Kojo Hamilton, MD, Daniel M. Sciubba M, Alexandra Soroceanu, MD, MPH, Amit Jain5, Peter G. Passias M, et al. Analysis of Successful versus Failed Radiographic Outcomes following Cervical Deformity Surgery [abstract]. *NASS 31st Annual Meeting Proceedings/The Spine Journal 16 (2016) S113–S250*.

[52] Han S, Hyun SJ, Kim KJ, Jahng TA, Lee S, Rhim SC. Rod stiffness as a risk factor of proximal junctional kyphosis after adult spinal deformity surgery: comparative study between cobalt chrome multiple-rod constructs and titanium alloy two-rod constructs. *Spine Journal*. 2017;17(7):962-968. doi:10.1016/j.spinee.2017.02.005

[53] Denis F, Sun EC, Winter RB. Incidence and risk factors for proximal and distal junctional kyphosis following surgical treatment for Scheuermann kyphosis: Minimum five-year follow-up. *Spine*. 2009;34(20):729-734. doi:10.1097/BRS.0b013e3181ae2ab2

[54] Cammarata M, Aubin CÉ, Wang X, Mac-Thiong JM. Biomechanical risk factors for proximal junctional kyphosis: A detailed numerical analysis of surgical

instrumentation variables. *Spine*. 2014;39(8):E500-E507. doi:10.1097/BRS.0000000000000222

[55] Maruo K, Ha Y, Inoue S, et al. Predictive factors for proximal junctional kyphosis in long fusions to the sacrum in adult spinal deformity. *Spine*. 2013;38(23). doi:10.1097/BRS.0b013e3182a51d43

[56] Ohtori S, Inoue G, Orita S, et al. Teriparatide accelerates lumbar posterolateral fusion in women with postmenopausal osteoporosis: Prospective study. *Spine*. 2012;37(23). doi:10.1097/BRS.0b013e31826ca2a8

[57] Oba H, Takahashi J, Yokomichi H, et al. Weekly teriparatide versus bisphosphonate for bone union during 6 months after multi-level lumbar interbody fusion for osteoporotic patients: A multicenter, prospective, randomized study. *Spine*. 2020;45(13):863-871. doi:10.1097/BRS.0000000000003426

[58] Bjerke BT, Zarrabian M, Aleem IS, et al. Incidence of Osteoporosis-Related Complications Following Posterior Lumbar Fusion. *Global Spine Journal*. 2018;8(6):563-569. doi:10.1177/2192568217743727

[59] Ebata S, Takahashi J, Hasegawa T, et al. Role of weekly teriparatide administration in osseous union enhancement within six months after posterior or transforaminal lumbar interbody fusion for osteoporosis-associated lumbar degenerative disorders: A multicenter, prospective randomized study. *Journal of Bone and Joint Surgery - American Volume*. 2017;99(5):365-372. doi:10.2106/JBJS.16.00230

[60] Wanderman N, Alvi M, Yolcu Y, et al. *Is Teriparatide Beneficial to Spinal Fusion Surgery in the Older Patient? A Narrative Review*.; 2019. www.clinicalspinesurgery.com

[61] Waltham MRHI 2017. *Tymlos™ (Abaloparatide) Injection, for Subcutaneous Use [Package]*. Accessed September 23, 2020. https://www.accessdata.fda.gov/drugsatfda_docs/label/2017/208743lbl.pdf

[62] Leder BZ, O'Dea LSL, Zanchetta JR, et al. Effects of abaloparatide, a human parathyroid hormone-related peptide analog, on bone mineral density in postmenopausal women with osteoporosis. *Journal of Clinical Endocrinology and Metabolism*. 2015;100(2):697-706. doi:10.1210/jc.2014-3718

[63] Bilezikian JP, Hattersley G, Fitzpatrick LA, et al. Abaloparatide-SC improves trabecular microarchitecture as assessed by trabecular bone score (TBS): a 24-week randomized clinical trial. *Osteoporosis International*. 2018;29(2):323-328. doi:10.1007/s00198-017-4304-9

[64] McCloskey E v., Odén A, Harvey NC, et al. A Meta-Analysis of Trabecular Bone Score in Fracture Risk Prediction and Its Relationship to FRAX. *Journal of Bone and Mineral Research*. 2016;31(5):940-948. doi:10.1002/jbmr.2734

[65] Bates DW, Saria S, Ohno-Machado L, Shah A, Escobar G. Big data in health care: Using analytics to identify and manage high-risk and high-cost patients. *Health Affairs*. 2014;33(7):1123-1131. doi:10.1377/hlthaff.2014.0041

[66] Passias PG, Klineberg EO, Jalai CM, et al. Hospital Readmission Within 2 Years Following Adult Thoracolumbar Spinal Deformity Surgery: Prevalence, Predictors, and Effect on Patient-derived Outcome Measures. *Spine*. 2016;41(17):1355-1364. doi:10.1097/BRS.0000000000001552

[67] Graat HCA, Schimmel JJP, Hoogendoorn RJW, van

Hessem L, Hosman A, de Kleuver M. Poor radiological and good functional long-term outcome of surgically treated scheuermann patients. *Spine*. 2016;41(14):E869-E878. doi:10.1097/BRS.0000000000001402

Section 5

Pediatric Neurosurgery

Chapter 12

Pediatric Skull Base Tumors

Usman A. Khan, Jillian H. Plonsker, Robert C. Rennert and Michael L. Levy

Abstract

Management of pediatric skull base tumors requires a multi-disciplinary team that integrates advances in neuro-imaging, radiation, medical and surgical treatments, and allied therapies. Tumors of the skull base harbor complex genetic and molecular signatures that have major implications on prognosis and quality of life. Individualized management requires a strong inter-disciplinary alliance amongst practitioners, as well as a strong therapeutic alliance with the patient and family to navigate the complex decision-making process of treatments. In this chapter, we present our experience managing surgical lesions of the pediatric skull base. General considerations to tumor pathology genetics and radiobiology, diagnostic imaging, rehabilitation of cranial neuropathies and cognitive function, surgical anatomy and reconstructive options, and quality of life should be applied to each case. We also present location- and tumor-specific considerations in the anterior, middle, and posterior fossa skull base with a focus on surgical approaches and complication avoidance. Special consideration is given to syndromic tumors, particularly those from neurofibromatosis type 2 (NF-2). Tumors can exist in multiple cranial compartments and as such some redundancy in concepts is unavoidable. Nevertheless, each patient presents with a unique clinical picture and tumor behavior. Knowledge and proficiency in skull base approaches is a necessary tool in every pediatric neurosurgeon's armamentarium.

Keywords: pediatric brain tumors, skull base tumors, pediatric neuro-oncology, pediatric neurosurgery

1. Introduction

Contemporary management options for skull base tumors include observation, stereotactic radiosurgery or radiotherapy, primary or adjuvant chemotherapy, and microsurgical resection. Factors influencing treatment decisions include patient age and medical condition, cranial neuropathies, tumor size, tumor genetics, and provider bias. Advances in imaging and treatment technologies have led to improved detection of small skull base tumors, a better understanding of the natural history of tumor growth, and reductions in post-operative morbidity and mortality.

We strongly advocate for a team-based approach to treat skull base tumors. Our program is led by a neuro-oncology and neurosurgery team, and composed of neurophysiologists, head and neck surgeons, radiation oncologists, ophthalmologists, plastic and reconstructive surgeons, as well as occupational- physical- and speech- therapists. Microsurgical resection is carried out in cases not amenable to observation or radiation therapy. Where applicable, and when neurologic function is not deteriorating, biopsy and individualized medical treatment is pursued in favor of radical resection. For example, advances in epigenetics and tumor expression profiles sensitive to *BRAF-V600E* confer favorable treatment response to kinase inhibitors in papillary craniopharyngioma [1]. In such cases, resection as index treatment is carried out in cases of neurologic deterioration, failed medical therapy, or favorable tumor handling at the time of biopsy.

Cranial nerve function takes priority when deciding to proceed with surgery. This is true both for extra-medullary lesions and intra-medullary lesions with exophytic components threatening cranial nerve function. The goals of resection should be considered when tailoring the surgical approach. For lower grade tumors, which comprise the majority of lesions, gross total resection with preservation of cranial nerve function is the standard of care. When cranial nerve function is threatened by poor tumor handling or adherence to adjacent neural or vascular structures, subtotal resection should be considered. This is especially relevant to lower cranial nerve function, which protects the airway and is associated with mortality when injured. Vision, oculomotor function, facial, and vestibulocochlear nerve function should also be considered.

Tumors that affect multiple cranial nerves together deserve special attention. This includes tumors that could affect all three oculomotor nerves, the fifth and seventh nerve together leading to insensate corneal abrasions and vision loss, and the lower cranial nerves together resulting in airway failure and death. Patients with contralateral cranial nerve dysfunction, such as in neurofibromatosis type 2 (NF-2), should also be given special consideration. In the case of bilateral acoustic neuromas, when contralateral hearing is absent, every attempt should be made to preserve ipsilateral hearing before attempting surgical resection. Bevacizumab has shown variable effect on tumor size and hearing function in such cases.

2. Anterior skull base

2.1 Introduction

The sellar and parasellar skull base contain several critical neurovascular structures. These include cranial nerves II through VI, the internal carotid arteries, the cavernous sinus, and the pituitary gland. Tumors in this area are likely to involve the olfactory nerves and the visual system in its orbital and cisternal course [2, 3]. Good pre-operative cranial nerve function predicts favorable neurologic outcome and pre-operative evaluation of cranial nerve function is essential. Anosmia in particular can herald the presence of a tumor [4]. Similarly, loss of olfactory function can significantly affect a patient's quality of life and should be taken into consideration when planning surgery. Ophthalmologic evaluation of visual function, including acuity, fundoscopy, and visual field testing may be useful in surgical planning. Evaluation by a multi-disciplinary team of neurosurgeons, ophthalmologists, and otolaryngologists is recommended for all anterior skull base tumors. We routinely obtain hi-resolution magnetic resonance imaging (MRI) and computed tomography (CT) during pre-operative evaluation. Constructive interference steady state (CISS) is especially useful in determining the course of cranial nerves involved in the tumor and surgical corridor. Gadolinium enhanced T1 weighted, and T2 weighted images help evaluate the extent of tumor invasion along the cranial nerves (peri-neural spread) as well as the bony skull base. MR or CT angiography is obtained in cases of suspected vascular encasement to determine the safety of surgical access and if bypass should be planned before resection. Formal angiography is performed in cases where bypass is planned. A detailed endocrinologic history and serologic workup should be completed for tumors involving the sellar and parasellar structures.

2.2 Regional anatomy

The anatomy of the anterior and parasellar skull base is complex and develops throughout childhood [5, 6]. Pathology that affects the skull base directly is relatively rare in children. Pathology and surgical intervention can significantly affect development of the pediatric skull base and potentially confer substantial morbidity. For this reason, surgical intervention is reserved for cases where neurologic or endocrinologic function are threatened or compromised, and where no other options for tumor control are possible. This should be determined by a multidisciplinary team.

We favor the endoscopic endonasal approach (EEA) for most pathology involving the anterior and parasellar skull base. Transcranial and transfacial approaches, or a combination of approaches are used for pathologies that span beyond the access of a single approach. Variability in the development of the pediatric skull base has relevance to all stages of the endonasal approach, including the (a) nasal phase (b) sphenoid phase (c) sellar and intradural phase and (d) closure and reconstruction. The anterior skull base and midfacies develop later than the posterior skull base and continue growing until 14 years of age.

The nasal aperture grows throughout childhood and can restrict access of endonasal instrumentation. We prefer to operate through a nasal aperture larger than 5 mm, which can be performed as early as 2 years [5]. The piriform aperture, limited by the nasal bones and maxilla, can limit the rostral-caudal extent of dissection. As a general rule, the working angle and distance to the sella from the piriform aperture increases with age. Endonasal approaches, particularly expanded approaches, may be more feasible in younger patients for this reason. The choanal aperture, limited by the middle and inferior turbinates, also has relevance to expanded approaches. We do not perform expanded approaches to the clivus in cases where choanal atresia is present, or where the choanal aperture is smaller than 10 mm [7].

The sphenoid sinus has conchal anatomy until 2 years of age [8, 9]. Pneumatization of the sphenoid sinus begins in the inferior-medial sphenoid bone and moves superiorly and laterally, ultimately determining the location of the carotid arteries. The inter-carotid distance is mature at 9 years, though pneumatization may continue beyond this age and affect the degree of protrusion of the carotid arteries into the sphenoid sinus [9]. Sellar lesions are best approached in sphenoid sinuses with greater than 10 mm between the cavernous carotid arteries. Pneumatization of the ethmoid sinuses begins anteriorly and moves posteriorly, with the posteromedial ethmoids pneumatizing last [9]. The degree of ethmoid sinus pneumatization has relevance to its communication with the maxillary sinus and the working trajectories available to the anterior skull base.

Growth of the nasal septum, and the potential use of a nasoseptal flap for reconstruction, lags behind the development of other anterior skull base structures [10]. Large defects in the anterior skull base may not be adequately covered by a nasoseptal flap before 10 years of age, and may limit the utility of the endonasal approach. Traditional sellar and tuberculum/planum approaches can be covered as early as 6 years, when needed. We do not routinely reconstruct with nasoseptal flaps, reserving their use only for cases where a high flow cerebrospinal fluid (CSF) leak is expected. Traditional reconstruction with fat, fibrin, collagen, and expandable polyvinyl acetate is performed routinely.

2.3 Regional pathology

The most common tumors involving the anterior skull base and parasellar space in children include meningiomas, fibrous dysplasia, craniopharyngiomas, pituitary adenomas, juvenile nasopharyngeal angiofibromas (JNA), dermoid and epidermoid tumors, and gliomas.

Meningiomas can arise from the dura of the olfactory groove, planum/tuberculum sphenoidale or anterior clinoid process [11, 12]. Pediatric meningiomas are rarer in children than adults and typically associated with NF-2 or prior radiation treatment. Some studies suggest that meningiomas in children are more aggressive than meningiomas in adults, but these findings have yet to be validated in large studies.

Adamantinomatous craniopharyngiomas are the most common craniopharyngiomas found in children [13]. The diversity of their clinical presentation reflects their relationship to the surrounding pituitary, infundibulum, hypothalamus, and optic apparatus (**Figure 1**). A majority of craniopharyngiomas have a suprasellar component, and approximately one third extend into the anterior or middle cranial fossa [13]. Extension into the third ventricle can contribute to hydrocephalus, which can produce nonspecific symptoms such as headaches, nausea, and vomiting. Visual field or acuity defects are commonly present, as are symptoms of endocrine dysfunction, of which growth hormone (GH) appears to be the most commonly affected. Some may have large cystic components (**Figure 2**). Adenomas can present similarly, but typically have a more benign clinical course than craniopharyngiomas with respect to cranial neuropathy and hydrocephalus. The specific clinical presentation depends on the secreting subtype of tumor, with prolactinomas occurring most commonly.

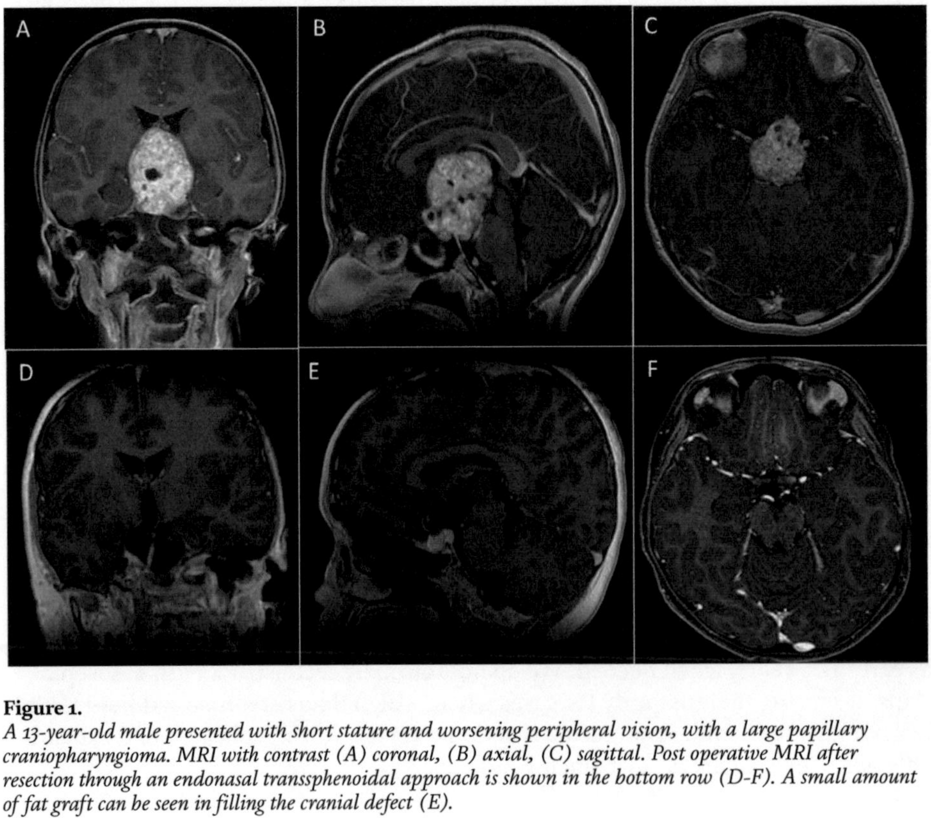

Figure 1.
A 13-year-old male presented with short stature and worsening peripheral vision, with a large papillary craniopharyngioma. MRI with contrast (A) coronal, (B) axial, (C) sagittal. Post operative MRI after resection through an endonasal transsphenoidal approach is shown in the bottom row (D-F). A small amount of fat graft can be seen in filling the cranial defect (E).

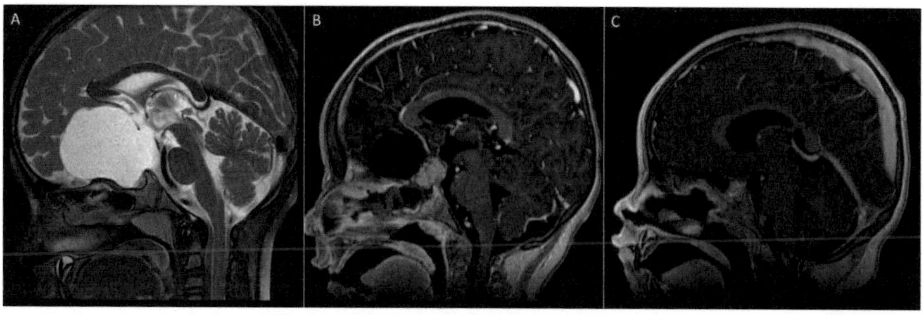

Figure 2.
This is a 4-year-old male who presented with vomiting and progressive vision loss with a suprasellar cystic papillary craniopharyngioma (A). An endoscopic trans-nasal, trans-cribriform approach was taken for resection. Fat graft is seen filling the craniotomy in the immediate post operative (B) and is partially resorbed with return of normal anatomic structure three months post-operatively (C).

JNAs classically occurs in adolescent boys and present with painless nasal obstruction and intermittent epistaxis [14]. They can originate in any part of the nasal cavity, but have a predilection for the posterolateral wall of the nasal cavity, adjacent to the sphenopalatine foramen. From here they can spread to the nasal cavity, nasopharynx, orbit, paranasal sinuses and intracranial compartment. The tumor often has a rich blood supply from the internal maxillary artery, which can serve as a target for pre-operative liquid particle embolization.

Dermoid and epidermoid cysts are indolent lesions that present with vague symptomatology related to intracranial hypertension and aseptic meningitis. Occasionally, they produce cranial nerve deficits, seizures, and behavioral changes. Dermoid cysts occur in the midline and epidermoid cysts occur in the parasellar spaces. Dermoid cysts are typically associated with a sinus tract, which are most commonly found at the glabella. Epidermoid cysts are classically associated with high intensity on diffusion-weighted images (DWI) [15].

Optic pathway gliomas (OPG) are prevalent in neurofibromatosis type 1 (NF1) and virtually all cases occur before 10 years of age. Sporadic OPGs have a more aggressive clinical course than NF1-associated OPGs, especially hypothalamic OPGs, which are less frequent in NF-1. Considered indolent, OPGs rarely progress after adolescence and optimal treatment remains controversial. When possible, visual function should be spared as long as possible before attempting resection [16].

2.4 Surgical approaches

The endonasal corridor can be used to access lesions in the anterior skull base via the classic trans-sellar/parasellar approach, the trans-tuberculum and trans-planum approach, and at its rostral extent the trans-cribriform approach. Each of these anatomic modules are delimited by critical neurovascular structures in the coronal plane.

All the endonasal approaches are performed with bi-nostril access and with a bimanual four-hand neurosurgery-otolaryngology team. Pre-operative evaluation of the paranasal sinuses with high resolution CT is essential, and care is taken to note deviated septum or bony spurs that may limit visualization or movement in the endonasal corridor. We do not routinely give peri-operative steroids, unless hypocortisolism is seen on preoperative workup. A microscope is always kept in the room and balanced with the observer scope on the left side of the primary surgeon.

A septal flap is raised before the sellar phase of the surgery only in cases where a high-flow CSF leak is expected. The posterior septum is resected before entering the sphenoid phase to facilitate visualization of the entire sella. The sella is expanded laterally to the lamina papyracea and anteriorly to the planum. Pneumatization of the sphenoid sinus aids in this phase of the exposure and identification of critical neurovascular structures surrounding the sella [17, 18]. Doppler ultrasonography can help identify the carotid artery where tumors may distort or encase vascular anatomy. The dura of the sella is then exposed between the cavernous sinuses. The medial optico-carotid recesses and tuberculum sphenoidale may also be resected for more lateral and rostral exposure, respectively, than is typically afforded by a trans-sellar approach.

Extension of this exposure rostrally can provide access to the posterior wall of the frontal sinus, between the medial orbital walls limited by the laminae papyracea. In this case, the nasal corridor described above is expanded with uncinetectomy, maxillary antrostomy, and ethmoidectomy. Care should be taken to avoid avulsing the ethmoidal arteries during ethmoidectomy, or coagulating the stumps of the ethmoidal arteries into the orbital wall, resulting in retrobulbar hematomas and orbital compartment syndrome. The lamina papyracea can be removed itself to provide access to the medial orbital wall [19].

2.5 Complication avoidance

Carotid artery injury is the most formidable complication of the EEA. Avoidance of carotid artery injury comes from meticulous planning, the use of stereotaxy, and adjunct tools including ultrasonography and fluorescence. Control of carotid artery injury can be achieved by an experienced two-surgeon team, and with coordination with anesthesiology and case support staff. We utilize a carotid artery injury "time out" to rehearse such a scenario in cases where the carotid artery may be encountered. This includes the possibility of endovascular sacrifice of the blood vessel, which is the safest immediate option in brisk bleeds. Endovascular sacrifice should only be attempted after hemorrhage is controlled.

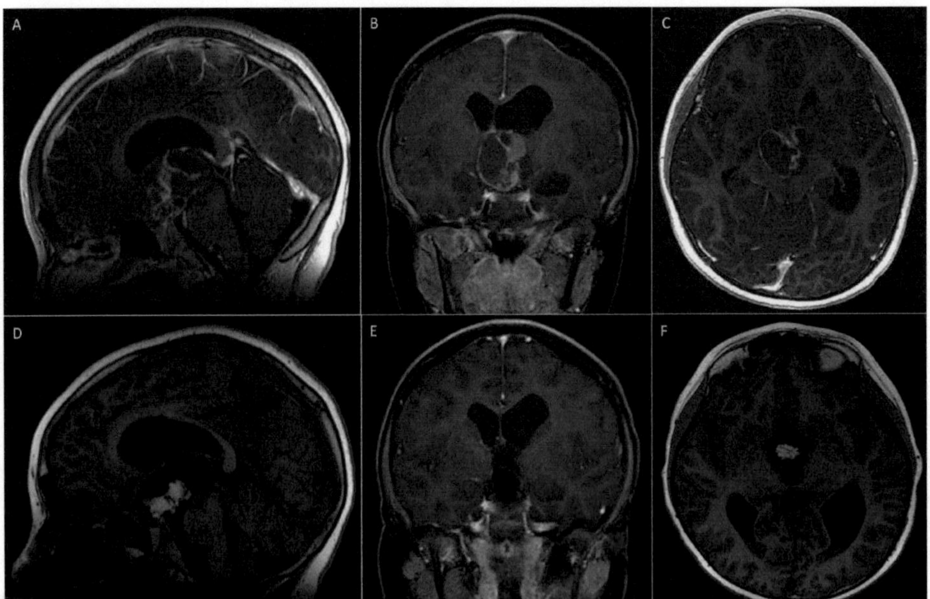

Figure 3.
A 7 year old male presented with vision changes and was diagnosed with craniopharyngioma on MRI with contrast (A) sagittal (B) coronal, (C) axial. This was resected by endonasal transsphenoidal approach. Post operative MRI (D-F) after gross total resection. A high flow CSF leak was identified intraoperatively, which was closed with a nasal septal flap and abdominal fat graft.

High flow venous bleeding should also be avoided, especially during exposure of the anterior intercavernous sinus. Bleeding from a robust intercavernous sinus can be brisk and is best avoided by isolating and dividing the sinus with cuts in the sellar and planum dura before moving forward in the exposure. Hemostatic agents and warm irrigation can aid in hemostasis from venous bleeding. Finally, while rare, carotid-cavernous fistula should be suspected in patients with mid-face or skull base trauma, and if present, treated before tumor resection is attempted.

CSF leaks are best avoided by respecting the arachnoid planes of dissection surrounding the tumor and sella. Entry into a subarachnoid cistern or ventricle can predict a CSF leak with confidence. We do not routinely use lumbar drainage for peri-operative care, unless such a leak is expected or encountered by misadventure. High flow CSF leaks can be addressed by raising a nasoseptal or turbinate flap for closure, though as described above, development of the septum and turbinates may lag behind development of the skull base and limit coverage of the flap (**Figure 3**).

Persistent leak can predispose a patient to developing tension pneumocephalus. Multi-layered closure can help prevent this rare complication, which is thought to arise from a ball-valve effect of air entry into the resection bed and intracranial compartment. CSF leaks can also confer a risk for meningitis and ventriculitis, and positive pressure ventilation (CPAP) is strictly avoided peri-operatively.

3. Middle fossa, infratemporal fossa, and petrous apex

3.1 Introduction

The middle fossa and petrous apex are at the center of the skull base and are surrounded by several critical structures. Tumors in this area grow from or envelope multiple cranial nerves, as well as deep venous and arterial structures with little collateral flow. The risks posed in the pre-pontine cistern are formidable, and surgical resection in this anatomically complex region should be performed by an experienced, multi-disciplinary skull base team. Most pathologies occurring in this area are benign, and gross total resection confers a benefit to the prognosis and quality of life of a child. Regardless of histology, maximum safe resection should be carried out. Outcomes are best in centers with experienced pediatric skull base, neuro-anesthesiology, critical care, and rehabilitation teams.

3.2 Regional anatomy

In our practice, resection of such tumors in the middle and infratemporal fossae, as well as the petrous apex is carried out by a combined neuro-otology and neurosurgery skull base team in all cases. A thorough understanding of the anatomy of the petrous temporal bone, anterior and posterior clinoid processes, and sphenoid bone is essential to safe removal of tumors in this area. Landmarks are neither constant nor readily apparent, and laboratory dissection is essential to familiarizing the surgeon with anatomy in this region.

The floor of the middle fossa is delimited by several key structures. Anteriorly, the middle meningeal artery can be identified as it enters foramen spinosum. An accessory meningeal artery is inconsistently seen in foramen ovale, anterior and medial to the middle meningeal artery [20]. A ridge of bone frequently obscures visualization of the foramen spinosum and can be drilled away for better exposure. The greater superficial petrosal nerve (GSPN) runs in a groove medial to the middle meningeal artery and enters the vidian canal under the mandibular nerve (V3). The GSPN is frequently dehiscent through the middle fossa floor in its course. The maxillary nerve (V2) enters the foramen rotundum superior and medial to foramen ovale. The area between V2 and V3 forms the lateral loop [21]. The sphenoid sinus and its invested vidian canal can be accessed through the lateral loop. The vidian canal is encountered laterally in patients with an over-developed sphenoid sinus, and medially when the sinus has conchal anatomy. The infratemporal fossa is accessed lateral to V3 at the floor of the middle fossa.

The arcuate eminence demarcates the location of the superior semicircular canal as well as the geniculate ganglion, which typically lies anterior to its lateral border [22]. The relationship of the arcuate eminence to both these landmarks is inconsistent, and drilling of the arcuate eminence is often necessary to clarify the anatomy of the middle fossa floor. Drilling to better visualize the anatomy of the middle fossa floor should be balanced against "blue-lining" the membranous labyrinth of the superior semi-circular canal, which may lead to inadvertent injury and hearing loss. Injury of the membranous labyrinth should be controlled with bone wax packing instead suction. The face of the superior semicircular canal invariably lies perpendicular to the two ridges of the petrous apex. These ridges cradle the superior petrosal sinus. Two important working windows are defined in this area. Kawase's rhomboid is bounded by the middle meningeal artery, mandibular nerve, GSPN, and petrous ridge. Glasscock's triangle (the posterolateral triangle of the cavernous sinus) is bounded V3, GSPN, and a line between the arcuate eminence and foramen spinosum. Drilling the bone in either of these spaces reveals the carotid artery, running deep to GSPN and medial to the eustachian tube. The cochlea has no external landmarks in this region, and its constant location medial to the genu of the carotid artery and the geniculate ganglion must be kept in mind during exposure of the internal auditory canal (IAC).

3.3 Regional pathology

Tumors affecting the skull base of the middle fossa include chordomas, meningiomas, and schwannoma.

Chordomas arise from the clivus and extend into the middle crania fossa in approximately one third of cases. They tend to grow locally but aggressively. Radical resection can be curative, but recurrence rates are high when subtotal resection is achieved, even with adjuvant proton beam therapy.

Meningiomas of the middle fossa are typically slow growing and most commonly present with headaches and visual disturbances. Tumors that invade the adjacent cavernous sinus may cause additional cranial neuropathies that affect extra-ocular movement. Meningiomas of the middle fossa typically arise from the medial sphenoid wing or the petrous ridge, and grow to span multiple cranial compartments (**Figure 4**).

Schwannomas in children are rare. Bilateral vestibular schwannomas are a hallmark of NF-2. Intracanalicular vestibular schwannomas can be resected via the middle cranial fossa approach, whereas larger lesions are typically resected via trans or retro-mastoid approaches. Observation is recommended for small or incidentally discovered trigeminal schwannomas. Small tumors show excellent control with radiosurgery in adults, but data is limited in children, and even stereotactic radiation in children may be linked to meningioma development later in life. For this reason, surgery is favored in our practice for schwannomas that show growth on surveillance imaging alongside cranial neuropathy or brainstem compression. Trigeminal schwannomas typically present with facial numbness. Trigeminal neuralgia tends to occur in lesions at and beyond the Gasserian ganglion, and involves all three divisions of the trigeminal nerve.

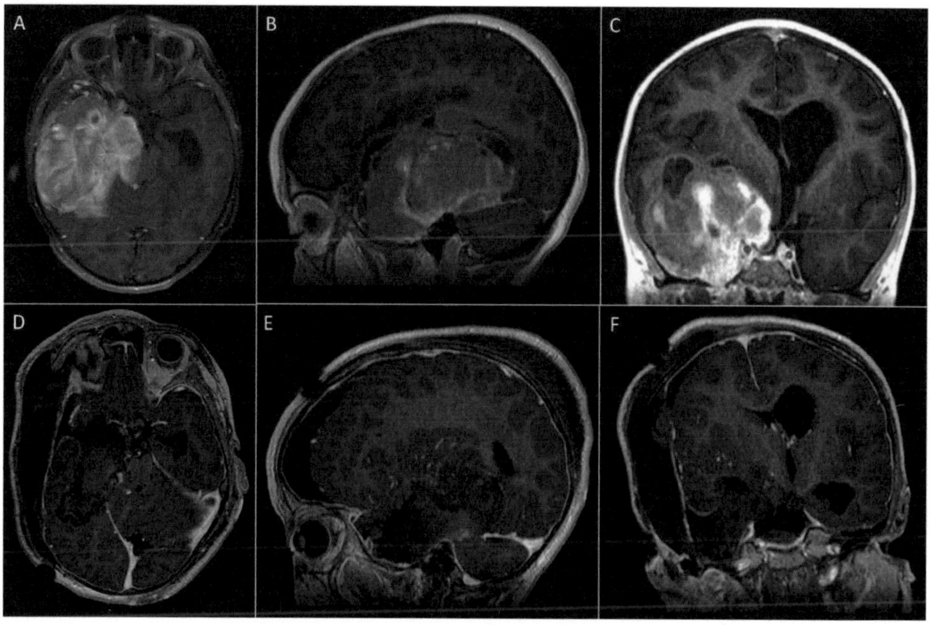

Figure 4.
A 4-year-old male presented with one month of nausea and headaches with a large cystic meningioma filling the temporal fossa and extending across the tentorium (A-C). Tumor was resected through a modified orbitozygomaticapproach. Immediate post-operative MRI (DF) with gross total resection and normal swelling.

3.4 Surgical approaches

We perform all middle cranial fossa, petrous ridge, and infratemporal fossa cases with a neurosurgery-neuro-otology skull base team. The middle fossa approach incision is a reverse question mark based at the root of the zygoma and extending to the superior temporal line. The muscle is elevated separately from the skin anteriorly and inferiorly. We use cutting and diamond burrs to drill a 5x5cm square craniotomy based 2/3rd anterior to the root of the zygoma, and 1/3rd posterior. Two points should be stressed in this exposure. First, the craniotomy should extend low, to the floor of the middle fossa, which is approximated by the root of the zygoma. Second, every attempt should be made to adequately expose the anterior petrous ridge to aid in deeper parts of the dissection. Failure to adequately expose the anterior floor of the middle fossa and petrous ridge places the neural structures (GSPN, IAC) in the exposure at risk.

The dura is elevated anteriorly until the middle meningeal artery (MMA) is identified. It is coagulated closer to the dural base than to the skull base, to prevent retraction and hemorrhage into the infratemporal fossa. Once the MMA is identified, elevation of the middle fossa dura proceeds in a posterior to anterior course, to avoid avulsion and injury to GSPN, which carries parasympathetic innervation to the lacrimal gland. Every attempt is made to avoid dividing the GSPN, as concomitant GSPN and V1 injury can lead to devastating insensate corneal abrasions and blindness. Elevation of the dura allows for identification of the arcuate eminence. This is followed medially to the petrous ridge, where the groove of the superior petrosal sinus is identified and divided. A shallow depression in the petrous ridge just above the porus acusticus can be used as a landmark for drilling.

The bone overlying the superior semicircular canal is drilled down and a House-Urban retractor is placed against the true petrous ridge. Care should be taken to avoid lacerating the dura during elevation and retraction, as seizure may occur.

Injury to the dominant temporal lobe can also result in aphasia, and is more likely when the vein of Labbe drains from an anterior position. Drilling begins at the pre-meatal petrous ridge, just anterior and medial to the IAC. Once saucerized, drilling of the post-meatal petrous ridge is done to expose a 270-degree arc of the IAC tunnel. All drilling is done with suction-irrigation to avoid thermal injury to the facial and cochlear nerves. Drilling laterally exposes the labyrinthine segment of the facial nerve, Bills bar, and the superior vestibular nerve. There is very low tolerance for a drilling misadventure in this area, as the labyrinthine segment of the facial nerve lies within 1 mm of the basal turn of the cochlea. The dura is opened along the length of the IAC, and on its posterior edge, to avoid injury to the expected location of the facial nerve anteriorly. Resection of inferior vestibular nerve tumors, the most common intracranial schwannoma, requires division of the superior vestibular nerve [23].

Access to the pre-pontine cistern, as well as the premeatal posterior cranial fossa can be accomplished through an extended middle fossa approach (eMFC). Drilling of the premeatal triangle in eMFC is generous, extending anteriorly to just under the Gasserian ganglion and V3, and laterally to the horizontal segment of the petrous internal carotid artery (C2) (**Figure 5**) [24].

Meckel's Cave, the lateral petrous apex, as well as the pterygopalatine and infratemporal fossae can be accessed through the endonasal corridor via a trans-maxillary, trans-pterygoid approach [25]. Bi-nostril access is required, with working access achieved through the contralateral nostril. This should be accounted for by the operative team and referral to experienced skull base teams is recommended for this approach. The posterior maxillary wall provides access to the pterygopalatine fossa. The pterygopalatine fossa is exposed in its entire anterior–posterior extent, taking care to protect the sphenopalatine ganglion, vidian nerve, palatine and orbital

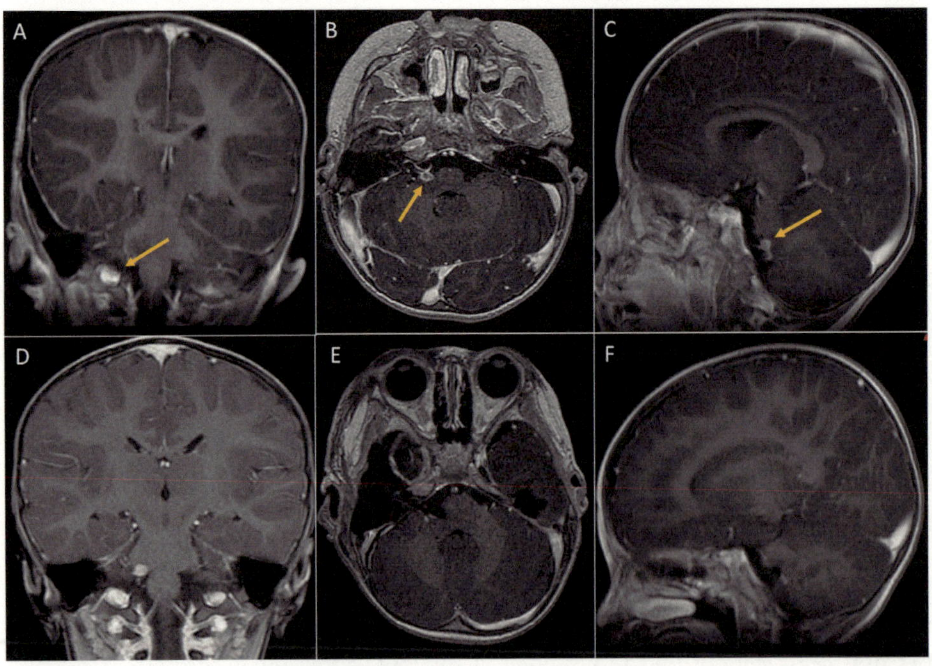

Figure 5.
A 21 month old female presented with right facial weakness since 5 months of age. A small meningioma in the right cerebellopontine angle was found(upper row A-C). This tumor was observed at first, but her weakness progressed and the lesion had grown. A middle fossa anterior petrosectomy was performed. Post-operative images are seen on the bottom row (D-F). Pathology demonstrated meningioma.

nerves. The inferior orbital nerve serves as a landmark for the perpendicular plate of the palatine bone [26]. Resection of the orbital process of the palatine bone exposes V2, near the sphenopalatine foramen. Dissection of the sphenoid process of the palatine bone exposes the vidian nerve at the pterygoid canal and the maxillary nerve at the foramen rotundum. It also exposes the base of the pterygoid process, which when resected allows for access to Meckel's cave through the quadrangular space bounded by V2, V3, cranial nerve VI, the and the transition of the petrous internal carotid artery to its laceral segment, in close proximity to the petrolingual ligament [27].

3.5 Complication avoidance

Cerebrospinal fluid leak is one of the most common complications of surgery to the middle fossa and petrous apex. CSF leak typically manifests two ways, as rhinorrhea or leakage from the surgical wound. Otorrhea is not commonly encountered through the middle fossa or trans-pterygoid approaches. We routinely obliterate communication between pneumatized air cells in the temporal bone with fat, to prevent leakage of CSF through the skin incision or the eustachian tube. Before doing so, the exposed air cells or dehiscence in the middle fossa floor are covered with wax or fascia. Incisional leaks are managed with wound oversewing and lumbar drainage. Rhinorrhea is managed with lumbar drainage. If either method fails to control the leak, wound exploration is performed.

Stroke can be a result of arterial or venous injury. We perform pre-operative CT or MR angiography on all patients with tumors adjacent to the arteries or veins of the skull base. If there is evidence of invasion or stenosis of the blood vessels of the skull base, formal cerebral angiography is performed. This helps evaluate the degree of collateral inflow and outflow from the resection site. A balloon occlusion test may help establish the feasibility of vessel sacrifice at the time of surgery. Whenever possible, sacrifice is avoided for benign lesions should be avoided.

4. Tumors of the cerebellopontine angle, jugular foramen, and craniovertebral junction

4.1 Introduction

The majority of pediatric brain tumors are located in the posterior fossa, with the most common pathologies being juvenile pilocytic astrocytomas, medulloblastomas, and ependymomas, all of which may require complex approaches when expansive. In this chapter, however, we will discuss primarily extra-axial tumors that specifically involve the skull base. Far lateral or ELITE (extreme lateral infrajugular transcondylar-transtubercular) for ventrolateral pathology, transpetrous approaches for access to the cerebellopontine angle, and anterior approaches can all be used in appropriate situations to maximize exposure to facilitate safe resection and preservation of critical neural structures. As above, we work closely with our otolaryngology partners to assist with transpetrous approaches when indicated and for endoscopic anterior approaches to the clivus and ventral brainstem.

4.2 Regional anatomy

A comprehensive knowledge of the relevant bony and vascular anatomy is required prior to performing approaches to the posterior fossa. The vertebral artery takes a lateral to medial course after exiting from the transverse foramen of C1 and travels in a groove along the superior edge of the posterior arch of C1 prior to entering the dura. The artery at this level is sheathed in an organized venous plexus which can bleed briskly but is easily stopped with hemostatic agents. If necessary, the vertebral artery can be mobilized by removing the posterior wall of the transverse foramen which further exposes the occipital condyle. Intradurally, the transverse and sigmoid venous sinuses frame the borders of the posterior fossa. Children less than two years old are more likely to have a persistent occipital sinus, and children with an occipital sinus are more likely to have an absent transverse sinus [28].

The occipital condyles form the connection of C1 to the foramen magnum laterally. The hypoglossal canal runs anterolaterally through the condyle and marks the border of the posterior and middle third of the condyle. Radiographic review of 50 pediatric CT scans demonstrated relative stability in the size and depth of the occipital condyle and hypoglossal canal throughout pediatric development. The jugular tubercle is located superiorly and anteriorly to the hypoglossal canal. Conversely, the jugular tubercle demonstrates significant growth during childhood and only measures 65% of adult size prior to puberty, therefore its removal may not confer as much benefit for lateral skull base approaches in younger children [29].

Laterally, the skull base is defined by the petrous pyramid located between the sphenoid and occipital bones, and houses the facial canal, the petrous carotid artery, and the osseous structures of the inner ear. The superior surface of the petrous bone forms the floor of the middle fossa, and the posterior wall of bone forms the anterior wall of the posterior cranial fossa. The internal auditory meatus houses the meatal segment of the facial nerve and the vestibulocochlear nerve as they exit the cerebellopontine angle and enter the middle of the petrous bone. The cochlea is located just anterior to the fundus and the otic capsule housing the bony labyrinth is located posterior to the internal auditory canal and above the jugular foramen, and can be easily delineated from the surrounding mastoid bone by its yellowish, hard cortical surface.

4.3 Regional pathology

The most common tumors of the cerebellopontine angle in pediatric patients are schwannomas (65%), meningiomas (5%), and epidermoid cysts (5%). Up to 10% of tumors of the cerebellopontine angle in pediatric patients may be malignant, which is significantly greater than in adults (**Figure 6**) [30]. Schwannomas are

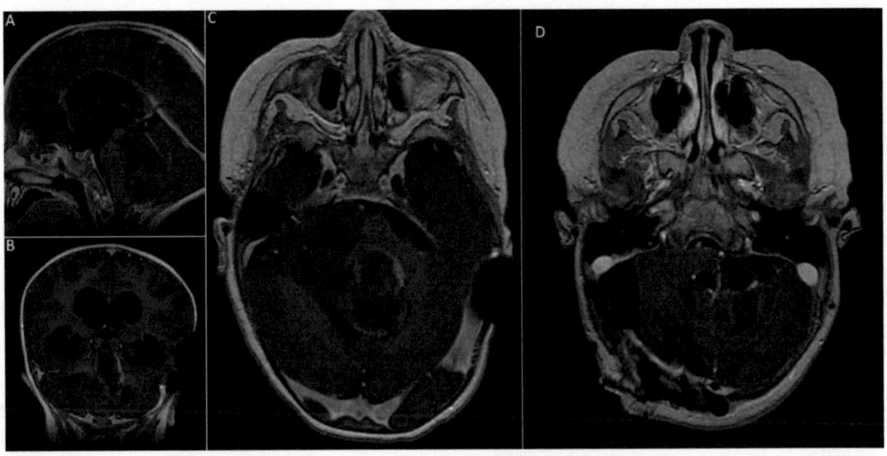

Figure 6.
A 21 month old male developed upgazepalsy and gross motor regression. MRI brain with contrast demonstrated large fourth ventricular ependymoma extending into the cerebellopontine angle (A-C). Gross total resection was achieved with a far lateral craniotomy (D).

rare tumors and rarer still in pediatric patients, with about 10% of cases diagnosed in patients younger than 21. These are considered benign masses that arise from Schwann cells of the nerve sheath and may be found anywhere in the body, with 16–45% reported to be in the head and neck [31]. The vestibular nerve is thought to be the most common location for intracranial schwannomas, though they can also occur on the trigeminal nerve, facial nerve, and lower cranial nerves in decreasing frequency.

Vestibular schwannomas present with unilateral hearing loss, tinnitus, headache, and disequilibrium, and they can cause cerebellar ataxia and brainstem compression with significant extension into the cerebellopontine angle [32]. Pediatric vestibular schwannomas tend to be diagnosed in adolescence and the tumors tend to be larger at presentation than in adults [32, 33]. Surgical resection, stereotactic radiosurgery, and observation are all valid treatment options for schwannomas, however the long life-span of pediatric patients argues for more aggressive definitive management. In one series of 148 pediatric vestibular schwannomas 82 (55.4%) patients were treated with surgery only, 45 (30.4%) with observation, 6 (4.1%) with radiation only, and 12 (8.1%) with surgery and radiation [33]. Residual tumors after surgery may grow at a faster rate than in adults, therefore the surgeon should safely attempt gross total resection or should consider radiosurgery in cases with significant residual tumor [32].

Sporadic schwannomas are rare in children, but they are the hallmark of genetic conditions, neurofibromatosis 2 (NF2) and schwannomatosis, with bilateral vestibular schwannomas affecting 95% of individuals with NF2 [34]. Overall treatment goals change in these patients due to the high lifetime number of tumors. Efforts should be made to avoid surgery unless necessary to preserve vital cranial nerve function and radiation should be avoided. Recent clinical trials have demonstrated hearing and quality of life improvement in both adult and pediatric NF2 patients with bevacizumab therapy. Pediatric patients did not demonstrate tumor regression unlike their adult counterparts in this trial [35].

Epidermoid cysts are rare dysontogenic lesions with a predilection for the cerebellopontine angle in 40–60% of cases and are the third most common lesion in the cerebellopontine angle. They tend to grow along arachnoid planes and frequently extend into neighboring compartments. These tumors tend to encase neurovascular structures and are quite adhesive. There is a characteristic appearance on MRI of a lesion filling and expanding the subarachnoid space that is dark on T1, bright on T2 and is avidly diffusion restricting. Patients present with cranial nerve impairments, most commonly of the trigeminal and the vestibulocochlear nerve.

Trigeminal neuralgia may be more common than sensory impairment when the trigeminal nerve is involved. Depending on the size of the tumor, almost all cranial nerve impairments have been described. Complete surgical excision can be curative; however, the surgeon must take great care to reduce morbidity and injury to cranial nerves. Complex or combined approaches may be necessary for tumors that span multiple compartments. Aseptic meningitis may occur post operatively and can be treated with a course of dexamethasone [36, 37].

At the craniocervical junction, chordomas are rare bony tumors that arise from notochordal remnants. These tumors are slow growing but locally aggressive. Only 5% of chordomas present in children, and they tend to be more aggressive in younger children. The most common location overall is the sacrum, with a minority of tumors occurring at the skull base. However, the more frequent location in pediatric patients is midline at the spheno-occipital synchondrosis of the clivus. Tumors present with headaches, other signs of increased intracranial pressure, diplopia, or mixed cranial neuropathies. Optimal treatment includes maximal safe resection followed by high dose radiotherapy, though there is still controversy regarding the type and dose of radiation. Proton beam may have benefits in pediatric patients over conventional radiotherapy due to a reduced radiation dose to neighboring structures. There is little role for chemotherapy due to the slow-growing nature of the disease [38, 39]. The future of chordoma treatment will likely be in molecular and targeted therapies and there are active clinical trials investigating a drug targeting programmed cell death ligand 1 (PD-L1), an immune checkpoint inhibitor expressed in over 90% of chordomas [40].

Chondrosarcomas are often grouped together with chordomas as they are both locally destructive, slow growing bony lesions, but they are a distinct histopathologic entity and have a better prognosis than chordomas. Chondrosarcomas are typically found in paramedian locations, arise from chondrocytes, and comprise 5–12% of cases found at the skull base. The most common location is the clivus followed by the temporal-occipital junction. There are four histologic subtypes: conventional, mesenchymal, clear cell, and dedifferentiated, and tumors are graded I-III based on the level of differentiation. The mesenchymal subtype tends to be the most aggressive. Radical surgical resection is again the mainstay of treatment with adjuvant radiation therapy, specifically proton beam, for most patients due to high rates of residual tumors and locoregional recurrence. Radiation has been shown to significantly decrease recurrence rates [41–43].

4.4 Surgical approaches

Pediatric tumors have a predilection for the posterior cranial fossa, specifically the cerebellar hemispheres and the fourth ventricle. A majority of these common intrinsic brain tumors such as medulloblastomas, juvenile pilocytic astrocytomas, and ependymomas do not require complex skull base approaches and can be accessed by a suboccipital craniotomy with or without a C1 laminectomy. However, many extrinsic tumors or large exophytic intrinsic tumors that extend to the cerebellopontine angle, the craniocervical junction, and the jugular foramen require knowledge of skull base approaches to maximize exposure.

The workhorse of posterior fossa approaches is the suboccipital craniotomy for dorsal midline lesions. The suboccipital craniotomy is performed by creating a dorsal midline window from the foramen magnum to the confluence of sinuses. There are many methods to perform this craniotomy including drilling bur holes, using a craniotome, a cutting and diamond bur, and Kerrison rongeurs. In children, we find it is safe and efficient to perform using a craniotome by stripping the dura from the foramen magnum and inserting the footplate under the lip of foramen magnum. This can be augmented by a C1 laminectomy for a more inferior to superior view. In rare cases, we have extended our craniotomy superior to the transverse sinus to perform a concurrent interhemispheric transtentorial approach to posterior fossa tumors.

For more inferior and lateral exposure than a standard suboccipital approach, the far-lateral, or extreme lateral transcondylar (ELITE), craniotomy may be required. This provides additional access to lower clival lesions, the craniocervical junction, and lesions of the upper cervical spine (**Figure 7**). In addition to a lateral suboccipital craniotomy, the ipsilateral occipital condyle is drilled extradurally until the hypoglossal canal is skeletonized. The hypoglossal canal generally is a marker that the posterior third of the condyle has been removed, which should not result in craniocervical instability. The lateral mass of C1 is also removed and the vertebral artery is sometimes mobilized. Though rarely necessary, the jugular tubercle can be drilled at this point to provide greater access to the lower cranial nerves and clivus.

The cerebellopontine angle (CP angle) is almost exclusively accessed by lateral skull base approaches, namely retrosigmoid and transpetrosal craniotomies. The

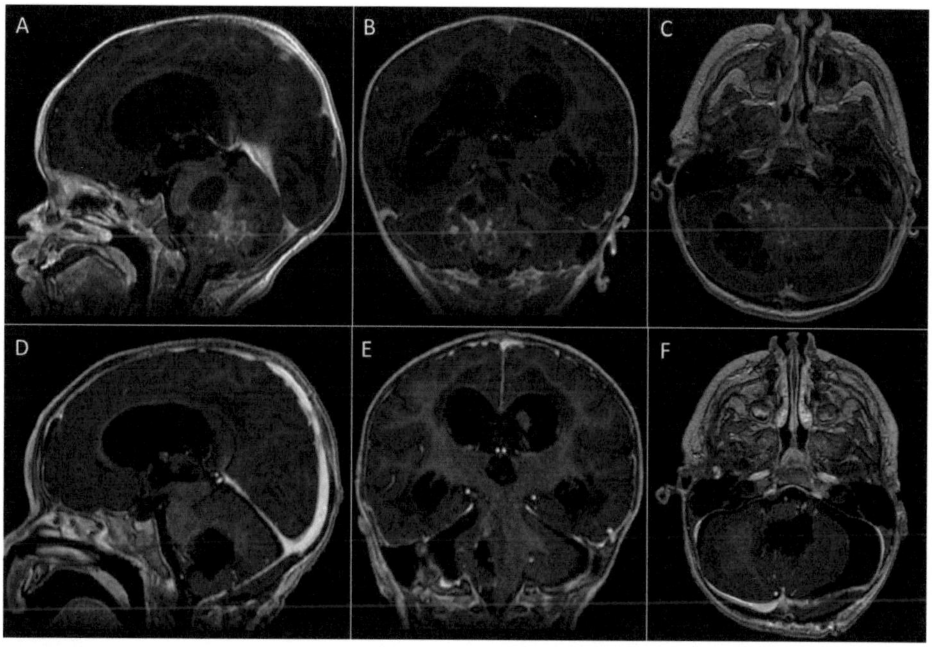

Figure 7.
A 13-month-old male presented to the emergency department with failure to thrive and eye movement abnormalities. A large atypical teratoid rhabdoid tumor (ATRT) was diagnosed with MRI brain (A-C). Tumor was resected using a suboccipital craniotomy with a modified far lateral approach to reach the tumor extending to the anteromedial brainstem.

retrosigmoid craniotomy is a standard neurosurgical approach. It is performed by creating a bony window just inferior and posterior to the transverse sigmoid junction. This can be performed with craniotome, bur holes and Kerrison rongeurs, or a cutting and diamond bur. Additional intradural drilling to open the internal auditory canal can be performed for vestibular schwannomas that extend from the auditory canal into the CP angle. The retrosigmoid craniotomy has immense flexibility, however it does rely on cerebellar retraction and therefore puts neural elements at some risk.

Transpetrosal approaches involve varying degrees of removal of the petrous temporal bone in order to expose the anterolateral brainstem from the tegmen to the jugular tubercle. With greater bony removal, there is increasing exposure of lesions of the anterior brainstem. However, the more extensive the petrosectomy, the greater the risk to cranial nerves, so the preoperative cranial nerve function and the goals of surgery are critically important when choosing an approach. Presigmoid retrolabyrinthine craniotomy preserves hearing and facial function. Translabyrinthine craniectomy sacrifices hearing but preserves the facial nerve well.

Transcochlear approaches sacrifice hearing by removing the labyrinth and closing the ear canal and puts the facial nerve at risk by mobilizing it from its canal. It is recommended that all these approaches are performed with a neurotology partner, as the mastoid is not well pneumatized in children and it can be difficult to identify the labyrinthine and facial recess. Any of these approaches can be combined with middle fossa approaches for combined exposure of lesions that span multiple compartments.

Transnasal, transmaxillary and transoral approaches provide access from the sella to odontoid process and upper cervical spine. These are generally reserved for midline extradural lesions such as chordomas and chondrosarcomas. The morbidity of these approaches is significantly decreased since the advent of endoscopic surgery.

4.5 Complication avoidance

As with other approaches to the skull base, cerebrospinal fluid leak is a common complication of posterior fossa surgery, especially because patients frequently have concomitant hydrocephalus. This is best avoided by multilayer water-tight closure and aggressive treatment of hydrocephalus either with an endoscopic third ventriculostomy, or temporary/permanent CSF diversion. Otorrhea or rhinorrhea after transpetrosal craniotomy can be treated again with CSF diversion, careful attention intraoperatively to packing of the middle ear, and external ear canal closure in persistent cases.

Sinus injury and sinus thrombosis are additional risks given their exposure in majority of posterior fossa approaches. It is advisable to use neuronavigation whenever possible to identify the location of the sinuses prior to performing the craniotomy and to study preoperative imaging to identify any aberrant anatomy such as persistent occipital sinuses or low-lying torcula, both of which may be present in children.

5. Conclusion

Brain tumors are the most common cancer in the pediatric population and often present late as presenting symptoms can be vague and children may not be able to communicate well. As targeted medical therapies develop the role for radical resections may decline, however when performed safely with appropriate execution of skull base approaches, surgical resection can provide excellent outcomes.

Author details

Usman A. Khan[1], Jillian H. Plonsker[1], Robert C. Rennert[1] and Michael L. Levy[1,2*]

1 Department of Neurological Surgery, University of California San Diego Health, La Jolla, CA, United States

2 Pediatric Neurosurgery Division, Rady Children's Hospital, San Diego, CA, United States

*Address all correspondence to: mlevy@rchsd.org

References

[1] Brastianos PK, Shankar GM, Gill CM, Taylor-Weiner A, Nayyar N, Panka DJ, et al. Dramatic Response of BRAF V600E Mutant Papillary Craniopharyngioma to Targeted Therapy. JNCI: Journal of the National Cancer Institute. 2015;108(2).

[2] J. W, Bidari S, Inoue K, Yang H, Rhoton. Extensions of the sphenoid sinus: a new classification. Neurosurgery. 2010;66(4).

[3] Ginsberg LE. Neoplastic diseases affecting the central skull base: CT and MR imaging. http://dxdoiorg/102214/ajr15931503031. 2013.

[4] Jm, A. EP, Lima C, da S. The human olfactory mucosa. European archives of oto-rhino-laryngology : official journal of the European Federation of Oto-Rhino-Laryngological Societies (EUFOS) : affiliated with the German Society for Oto-Rhino-Laryngology - Head and Neck Surgery. 2009;266(11).

[5] M. W, Takeno S, Hawke. The early development of sino-nasal mucosa. The Laryngoscope. 1994;104(7).

[6] Sinonasal Development and Anatomy | K.J. Leeâs Essential Otolaryngology: Head and Neck Surgery, 12e | AccessSurgery | McGraw-Hill Medical 2020 Available from: https://accesssurgery.mhmedical.com/content.aspx?bookid=2666&sectionid=219825879.

[7] G. W, Anderhuber W, Kuhn. Development of the paranasal sinuses in children: implications for paranasal sinus surgery. The Annals of otology, rhinology, and laryngology. 1993;102(9).

[8] Ee, K. SR, Dhingra JK, Carter BL, Rebeiz. Paranasal sinus development: a radiographic study. The Laryngoscope. 2003;113(2).

[9] Vidić. The postnatal development of the sphenoidal sinus and its spread into the dorsum sellae and posterior clinoid processes. The American journal of roentgenology, radium therapy, and nuclear medicine. 1968;104(1).

[10] Hl, D. VC, Verwoerd V. Rhinosurgery in children: developmental and surgical aspects of the growing nose. GMS current topics in otorhinolaryngology, head and neck surgery. 2010;9.

[11] DeMonte. Surgical treatment of anterior basal meningiomas. Journal of neuro-oncology. 1996;29(3).

[12] Pm, J. DK, Zhu JJ, Black. Meningiomas: updating basic science, management, and outcome. The neurologist. 2004;10(3).

[13] Jh, E. ER, Jane JA, Wisoff. Surgical management of craniopharyngiomas in children: meta-analysis and comparison of transcranial and transsphenoidal approaches. Neurosurgery. 2011;69(3).

[14] H. SC, Pant H, Carrau RL, Gardner. A new endoscopic staging system for angiofibromas. Archives of otolaryngology--head & neck surgery. 2010;136(6).

[15] Jt, I. A, Auguste KI, Vachhrajani S, Dirks PB, Drake JM, et al. Neurosurgical management of intracranial epidermoid tumors in children. Clinical article. Journal of neurosurgery Pediatrics. 2009;4(2).

[16] Ml, J. BM, Liu JK, Kestle JR, Brockmeyer DL, Walker. Optic pathway gliomas: a review. Neurosurgical focus. 2007;23(5).

[17] J. N, Schupper AJ, Deconde A, Levy. Pediatric Endoscopic Endonasal Approaches for Skull Base Lesions in the Very Young: Is It Safe and Effective?

Journal of neurological surgery Part B, Skull base. 2018;79(6).

[18] Dj, S. GC, Perry A, Link MJ, Daniels. Pediatric Craniopharyngiomas: A Primer for the Skull Base Surgeon. Journal of neurological surgery Part B, Skull base. 2018;79(1).

[19] Sk, H. KY, Wang KC, Phi JH, Kim. Endoscopic Endonasal Approach for Suprasellar Lesions in Children: Complications and Prevention. Journal of Korean Neurosurgical Society. 2017;60(3).

[20] Surgical exposure of the internal auditory canal and its contents through the middle, cranial fossa - House - 1961 - The Laryngoscope - Wiley Online Library. 2020.

[21] Krisht A, Kadri P. Microsurgical Anatomy of the Cavernous Sinus. Techniques in Neurosurgery. 2003;8:199-203.

[22] Kl, F. HW, Hitselberger WE, Horn. The middle fossa transpetrous approach to the anterior-superior cerebellopontine angle. The American journal of otology. 1986;7(1).

[23] Friedman RA, Brackmann DE. The middle cranial fossa approach to vestibular schwannomas. Operative Techniques in Neurosurgery. 2001;4(1):30-35.

[24] Sweeney AD, Carlson ML, Ehtesham M, Thompson RC, Haynes DS. Surgical Approaches for Vestibular Schwannoma. Current Otorhinolaryngology Reports. 2014;2(4):256-264.

[25] Truong HQ, Sun X, Celtikci E, Borghei-Ravazi H, Wang EW, Snyderman CH, et al. Endoscopic Transmaxillary Trans-Alisphenoid Approach to the Meckel's Cave: An Anatomical Study. J Neurol Surg B Skull Base. 2017;78(S 01):P003.

[26] We, Bolger. Endoscopic transpterygoid approach to the lateral sphenoid recess: surgical approach and clinical experience. Otolaryngology--head and neck surgery : official journal of American Academy of Otolaryngology-Head and Neck Surgery. 2005;133(1).

[27] Kassam AB, Gardner P, Snyderman C, Mintz A, Carrau R. Expanded endonasal approach: fully endoscopic, completely transnasal approach to the middle third of the clivus, petrous bone, middle cranial fossa, and infratemporal fossa. Neurosurg Focus. 2005;19(1):E6.

[28] Widjaja E, Griffiths PD. Intracranial MR Venography in Children: Normal Anatomy and Variations. American Journal of Neuroradiology. 2004;25(9):1557.

[29] Rennert RC, Hoshide R, Brandel MG, Steinberg JA, Martin JR, Meltzer HS, et al. Surgical relevance of pediatric skull base maturation for the far-lateral and extreme-lateral infrajugular transcondylar–transtubercular exposure approaches. Journal of Neurosurgery: Pediatrics PED. 2019;24(1):85.

[30] Holman MA, Schmitt WR, Carlson ML, Driscoll CL, Beatty CW, Link MJ. Pediatric cerebellopontine angle and internal auditory canal tumors: clinical article. J Neurosurg Pediatr. 2013;12(4):317-324.

[31] Hawkins DB, Luxford WM. Schwannomas of the head and neck in children. Laryngoscope. 1980;90(12):1921-1926.

[32] Malina GEK, Heiferman DM, Riedy LN, Szujewski CC, Rezaii EG, Leonetti JP, et al. Pediatric vestibular schwannomas: case series and a systematic review with meta-analysis. J Neurosurg Pediatr. 2020:1-9.

[33] Janz TA, Camilon PR, Cheung AY, Nguyen SA, Meyer TA, McRackan TR, et al. Characteristics and Outcomes of Pediatric Vestibular Schwannomas. Otol Neurotol. 2019;40(8):1047-1053.

[34] Ardern-Holmes S, Fisher G, North K. Neurofibromatosis Type 2. J Child Neurol. 2017;32(1):9-22.

[35] Plotkin SR, Duda DG, Muzikansky A, Allen J, Blakeley J, Rosser T, et al. Multicenter, Prospective, Phase II and Biomarker Study of High-Dose Bevacizumab as Induction Therapy in Patients With Neurofibromatosis Type 2 and Progressive Vestibular Schwannoma. J Clin Oncol. 2019;37(35): 3446-3454.

[36] Caldarelli M, Massimi L, Kondageski C, Rocco CD. Intracranial midline dermoid and epidermoid cysts in children. Journal of Neurosurgery: Pediatrics. 2004;100(5):473.

[37] Safavi-Abbasi S, Di Rocco F, Bambakidis N, Talley MC, Gharabaghi A, Luedemann W, et al. Has management of epidermoid tumors of the cerebellopontine angle improved? A surgical synopsis of the past and present. Skull Base. 2008;18(2):85-98.

[38] Beccaria K, Sainte-Rose C, Zerah M, Puget S. Paediatric Chordomas. Orphanet J Rare Dis. 2015;10:116-.

[39] al-Mefty O, Borba LA. Skull base chordomas: a management challenge. J Neurosurg. 1997;86(2):182-189.

[40] Connors SW, Aoun SG, Shi C, Peinado-Reyes V, Hall K, Bagley CA. Recent advances in understanding and managing chordomas: an update. F1000Res. 2020;9.

[41] Bloch OG, Jian BJ, Yang I, Han SJ, Aranda D, Ahn BJ, et al. Cranial chondrosarcoma and recurrence. Skull Base. 2010;20(3):149-156.

[42] Weber DC, Badiyan S, Malyapa R, Albertini F, Bolsi A, Lomax AJ, et al. Long-term outcomes and prognostic factors of skull-base chondrosarcoma patients treated with pencil-beam scanning proton therapy at the Paul Scherrer Institute. Neuro Oncol. 2016;18(2):236-243.

[43] Kremenevski N, Schlaffer SM, Coras R, Kinfe TM, Graillon T, Buchfelder M. Skull Base Chordomas and Chondrosarcomas. Neuroendocrinology. 2020;110(9-10):836-847.

Chapter 13

Will CSF Diversion in Patients with Idiopathic Intracranial Hypertension (IIH) Lead to Long-Lasting Shunt Dependency?

Tryggve Lundar and Bernt Johan Due-Tønnessen

Abstract

Long-term shunt dependency rates in patients treated for IIH with CSF diversion have not been established. We therefore present our experience with 5 children shunted for IIH during the years 1984–2000 with very long-time follow-up. Three out of these patients have experienced late or very late episodes of severe shunt failure during the second or third decade after initial shunt treatment. They were all boys and may not be representative for IIH patients as a whole. Three of them appear, however, to be permanently shunt dependent, indicating that long-term shunt-dependency in children treated for IIH with CSF diversion may be more common than previously expected.

Keywords: idiopathic intracranial hypertension (IIH), children, CSF diversion, shunt dependency

1. Introduction

Main topics

i.e. Shunt failure
Shunt revision
Shunt dependency/independency
Overdrainage
Shunt surviva

In 1937 Walter Dandy published a series of 22 patients treated surgically for intracranial hyper-tension without a tumor [1]. Among his cases treated with subtemporal decompression during a period of 10 years, there were 3 children. Later on, this condition with papilledema, headache and visual disturbances was called benign intracranial hypertension, and many of them could be managed favorably by medical treatment [2]. In more severe cases, it soon became clear that this obscure disease is not always that benign [3]. In severe cases the term malignant pseudotumor was introduced [4]. Later on the term Idiopathic Intracranial Hypertension (IIH) was introduced [5].

Neurosurgical treatment with CSF diversion has been performed in severe cases where the response to medical treatment has been unsatisfactory, or as primary treatment in patients with severe visual affection [6, 7]. Unlike the situation for hydrocephalic children treated with CSF shunts who for the most become shunt dependent, clinical results on long term shunt dependency in IIH are unavailable.

Modified Dandy criteria:

Symptoms and signs of raised intracranial pressure (headache or papilledema).
No localizing signs in neurological examination (except abducent nerve palsy).
Normal neuroimaging.
Increased intracranial pressure as measured by lumbar puncture.
Normal CSF composition.
Alert and awake patient.
No other cause of raised intracranial pressure.

1.1 Diagnostic work-up

Idiopathic intracranial hypertension is a diagnosis where other causes I leading to increased intracranial pressure have been excluded by CT or MRI, including unobstructed venous outflow. Normal CSF composition rules out infection. The diagnosic procedure of intracranial hypertension itself is usually performed by a simple lumbar puncture. This gives CSF for analysis, and fluid may spurt out in cases of severe IIH. When the Intracranial pressure (ICP) is measured via the lumbar route, the patient is posisioned flat with the puncture site in equal hight as the IIIrd ventricle. The needle seize should not be very thin (G19), to obtain a presice manometric pressure reading. Loss of fluid should be avoided, since the pressure falls rapidly unless ICP is very high. Pathological elevated ICP is above 25 cm H_2O (15–20 in children). ICP is,however, influenced by a number of factors that may give misleading results when ICP is evaluated by the lumbar route.

Firstly, the patient should be cooperative and relaxed. Furthermore ICP is highly influenced by changes in $PaCO_2$. If the patient is anxious and hyperventilate, ICP will fall rapidly. The pressure recording can also be performed by the use of standard fluid pressure transduces and may be combined by other diagnostic work-up, such as lumbar infusion tests. In children, these diagnostic procedures must be undertaken during general anesthesia and normocapnia.

When patients with severe headache but without papilledema or visual affection, are given a IIH diagnosis, correct evaluation of the CSF hydrodynamic situation is pertinent. If CSF pressure is observed under unstable conditions or is influenced rapid changes in the central venous pressure, misinterpretations may take place. Queckensteds test (venous compression in the neck) demonstrates this effect on the CSF pressure, and was previously used to exclude a spinal block. Lumbar infusion tests can be used to explore the need for therapeutic CSF diversion, and of course demonstrate that an indwelling shunt is patent (LP-shunt or VP-shunt). A simple lumbar puncture will of course also be helpful to exclude severe shunt failure, as well as shunt infection.

It should be pointed out that the lumbar puncture itself will give an opportunity to explore the possibilities for a good result in IHH patients. After puncture with a 19G cannula, CSF will leak during the following three weeks, especially in true IIH patients with increased CSF pressure. This is why some individuals without IIH, will experience post-puncture headache due to intracranial hypotension. The beneficial effect of LP and CSF removal on severe headache and visual affection, is often temporary and repeated punctures or shunt implantation will be needed.

2. Methods

All children (0–19 years old) who underwent a shunt implantation for IIH during the years 1980–2000 in our institution were identified from the surgical protocols. Ethical approval was obtained from the medical ethics committee of Norway, the Regional Committee of Medicine and Heath.

We present our experience with these pediatric patients shunted for IIH during the years 1984 to 2000; and therefore have long-term follow-up.

3. Results

Five pediatric patients aged 0–19 years presented with clinical signs and symptoms of increased ICP.

They had small ventricles, no venous outflow obstruction, high opening pressure on LP and normal CSF composition.

They were all males, four were in the first decade (age: 1,3,4,5 and 18 years). All had bilateral papilledema, headache and visual disturbances in spite of medical treatment (Acetazolamide, corticiosteroids, furosemide). They all had normal weight for age. The results are summarized in **Table 1**.

Patient number Age/sex	Year	Shunt procedure	Number of shunt proce-dures	Follow-up years	Shunt depend?	Clinical presentation
1 M 18	1984	LP	3	36	Yes	Headache, visual loss, papilledema
	2003	LP(rev)				Headache, blurred vision
	2013	VP				Headache
2 M 4	1988	CA		32	No	Papilledema, VIth n. palsy, visual loss
	2016	Remove				Overdrainage symptoms
3 M 3	1989	CP	3	31	Yes	Papilledema, visual loss
	2006	LP				Headache, vomiting, High CSF pessure
	2009	LP(rev)				Headache
4 M 5	1991	CP	5	29	Yes	Hedache, papilledema, ataxia, blurred vision, unstable level of consciousness
	1994	revCP				Headche, vomiting
	2004	VP				Headache, vomit, diplopia,papilledema
	2006	LP				Episodes of vislual loss, high ICP
	2009	Remove P-kat				Abdominal disability
5 M 1	2000	LP	1	18	?	Blilat. VIth nerve palsy, papilledema

LP – lumboperitoneal; VP – ventriculoperitoneal; CA – cisterno(Magna)atrial; CP - cisternoperitoneal.

Table 1.
Clinical details.

3.1 Case 1

The first patient was a 18 year-old boy. In spite of medical treatment and LP every 4 weeks, the headache was troublesome and his vision was partly lost (0,5) during six months in spite of the repeated taps. A lumboperitoneal shunt (mini Holter high valve) was therefore implanted in January 1984. The symptoms resolved and his vision improved but not completely during the next year. After many years, in 2003, he once more experienced headache and blurred vision. There was no papilledema, but high opening pressure on LP. The LPshunt was found blocked and after revision he once more was symptom free.

In 2013 another episode of clinical shunt failure took place, and the symptoms again responded favorably after implantation of a VP shunt. Today, with 36 years follow-up, he is in full-time work as a diary worker.

3.2 Case 2

The second patient was a 4 year-old boy presenting with VIth nerve palsy, bilateral papilledema, headache and visual affection in spite of treatment with furosemide for some weeks. After implantation of a cisterno-atrial shunt (mini-Holter high valve), the symptoms resolved (slight binasal visual defect). After many good clinical years until about 2012, he thereafter during the next years experienced increasing overdrainage-symptoms (headache, dizziness, sometimes also subjective affection of vision and hearing) when rapidly changing to the upright position. The symptoms were reversed effectively in the recumbent position. In 2016 the shunt was removed and ICP was monitored in 4 days along with clinical observation. He clearly improved, and his clinical symptoms related to change in body position disappeared. He now appears to be shunt independent for more than three years.

3.3 Case 3

The third patient was a 3 year-old boy admitted with a short history of lost vision for 36 hours, reduced pupil reactivity, ataxia and poor general condition. Fundoscopy demonstrated choked discs and cerebral MRI was normal including unobstructed venous outflow. Lumbar puncture revealed normal CSF composition and increased CSF pressure, but the ICP level was difficult to measure due to lack of cooperation. A lumbar infusion test during general anesthesia demonstrated increased CSF opening pressure as well as slightly increased outflow resistance.

Due to the dramatic clinical symptoms with complete visual loss, corticosteroid treatment was implemented and an acute shunt procedure was performed during the same general anesthesia. A proximal catheter was introduced into cisterna Magna and connected to a low pressure Holter valve with diversion to the peritoneal cavity.

His vision gradually reappeared within days, and after one week there was normal vision and pupillary reactivity to light. Some ataxia and clumsy motor function persisted for weeks, but after 6 months his clinical condition was quite normal. During the first two years of treatment he experienced a few episodes with headache, ataxia and diplopia (VIth nerve paresis) which resolved spontaneously within a couple of days or after pumping on the Holter valve. At the age of 5 years (1991) he demonstrated episodes of overdrainage in the upright position, which subsided after implementation of an ASD (anti-syphon-device) distal to the valve.

Thereafter his clinical condition was uneventful for many years. During his university studies (in 2006), he became acutely ill with signs of increased ICP (headache and vomiting). There was no choked discs, but lumbar puncture revealed markedly increase CSF pressure level (50 cm H_2O) and no signs of infection. Once more MRI was normal (**Figure 1**). After a shunt revision (LP-shunt), his clinical condition normalized within a few days. In 2009, he experienced shunt failure once more, again followed by rapidly improvement after shunt revision.

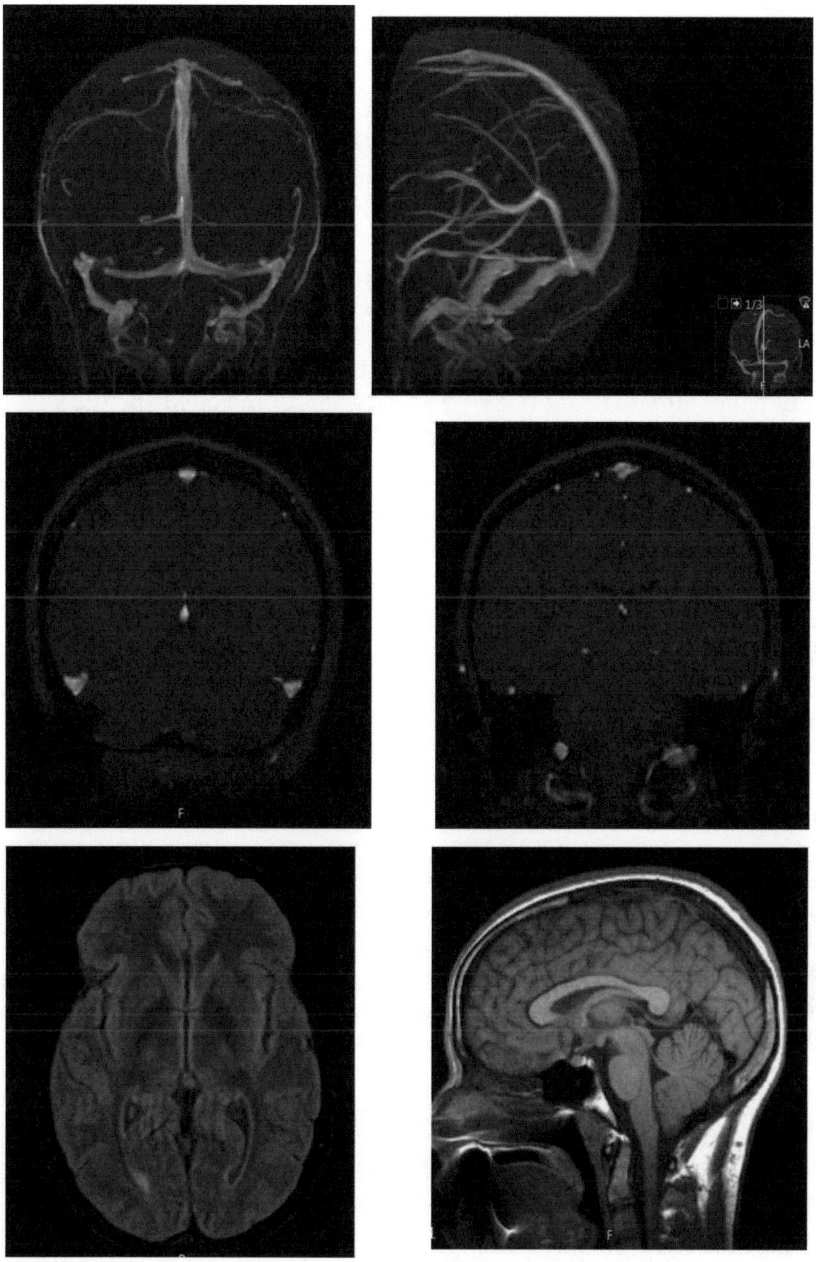

Figure 1.
(Case 3) demonstrates normal intracranial structures during the episode of shunt failure in 2006 (lower row) including unobstructed venous outflow (upper and middle row).

Thereafter he has been working full time, and has been clinically quite well for another 11 years.

This case with a very rewarding clinical result indicate that this 35 year-old man in excellent condition most likely is permanently shunt dependent.

3.4 Case 4

The fourth patient was a 4 year-old boy presented with headache, bilateral papilledema, ataxia, and unstable level of consciousness and episodes of blurred vision. The ventricles were small, venous outflow was unaffected and a lumbar infusion test during general anesthesia (normocapnia) revealed ICP of 24 mm Hg and increased resistance to outflow of CSF. A medium Holter shunt was implanted from cisterna Magna to the peritoneal cavity and the symptoms normalized. Three years later he experienced acute shunt failure(disconnection) with headache, papilledema, vomiting and a lumbar pressure of 45 mm Hg. After revision, the situation once more normalized. Ten years later, in 2004, he experienced another episode of shunt failure with headache, vomiting, diplopia and bilateral papilledema. Lumbar pressure was highly increased. A VPshunt (Codman Medos) was now implanted. During the next two years the situation was more unstable, with episodes of clinical symptoms related to over- as well as underdrainage. In 2006, he experienced episodes of visual loss, and ICP monitoring revealed pathological ICP. A lumboperitoneal shunt (OSV II) was therefore implanted and the VPshunt removed. During the subsequent 12 years he has been clinically well and fulfilled a master degree at the university.

3.5 Case 5

The fifth patient was a one-year-old boy with bilateral papilledema, bilateral VIth nerve paresis and a LPshunt was implanted in 2000 with good clinical response. His development during the following years has been uneventful. He is now working as an electrician, climbing in poles and without any clinical symptoms of ICP disturbances.

4. Discussion

Clinical series of patient with IIH are heterogenous with respect to age, sex and the severity of disease. When Dandy presented his series of 22 cases in 1937, he gave an individual and detailed overview of clinical history, symptoms and signs of his patients [1]. They illustrate the severity of the problems these patients were faced with when they sought neurosurgical treatment 80–90 years ago. One of 3 children in Dandys` series was:

4.1 Dandy's case 12

Female Age 13 –January 21 to February 1936.

Complaints. – Failing vision, diplopia and headache.

Present illness – Seven months ago pain developed in her left hip causing her to limp. The pain progressed steadily for three months when she was no longer able to walk. Roentgenograms were taken and were said to have been negative. A month later a second roentgenologic examination revealed an abnormality about the epiphysis of the femur and atrophy of its neck. The leg was placed in a plaster spica. The pain immediately disappeared. She felt better, ate heartily and gained some weight. A month later, i.e., two months ago, she had an attack of vomiting. One month later, i.e., one month ago, she complained of dizziness and headache over both eyes. Within a week her eyesight became blurred, there was double vision and the headache had become much more severe. It was then located in the occipital as well as the frontal region. There were pain and stiffness in the neck. Vomiting became more severe, occurring several times a day. Three weeks ago the plaster spica was removed and an appendicectomy performed because of the vomiting. There was no upset following the operation, and although her headache continued, the vomiting ceased. One week ago her vision had become so poor that she could only recognize light with the left eye. She was still able to read with the right eye. For the past three or four weeks there have been attacks of numbness in the right (not the leg in the spica).

Examination.- Patient is a sallow, fairly well nourished, young girl suffering severely with headache. Temperature normal; pulse 110; respirations 24; blood pressure 120; W.B.C. 7,800. There is a definite cracked-pot sound (Maceven's sign) on tapping the frontoparietal suture line. Moreover, roentgenologic examination showed separation of the sutures – unusual at the age of 13, and indicative of an extreme degree of intracranial pressure. There is only light perception in the left eye. She can read ordinary print with the right eye. Being bedfast and in a plaster spica, a more detailed eye examination is not possible. There is papilledema of five to six diopters in the right eye; two to three diopters in the left (the blind eye). The disk and surrounding retina are filled with large flame-like hemorrhages; these are more pronounced on the right side. There is weakness of the external rectus muscle on the left, but the parents say this has always been present. The knee jerks on the right could not be elicited; The left leg is in a plaster spica. Babinski is negative; no clonus.

Diagnosis. – Although I had suspected a tuberculous hip and a metastatic infection of the brain, Dr. George Bennett, who saw her with me, excluded tuberculosis from the study of the roentgenograms. The coexistence of the two lesions made us suspect a relationship between the two, but the only positive finding in the hip was the epiphyseal separation and atrophy of the neck and upper part of the shaft. There was no positive infective process.

Trephine and Air Injection. – January 22, 1936. The right ventricle was tapped. Fluid spurted out under tremendous pressure – at least a distance of three feet. About 15 cc. of fluid escaped and then the flow shut down abruptly. Ten cubic centimeters of air were injected under pressure to replace the fluid. The ventriculograms showed a perfectly normal ventricular system. The fluid showed four cells, all lymphocytes. A guinea-pig was inoculated with the fluid, because of the suspicion of tuberculosis; it had no effect upon the animal.

A right subtemporal decompression was performed immediately after the ventriculograms had been interpreted. The dura was exceedingly tense. A small nick was made in the dura, hoping that fluid might be encountered and thus reduce the terrific tension. A large amount of fluid did escape, but it seemed to make little, if any, impression upon the tension of the dura. The dura was rapidly opened but the pressure was still so extreme that the cortex ruptured inferiorly. The intracranial pressure has just about reached its limit.

Following the operation the decompression was exceedingly tense. A spinal puncture on the third day after operation registered 460 Mm of water; this, in spite of decompression. With this great pressure it looked as though the decompression would be futile. A lumbar puncture was performed on each of the following seven days; about 30 cc. of fluid being removed each time. On the eighth day after operation the spinal fluid pressure registered 350 Mm. The tension of the decompression gradually decreased during the next five days. On the fourteenth day the decompression was flat and the spinal fluid pressure measured 160 Mm. Patient remained in the hospital a week longer. The decompression remained perfectly flat throughout that time.

For a few days after operation patient was unable to se with either eye. As the pressure became less her vision returned and at the time of her discharge she was able to read fine print with the right eye, but the left eye still remained blind. Her general condition had changed entirely, her color was better, and she was very much more alert and active mentally.

Subsequent Course. – When examined by me three months later, she was totally blind, had severe headaches, and the decompression was full and as tense as it could possibly be. The left optic disk showed extreme optic atrophy with sharply defined disk and normal sized veins. The right had much the same appearance but slightly less advanced. It did not look as though vision could ever return. Within two weeks the decompression was again flat, and vision returned on the right eye,

February 12, 1937. 13 months after the operation, she was well; had no more evidence of increased pressure, the decompression had remained soft; her vision was 20/70 in the right eye and there was a fairly normal field of vision. Her femur has healed and gives no trouble; there is no limp.

4.1.1. Historical perspective on IIH management

Patients with extreme presentations in terms of visual disturbancies and headache underwent subtemporal decompression procedures in small volumes during the following decades. Although positive clinical responses were obtained in shortly after decompression in many of them, the procedures were dangerous and serial lumbar punctures had to be performed to achieve more long lasting relief from the decompression. When lumbo-peritoneal shunting was introduced in the treatment of hydrocephalus in the 1950ies, it was therefor natural to explore this treatment also in severe cases of pseudotumor. When other CSF diversion procedures for HC were established in the 1960ies (VA-shunts) [8], and later on VP-shunts [9], they were also found applicable in treatment of iIH.

Although shunt procedures are generally effective in relieving the CSF pressure in IIH, these CSF procedures have a substantial number of complications. When medical treatment for IIH became available (Diamox, Furosemide etc), non-surgical treatment would be preferred by many, since shunt failure, shunt infection and shunt dependency could therefore be omitted.

During the 1980ies and 1990ies, the number of patients with IIH increased rapidly, especially among people with severely increased body mass index, with a clear female dominance [10].

In some of these patients bariatric surgery has been introduced to reduce the weight problem and may also solve the IIH or alt least reduce the need for CSF diversion procedures [11]. It also seems that morbid overweight increases the problems with CSF diversion to the peritoneal cavity.

Several studies have compared lumboperitoneal shunts versus ventriculoperitoneal shunts in the treatment of IIH [12]. Both types of CSF are highly effective in the acute stage, but there are more revisions during the following years in patients treated with LP-shunts [13]. McGirt and coworkers furthermore underscore that while CSF diversion is effective in the acute stage, several patients experience that headaches returns. The found that this happens more often in patients without papilledema and long-standing symptoms before shunt treatment.

In early years LP shunts were considered applicable since it was technically easy to achieve CSF from the lumbar CSF reservoir, compared to get ventricular access in patients with small or slit ventricles.

In recent decades modern imaging (MR,CT) and stereotactic placement of ventricular catheters have resulted in ventriculo-peritoneal CSF shunting as the most used procedure, at least in adults. In patients with severe overweight, distal end problems with abdominal complaints is common.

Pediatric IIH is a rare disease [14] and pediatric cases are often presented in series of institutional IIH patients of all ages, where females of reproductive age dominate. Another problem is that clinically IIH covers a wide spectrum of symptoms and signs. When patients without papilledema or frank visual affection are included, non-surgical management is preferred and may lead to satisfactory outcomes. Long-term follow-up of IIH-children treated conservatively (with papilledema) has demonstrated that some are left with visual defects [15]. In recent years focus has been directed to the small group of IIH patients where troublesome headaches are not the main threat, but visual affection. If treatment over time is not efficient in reducing papilledema and visual affection, permanent reduction in visual acuity, visual field defects and even blindness may take place [16, 17].

This was the case in our Case 1, where serial lumbar taps gave excellent symptomatic relief of headache for 3 weeks, but during the fourth week the symptoms built up. When a LP-shunt eventually was implanted after 6 months, his visual acuity was reduced by 50%, and only improved slightly during the subsequent year. He obviously should have been shunted earlier. The visual threat also have a strong time component, implying that when visual deterioration is rapid or abrupt, surgical intervention is imminent (CSF-diversion or optical nerve sheath fenestration). Progression of visual affection over weeks have been considered a strong indication for surgery, with the prospect of avoiding further visual affection. Our Case 3, demonstrates that frank blindness can be treated successfully with restoration of vision, but this raises the question of emergency surgery in such rare cases. A number of publications point to this problem when patients with IIH are faced in emergency departments [6, 18,–20]. These rare, but very important experiences are in accord with the eminent and detailed clinical observations made by Walter Dandy 80 years ago.

Over-night blindness has even been reported after shunt failure in IIH [21]. Shunt failure may result in reoccurrence of sever headache and visual affection, and even lead to CSF leak [22].

Thus, neurosurgical treatment by CSF diversion is well established in IIH patients with severe visual affection as well as in cases with unsatisfactory response to medical treatment [23]. When the clinical result is good over years, as in our patient 5, it is difficult to know if the shunt is still functioning or the underlying condition has normalized spontaneously [24].

However, our five cases with very long-term follow up (20–36 years) demonstrate episodes of shunt failure in three of them, up to 29 years after initial shunt treatment. All together 7 episodes of shunt failure requiring shunt revision were observed. Only one of these distinct shunt failures took place during the first decade after implantation (after 3 years, disconnection). The others occurred from 13 to 29 years after implantation. All the shunt failures were restricted to 3 out of the 5 patients, and all of these 3 experienced repeated delayed shunt failures (in the second or third decade after initial treatment). There are few pediatric series with shunt treated IIH children reported. Niotakis and coworker report on 7 cases who underwent lumbar CSF shunt surgery. There was 2 acute procedures due to severe visual affection, but 3 patients presented with severe headache without papilledema. All patients had shunt revisions, due to symptoms of overdrainage or obstruction. An adult series from Dublin [25] reported low failure rates both in LP-shunts (11%) and VP shunts (14%), nevertheless revision rates were 60% in LP shunts and 30% in VP shunts. Bjørnson and coworkers report a lower revision rate (11%) in VP-shunted IIH adults. The follow-up periods in these studies are restricted, and late shunt failures have not been reported in adults (beyond 7 years).

Since IIH has been considered a benign and perhaps self restoring condition, this might explain the lack of long-term follow-up studies. Good long-term results can therefore both be explained by a no-longer existing CSF diversion demand andsome of the well functioning shunted patients may in fact have functioning shunt. This question has not been addressed, but very late shunt failure has not been reported. Many revisions in reported in IIH shunted individuals, describe other problems than shunt failure (obstruction or hypofunction); i.e. overdrainage, shunt infection or unstable diversion.

Shunt implantation in children with severe IIH raises the question of making these children permanently shunt dependent [3]. While some authors have addressed this question, no cases with late or very late shunt failure has been reported, until our case 3, published in 2017 [26]. Four of our pediatric cases have been published previously [27], and our case 1 was not included since his age of 18 did not fit with the series (reviewers opinion).

This case with 30 years follow-up, indicate that individuals shunted for IIH can be persistently dependent on their shunt, and may experience acute shunt failure even after many years of treatment. We also consider our patient 1, with shunt failures 19 and 29 years after initial treatment to be permanently shunt dependent. Also patient 4 with shunt failure after 15 years is most likely in the need for life-long shunt treatment.

The last two patients tell a different story. Patient 2 had a good clinical response to shunt treatment in 24 years and thereafter experienced progressive symptoms from overdrainage. His shunt was therefore removed under ICP observation for 4 days, and he responded well. After 3 years further follow-up, we consider him shunt independent.

Our small group of shunt treated IIH children is peculiar since they are all boys, compared to the well known female dominance in IIH patients as a whole. It is, however, also known that females do not outnumber males in the first decade in IIH treated children [28]. In a report from a large pediatric emergency unit, children with papilledema and visual affection diagnosed with IIH, were twice as common in boys compared with girls in the first decade of life, while the opposite was found in the second decade [19]. It is unclear if our small study group is representative for all pediatric IIH patients and for the large group of adult IIH patients, many with high body mass index (BMI).

Clinical studies describing adult IIH cohorts illustrate the female dominance, often up to 90 per cent.

Comparison of treatment strategies as well as results is troublesome because inclusion criteria may vary. In the United States a rapidly rising incidence of cerebrospinal fluid shunting procedures for idiopathic intracranial hypertension was described for the years 1988–2002 [10]. The increase seemed to correlate with the rapid rise in morbid obesity. The increase was 320% for the population as a whole, but only 38% for males, and 52% for pediatric cases (<13 yrs., both sexes).

Bariatric surgery is considered to be beneficial for overweight IIH patients, and may reduce the need for shunt treatment. Bariatric surgery has been used as primary treatment as well as additional surgical procedure in IIH patients after CSF shunt procedures. The are a number of reports on multiple shunt procedures in such patients. In a group of 6 patients where bariatric surgery was performed in shunted IIH individuals, the shunt was externalized and clamped. Due to severe overdrainage symptoms, shunt removal was planned, but the shunt had to be acutely reestablished due to unexpected and clear shunt dependency [29].

This points to another problem, namely that evaluation of shunt function in IIH patients can be difficult. When headache is the dominating clinical problem, differentiation between high-pressure symptoms (shunt failure), visual affection; and low-pressure symptoms (over drainage) may be challenging. It is easy when overdrainage-symptoms in terms of headache and dizziness are rapidly reversed in recumbent position, but if the CSF drainage is unstable the clinical picture may include both. In such situations ICP-monitoring or use of lumbar or ventricular infusion tests may be helpful [27, 30], and additional shunt revisions and increased risk of shunt infection can be reduced.

Although the report from Roth and coworkers [20] presented 6 aldults that were unexpectedly shunt dependent, it is remarkable that long-term shunt dependency has not been a topic. Since benign intracranial hypertension has been considered a self-solving condition, long lasting shunt dependency may therefore have been unexpected, but perhaps also overlooked. In research on shunt patency in hydrocephalic patients, the term *shunt survival* has been used; meaning the time from the initial shunt procedure to the first shunt revision. This has been a kind of quality measurement in management of hydrocephalic patients, and presented in per cent for the first, second or five years.

The proportion of patients still having their initial shunt unrevised was anticipated to represent individuals with persistent shunt dependency, but harboring still functioning shunts.

In our long-term follow-up of children shunted for hydrocephalus I the 1960is and 1980 we have found shunt dependency rates of about 90% [2, 11]. That is why ETV is now a preferred treatment when feasible in primary management of hydrocephalus. The other 10% are for sure not shunt dependent, since their shunt has been explanted, in some of them in combination with an ETV procedure. The correct description would therefore be that up to 90% still are or can be more or less shunt dependent.

5. Conclusion

The shunt dependency rates for pediatric IIH treated with CSF diversion are actually not known, and long-term follow-up reports are scarce. Our limited experience, however, indicate that permanent shunt dependency may be more common than previously expected. In adults this topic has hardly been addressed.

Conflict of interest

None.

Abbreviations

CSF	cerebrospinal fluid
LP	lumbar puncture
IIH	idiopathic intracranial hypertension

Author details

Tryggve Lundar[1,2*] and Bernt Johan Due-Tønnessen[1]

1 Department of Neurosurgical, Oslo University Hospital, Oslo, Norway

2 Department of Neurosurgical, University of Oslo, Oslo, Norway

*Address all correspondence to: tryggve.lundar@gmail.com

References

[1] Dandy WE. Intracranial pressure without brain tumor. Ann Surg 106(4): 492-513, 1937.

[2] Foley J. Benign forms of intracranial hypertension; toxic and otitic hydrocephalus. Brain 78(1): 1-41, 1955.

[3] Johnston I, Besser M, Morgan MK. Cerebrospinal fluid diversion in the treatment of benign intracranial hypertension. J Neurosurg 69:195-202, 1988.

[4] Kidron D, Pomeranz S. Malignant pseudotumor cerebri. Report of two cases. J Neurosurg 71:443-445, 1989.

[5] Karsy M, Abou-Al-Shaar Haussam, Bowers CA, Schmidt RH. Treatment of idiopathic intracranial hypertension via stereotactic placement of biventriculoperitoneal shunts. J Neurosurg 130:136-144, 2019

[6] Bhandohal JS, Mirza T. BLIND OVERNIGHT: A case of fulminant idiopathic intracranial hypertension. American Journal of Emergency Medicine 35 (2017): 1581.e1-1581.e2

[7] Bjørnson A, Tapply I, Nabbanja E, Lalou A-D, Czosnyka M, Czosnyka Z, Muthusamy B,Garnett M. Ventriculo-peritoneal shunting is a safe and effective treatment for idiopatic intracranial hypertension. British Journal of Neurosurg 33:62-70, 2019.

[8] Paulsen AH, Due-Tønnessen BJ, Lundar T, Lindegaard K-F. Persistent shunt dependency and very late shunt failure in a 3-year-old boy with idiopathic intracranial hyoertension (IIH) Childs Nerv Syst 33:213-215, 2017.

[9] Paulsen AH, Lundar T, Lindegaard K-F. Pediatric hydrocephalus: 40-year outcomes in 128 hydrocephalic patients treated with shunts during childhood. Assessment of surgical outcome, work participation, and health-related quality of life. J Neurosurg Pediatr 16:633-641, 2015.

[10] Curry WT, Butler WE, Barker FG. Rapidly Rising Incidence of cerebrospinal fluid shunting procedures for idiopathic intracranial hypertension in the United States, 1988-2002. Neurosurgery 57:97-108, 2005

[11] Hoang KB, Hooten KG, Muh CR. Shunt freedom and clinical resolution of idiopatic intracranial hypertension after bariatric surgery in the pediatric population: report of 3 cases. J Neurosurg Pediatr 20:511-516, 2017

[12] Kalyvas A, Neromyliotis E, Koutsarnakis C, Komatis S, Drosos E, Skandalakis GP, Pantazi M, Gobin YP, Stranjalis G, Patsalides A. A systematic review of surgical treatments of idiopathic intracranial hypertension (IIH), Neurosurgical Review https://doi.org/10.1007/s10143-020-01288.1

[13] Lundar T, Due-Tønnessen BJ: Persistent shunt dependency in children treated with CSF diversion for Idiopathic Intracranial Hypertension (IIH). Acta Neurochir (Wien) 162:39-42, 2020

[14] Amacher LA, Spence JD. Spectrum of benign intracranial hypertension in children and adolescents. Childs Nerv Syst 1:81-86, 1985

[15] Baker RS, Carter D, Hendrick EB, Bunic JR. Visual Loss in Pseudotumor Cerebri of Childhood.A Follow-up Study. Arch Ophtalmpl 103:1681-1686, 1985

[16] Lim M, Kurian M, Calver D, Lin J-P. Visual failure without headache in idiopatic intracranial hypertension. Arch Dis Child 90:206-210, 2005

[17] Shaia JK, Elzie C. Acute presentation of idiopathic intracranial hypertension

with severe vision deficits. SAGE Open Medical Case Reports 8:1-4, 2020

[18] Bouffard MA. Fulminant Idiopathic Intracranial Hypertension. Current Neurology and Neuroscience Reports 20:8, 2020. https//doi.org/10.1007/s11910-020-1026-8

[19] Glatstein MM, Oren A, Amarilyio G, Scolnik D, Tov AB, Yahav A, Alper A, Reif S. Clinical Characterization of Idiopathic Intracranial Hypertension in Children Presenting to the Emergency Department. The Experience of a Regional Tertiary Care Pediatric Hospital. Pediatric Emergency Care 31:6-9, 2015

[20] Roth J, Constantini S, Kessler A. Over-drainage and persistent shunt-dependency in patients with idiopathic intracranial hypertension treated with shunts and bariatric surgery. Surg Neurol Int 6:S655-60, 2015

[21] Liu GT, Volpe NJ, Schatz NJ, Galetta SL, Farrar JT, Raps EC. Severe Sudden Visual Loss Caused by Pseudotumor Cerebri and Lumboperitoneal Shunt Failure.Am Journal of Ophtalomology 122:129-131, 1996

[22] Paulsen AH, Lundar T, Lindegaard K-F. Twenty-year outcome in young adults with childhood hydrocephalus: assessment of surgical outcome, work participation, and health-related quality of life. J Neurosurg Pediatrics 6:527-535, 2010.

[23] McGirt MJ, Woodworth G, Thomas G, Miller N, Williams M, Rigamonti D. Cerebrospinal fluid shunt placement for pseudotumor cerebri-associated intractable headache: predictors of treatment response and ananalysis of long-term outcomes. J Neurosurg 101:627-632, 2004

[24] Ransom ER, Komotar RJ, Mocco J, Connolly ES, Mullins KJ. Shunt failure in idiopathic intracranial hypertension presenting with spontaneous cerebrospinal fluid leak. Case reports/ Journal of Clinical Neuroscience 13:598-602, 2006.

[25] Abubaker K, Ali Z, Raza K, Bolger C, Rawluk D, O'Brien D. Idiopathic intracranial hypertension: lumboperitoneal shunts versus ventriculoperitoneal shunts – case series and literature review. British Journal of Neurosurgery 25: 94-99, 2011

[26] Niotakis G, Grigoratos D, Chandler C, Morrison D, Lim M. CSF diversion in refractory idiopatic intracranial hypertension: single-center experience and review of efficacy. Childs Nerv Syst 29:263-269, 2013.23.

[27] Lundar T. Shunt removal or replacement based on intraventricular infusion tests.Child's Nerv Syst 10: 337-339, 1994.

[28] Nadakarni TD, Rekate HL, Wallace D. Concurrent use of lumboperitoneal shunt with programmable valve and ventricular access device in the treatment of pseudotumor cerebri: review of 40 cases. J Neurosurg Pediatrics 2:19-24, 2008

[29] Rosenberg ML, Corbett JJ, Smith C, Goodwin J, Sergott R, Savino P, Schatz N. Cerebrospinal fluid diversion procedures in pseudotumor cerebri NEUROLOGY 43:1071-1072, 1993

[30] Woodford J, Saunders RL, Sachs E. Shunt system patency testing by lumbar infusion. J Neurosurg 45:60-65, 1976